Clinical Psychology in the Mental Health Inpatient Setting

This ground-breaking volume pr… account of clinical psychologists' … …ic ward in mental health inpatient set… …llection of clinical psychologists describe challe… …vements inherent to their work, illustrating the application …ablished, state-of-the-art, and cutting-edge methods and modes of intervention, assessment, therapeutic work, training, and leadership roles currently practiced in these settings.

Chapters present numerous examples of psychologists' ability to contribute in multiple ways, benefiting patients, staff, and the overall functioning of the ward. Each of the book's four sections is dedicated to a specific domain of the clinical psychologist's work within the psychiatric inpatient setting. These include systemic modes of intervention; psychotherapeutic interventions; assessment and psychodiagnosis; and internship and supervision.

From novice to experienced practitioners, psychologists will gain insight from the innovative and creative ideas this book brings to the practice of clinical psychology, as well as the practical suggestions that will enhance the varied interventions and therapeutic work they do in such settings.

Meidan Turel, MA, is a licensed Clinical Psychologist in Israel and Director of psychological services in a public inpatient and outpatient mental health center.

Michael Siglag, PhD, is a Clinical Psychologist with over 30 years of experience working in inpatient civil psychiatric and forensic settings, both in direct service and leadership positions.

Alexander Grinshpoon, MD, PhD, MHA, is a specialist in psychiatry and the Director of a public mental health center in Israel, as well as the head of the psychiatry department in the Rappaport Faculty of Medicine, Technion, Israel Institute of Technology.

Clinical Psychology in the Mental Health Inpatient Setting

International Perspectives

Meidan Turel, Michael Siglag, and Alexander Grinshpoon

Routledge
Taylor & Francis Group
NEW YORK AND LONDON

First published 2020
by Routledge
52 Vanderbilt Avenue, New York, NY 10017

and by Routledge
2 Park Square, Milton Park, Abingdon, Oxon, OX14 4RN

Routledge is an imprint of the Taylor & Francis Group, an informa business

Library of Congress Cataloging-in-Publication Data
A catalog record for this title has been requested

ISBN: 978-1-138-61271-6 (hbk)
ISBN: 978-1-138-61273-0 (pbk)
ISBN: 978-0-429-46458-4 (ebk)

Typeset in Goudy
by Swales & Willis, Exeter, Devon, UK

Contents

Foreword

I feel very honored to have been asked by the editors of this rich and informative volume, Meidan Turel, Michael Siglag, and Alexander Grinshpoon, to write this Foreword. Particularly, in our current zeitgeist in which the role of genes are hyped, and clinicians fail to realize that 'symptoms' can work through genes and the brain, but perhaps not because of them. Genome-wide association studies reveal weak risk alleles, i.e., genes of low penetrance and effects, for many psychiatric disorders, quite discrepant with family studies. Epigenetics (e.g., the study of environmental control of gene expression) and biological embedding of adverse social experiences (e.g., of adverse childhood experiences, ACEs) are just beginning to make their way into the consciousness of clinicians.

I began my career as a psychologist as a young boy watching a middle-aged woman in my neighborhood walk down the street. She would suddenly stop walking, turn to the building on her left, stay still for some time with a fixed gaze at the wall, and then just as suddenly begin skipping down the street. I still remember her over a half century ago. My psychological career was also initiated by having a fourth-grade teacher, a very loveable older woman, quite lonely I believe, tell the class that Australia was really named after her. On a more intimate level, I believe, my professional choice was also forged by witnessing the sometimes painful emotional conflicts between my parents, resulting in my fear that our family might be suddenly rent asunder.

Fast forward about 12 years, and I volunteered at a state-run psychiatric hospital for children, in particular, an autism service. My job was to initiate social interaction and play with the children. I was both scared and emotionally moved by what I saw. Children banging their heads, biting their own hands, all within a terribly depressing and sterile ward environment. The children were locked into their rooms at night. I instinctively knew there must be a better way. Around the same time, in the early 1970s, I started volunteering at a private homeless shelter, The Catholic Worker, on East First Street in the Lower East Side of Manhattan, later referred to as the East Village. There I encountered persons who were overwhelmed by the tragedies of life, human existence, and social injustice. I remember one day being chased by an older woman who claimed I was the devil. I began my experience as a psychology extern in a teaching hospital in New York City, on a child and adolescent psychiatric inpatient unit in the mid-1970s. My study of psychology in undergraduate and graduate school was of little help in my encounters with children who had just tried to hang themselves, who were hearing chronic persecutory voices, or who had killed people. I considered going to medical school, encouraged by the chief of the child and adolescent psychiatry department, a lovely and caring psychiatrist who I still fondly remember. I decided against it for many reasons, not least of which was that I wanted to concentrate on learning neuroscience and most of all, I wanted to become a psychotherapist. I believed clinical psychology was the best fit for me. Neuroscience was just beginning as a field in the mid-1970s and it fit with my strong interest in biology which I had since high school. I found a program that embraced both disciplines. My field experience in the doctoral program included a placement in a local state psychiatric hospital, in an outpatient psychosocial club. I began working in intensive psychotherapy with a middle-aged man who had a history of violence, long term psychiatric hospitalizations, ECT, and antipsychotic medications. This person taught me a great deal about the meanings encoded in seemingly incomprehensible 'psychotic symptoms'. The Jasperian legacy of diagnostic incomprehensibility shifted in my mind to the real issue of our 'failing their feast' (Macbeth, William Shakespeare), of our not tuning in enough, perhaps because of our own areas of dissociation, conflict, etc. After graduation and an internship doing psychotherapy in an outpatient community health clinic in a New York City neighborhood, I eventually began working on a psychiatric inpatient unit in the Bronx, NY. I learned a great deal there: teaching psychiatric residents and medical students how to do psychotherapy, organizing and chairing psychology grand rounds, and engaging in individual psychotherapy with a wide range of persons. I learned a great deal about human illnesses of all kinds and how to faithfully encounter suffering persons with respect, recognition, and acknowledgment, and a deep and sustained form of listening which psychotherapy affords us. I learned more there about our human condition from the persons who entrusted their stories to me than from my doctoral graduate training and research.

Manfred Bleuler, son of Eugen Bleuler who coined the term 'the group of schizophrenias'. stated that psychotherapy was the soul of psychiatry. During this time, the average length of stay in community inpatient services was shrinking to just a few weeks. I wished to have more continuity with the people I was working with, so I went to work in a local New York State psychiatric hospital. The living conditions for the persons hospitalized there deeply affected me: no air conditioning in summer (until the mid to late 1990s), no organized psychotherapeutic programs, little ongoing or intensive psychotherapy for persons who were on the so-called 'back wards'. Fortunately, the chair of the psychology department, a humanistically oriented administrator, gave me the opportunity to engage primarily in group and individual psychotherapy with many of the persons living there for years, as well as with new admissions. Over the years there, I saw the importance of offering a sustaining, empathic, and reliable relationship to persons who often gave up on relatedness because of histories of betrayals, abandonment, childhood adverse experiences, transgenerational transmission of traumas, social adversities, and injustices. With permission from the hospital ethics committee, I continued working with some of these individuals in my private practice once they left the state hospital (none of them ever returned to the state hospital). I am still working with one of these persons for decades now and feel quite honored to have this opportunity.

I have learned a great deal from neuroscientists and geneticists about the neurobiological and genetic/epigenetic correlates/mediators of what we call psychosis, but what I have learned from people with lived experience, clinical psychologists, psychoanalysts, and psychotherapists has had more of a positive impact on the lives of my psychotherapy partners. My study of neuroendocrinology and neurobiology led me to propose in the 1990s that the neuroscience of what we call 'schizophrenia' (certainly a heterogeneous group of persons) overlaps significantly with the neuroscience of early life and chronic stress, adverse childhood experiences (ACEs), social isolation and social defeat, and stigma. My training in and ongoing exposure to clinical psychology, psychoanalysis, and cognitive behavior therapy for psychosis, and most importantly listening to the life stories of the persons I work with as well as the stories of persons in the peer movement ('nothing about us, without us'), have helped me see meaning and coherence in what we call delusions, voices, etc.

Many of the values and perspectives that have shaped my career as summarized in this Foreword are shared and reflected in work described by the authors of the chapters of this book, through their own experiences and work. Though psychologists here describe a variety of theoretical approaches, the healing power and value of listening and working to establish therapeutic relationships comes across throughout the chapters here. The centrality of these interactions, particularly in the context of psychotherapy, but also during assessment, is described in many settings in which the psychologists represented here carry out their work. These unique characteristics of clinical psychologists' work and contribution within the mental health inpatient settings are importantly brought together and collected into this volume, a first of its kind.

I would like to end this Foreword with the words of Charles Dodgson (Lewis Carroll): 'If there's no meaning in it', said the King, 'that saves a world of trouble, you know, as we needn't try to find any. And yet I don't know', he went on, spreading out the verses on his knee and looking at them with one eye. 'I seem to see some meaning in them, after all' (Carroll, 1960).

Brian Koehler, PhD, MS, New York University and TC, Columbia University

Reference

Carroll, L. (1960). *Alice's adventures in wonderland*. New York: Signet Classics.

Acknowledgments

The editors would like to extend their heartfelt gratitude and thanks to Mrs. Rena Kurs, former medical librarian at Sha'ar Menashe Mental Health Center, for her continuous and unceasing support and help in preparing this manuscript for publication. From the early days of this project several years ago, and until its present fulfillment and publication, Rena persisted in providing sound advice and practical help on innumerable issues and aspects concerning the writing, editing, and publication of this volume. Without her unwavering devotion and effort in accompanying us in this process, this book would not have materialized.

We would like to thank each of the book's contributors for their participation in this project. This book would not have been possible without the many psychologists who wanted to share and describe their work.

Special thanks to our Routledge editor, Ms. Nina Guttapalle and assistant editor Ms. Olivia Powers. Their constant availability and help in working through the many issues and stages involved in bringing this book to press was a pleasant and rewarding experience for us.

The Editors

I would like to thank my two co-editors, Dr. Mike Siglag and Professor Alexander Grinshpoon, for the pleasurable and creative process we jointly held together in bringing this book through all its many stages from inception to publication. Our pleasant cooperation and hard work together inspired and supported me throughout this process.

I am indebted to Ms. Naomi Schwartz, retired head of psychological services at my hospital, for supporting me through all of my many years of work there. Many of my ideas and understandings concerning psychologists' work and involvement within mental health inpatient settings, and that have come through in my writing and editing of this volume, originated in our joint work and many discussions throughout these years.

Many thanks to Dr. Aviva Mazor who gave me important and sound advice on various material in this book.

To my children, Rohan and Anveh, thank you for being a continuous source of strength for me throughout this project.

To my wife Avishag, I owe the most. Her continuous encouragement and belief in the importance and worthiness of this project, as well as her wise advice generously provided whenever challenging difficulties had to be resolved, were a tremendous source of support enabling me to persevere and bring this project to its fulfillment.

Meidan Turel

I am grateful for both the unique opportunity and great professional challenge this project posed. The chance to work with my co-editors Meidan Turel and Alexander Grinshpoon over the course of this project was a pleasure. The personal and professional collaboration with Meidan Turel, and the many hours spent discussing this project and wide-ranging ideas about psychological work in inpatient settings, were particularly enriching, rewarding, and enjoyable.

To my friends Judith Carr and John Urich, who provided much-appreciated and important input that influenced my writing, thank you.

To my former professors, supervisors, colleagues, and supervisees, and the many individuals I have worked with in treatment over the years, I am grateful for what you have taught me. You provided the academic and experiential foundation for my contribution to this project.

Many thanks to my wife Corinne for your ever-present support, and invaluable suggestions and input throughout my participation in this book project. To my children, Ian and Amelia, I appreciate you sharing me during the many hours I spent working on this project.

Finally, I want to thank my parents, whose support helped make it possible for me to follow the path I chose, to become a psychologist, and to do the kind of work described in this book by myself and others.

Michael Siglag

I would like to extend my sincere thanks to my two co-editors, Meidan Turel and Michael Siglag, for the opportunity to work together on this project. Working with them has been an immensely rewarding and interesting experience. Special thanks to Mrs. Rena Kurs, for her continuous help in numerous tasks along the way and for our work together, as co-authors, in writing our part of the introduction to this book. I am grateful to my family, my wife Alla, and children Miri, Koren and Alon, for their support and patience during my work on this project.

Alexander Grinshpoon

Contributors

Christina Biedermann, PsyD, ABAP, is a Clinical Psychologist board-certified in assessment psychology. She is a Senior Psychologist at the ARC Professional Group in Chicago, Illinois, and an Adjunct Faculty member at the Illinois School of Professional Psychology at Argosy. She is a member of the Chicago Center for Psychoanalysis. drbiedermann@northsidechicagopsychology.com

Spencer Biel, PsyD, is a Clinical Psychologist and Supervisor in private practice with the Wellington Counseling Group in Chicago, Illinois. At the time the chapter was being written, Spencer was a Staff Psychologist, Supervisor of Psychological Testing, and the Associate Director of the Therapeutic Community Program at the Austen Riggs Center. sbiel@wellingtoncounselinggroup.com

Heidi Camerlengo, EdD, is a licensed Psychologist working in an outpatient forensic evaluation program at Ann Klein Forensic Center in West Trenton, New Jersey, USA. Prior to this appointment, Dr. Camerlengo worked as a Clinical Psychologist for over 17 years at Ancora Psychiatric Hospital in Hammonton, New Jersey. Heidilyn-nc55@yahoo.com

Marilyn Charles, PhD, ABPP, is a Clinical Psychologist and Psychoanalyst at the Austen Riggs Center in Stockbridge, Massachusetts, USA. She is also affiliated with the Chicago Center for Psychoanalysis, Harvard University, Boston Graduate School of Psychoanalysis, and Universidad de Monterrey. Email: mcharlesphd@gmail.com

Beatriz Sanchez Curtis, CPsychol AFBPsS, is a Consultant Clinical Psychologist in the UK. Beatriz is currently working for the Cambian Group. Previously, Beatriz has headed the Psychology department on a secure inpatient unit in London which provided services across general psychiatry, forensic psychiatry, and neuropsychiatry. beatriz-sanchez@bspsychology.com

Peter J. D'Amico, PhD, ABPP, is a Clinical Psychologist and Director of Child and Adolescent Psychology at the Long Island Jewish (LIJ) Medical Center of Northwell Health, New York. Dr. D'Amico has held various positions across three major medical centers spanning roughly 25 years including inpatient, day hospital, and school-based mental health programming. He is an Associate Professor at Donal and Barbara Zucker School of Medicine at Hofstra/Northwell. PDAmico@northwell.edu

Patricia Daza, PhD, is a Clinical Psychologist and Program Director of the Compass Young Adult Program, The Menninger Clinic, Houston, Texas, USA. Dr. Daza is Associate Professor at the Baylor College of Medicine. pdaza@menninger.edu

Amit Fachler, PhD, is a Clinical Psychologist and Supervisor in Israel. Dr. Fachler is the Head Psychologist in the outpatient unit in 'Geha' Mental Health Center, Israel. Amit teaches at the Center for Academic Studies, Or Yehuda, as well as at the Independent and Relational Tracks, Psychotherapy Postgraduate Program, Tel Aviv University. He is the author of the book: *Fatherless Fathers: Love, Guilt, and Reparation*, Carmel Publishing House (Hebrew). At the time of writing the chapter, he held the positions of Head Psychologist in the Adult Inpatient Unit in 'Geha' MHC; and Manager of the Psychotherapy Unit, the Interdisciplinary Clinical Center, Haifa University. fachler@012.net.il

Jim Geekie, PhD, is a Clinical Psychologist currently working in Scotland for National Health Service (NHS) Lothian and NHS Education for Scotland, as a Clinical Tutor on the University of Edinburgh training program. At the time of writing his chapter for this book, Jim was working as Principal Clinical Psychologist in an acute inpatient unit in Essex, England. jim.geekie@ed.ac.uk

Hannah Green, DClinPsyc, MSc, BA, is a Clinical Psychologist working on an adult acute inpatient unit and in adult community mental health teams in South East London, Oxleas NHS Foundation Trust. She has worked in adult mental health since 2010 and has a special clinical interest in systemic family therapy. Hannah.green18@nhs.net

Kim Griffiths, DClinPsyc, PGDip, BSc, is a Lead/Principal Clinical Psychologist working on an adult acute inpatient unit and in adult community mental health teams in South East London, Oxleas NHS Foundation Trust. He has worked as a Clinical Psychologist in adult mental health since 2007 and has a special interest in acute inpatient clinical psychology as well as a special clinical interest in mindfulness-based approaches. Kim.Griffiths@nhs.net

Dione Johnson-Williams, PhD, is a licensed Clinical Psychologist. Dr. Johnson-Williams worked at Trenton Psychiatric Hospital on an all-male forensic unit in Trenton, New Jersey. Currently, she is the CEO of Juvenile & Adult Re-Entry Connections, an outpatient behavioral health company which provides services for at-risk juveniles and juvenile and adults post-release from correctional and residential settings in New Jersey. drj@jarchealth.org

Jimmy I. Kim, PsyD, is a Senior Psychologist at the Zucker Hillside Hospital of Northwell Health in Glen Oaks, New York, USA. Dr. Kim has been working on the acute care psychiatry service for more than 11 years. He is also an Assistant Professor at the Donald and Barbara Zucker School of Medicine at Hofstra/Northwell. jkim@northwell.edu

Rena Kurs, MA, is a former Medical Librarian at the Sha'ar Menasheh Mental Health Center, Israel. She has over 25 years' experience as an information specialist in psychiatry and the social sciences. She is also associate editor of the *Israel Journal of Psychiatry*. renakurs@gmail.com

Suzie Lemmey, DClinPsyc, MSc, BSc, at the time of writing the chapter, was an Assistant Psychologist in Oxleas NHS Foundation Unit and then a Trainee Clinical Psychologist at Salomons Centre for Applied Psychology, University of Christ Church Canterbury, Tunbridge Wells, Kent, UK. She has since qualified with a doctorate in Clinical Psychology and works in Learning Disability Services. suzie.lemmey@nhs.net

Sophie H. Li, PhD, is a Clinical Psychologist in Australia. She is a Postdoctoral Fellow in the School of Psychology, University of New South Wales, Sydney; prior to that was a Clinical Psychologist at Early Intervention for Psychosis, Camperdown Mental Health Service, Sydney Australia. s.h.li@unsw.edu.au

Daria Mamon, PsyD, is a Clinical Psychologist. At the time of writing her chapter, Daria was an intern at the Colorado Mental Health Institute at Fort Logan in Denver, Colorado, USA. She completed two APA-accredited postdoctoral fellowships specializing in the treatment of Veterans. Currently, she is serving as a Staff Psychologist at the Massachusetts General Hospital and as an instructor in Psychiatry at Harvard Medical School. Dmamon@mgh.harvard.edu

Mark Andrew McFetridge, DClinPsychol, MSc, PGDip, BSc, is a Senior Consultant Clinical Psychologist at the Retreat York UK; Clinical Lead for the Tuke Centre York. Honorary Lecturer, University of Leeds and University of Hull. Board Member and Research Officer of the UKPTS (UK Psychological Trauma Society).

Associate Fellow of the BPS. Senior Fellow of the Institute of Mental Health. mmcfetridge@btinternet.com

Enav Or-Gordon, MA, is a licensed Clinical Psychologist in Israel and in the Czech Republic, and former Head Psychologist in the forensic ward of Bounce Hospital, Prague, the Czech Republic. Currently practicing Clinical Psychology in Alivio Centre, Prague. enavorgordon@gmail.com

Manish Parswani, PhD, MPhil and MA (Clin psy), is a Clinical Psychologist at East Auckland Psychology and practices at Pakuranga Medical Centre, Auckland, New Zealand. He was formerly Senior Clinical Psychologist for the Adult Acute Inpatient Mental Health Unit, Middlemore Hospital Auckland for 7 years. He has previously worked in a wide range of settings including hospital, university, and corporate settings with teaching, clinical, and research positions. manishparswani@gmail.com

Hilik (Yechiel) Peri, MA, is a Supervising Clinical Psychologist in Israel. Hilik works as a Senior Clinical Psychologist in a maximum security forensic ward in Sha'ar Menasheh, an Israeli state inpatient psychiatric facility where he also conducts research on the assessment of malingering. In his private practice, he is also a child and adolescent psychotherapist. hilikperi@hotmail.com

Karin Reddie, MA, is a licensed Clinical Psychologist in Israel. At the time of writing her chapter, Karin was a Clinical Psychology Intern working in an acute closed unit in Sha'ar Menasheh, an Israeli state psychiatric facility. karinoss20@gmail.com

Jeremy M. Ridenour, PsyD, is a Clinical Psychologist, Psychoanalyst, and Director of Testing, Austen Riggs Center, Massachusetts, USA. Dr. Ridenour is a Psychologist and Psychoanalyst whose research interests include the psychotherapeutic treatment of individuals with schizophrenia-spectrum disorders. He has written and presented on schizophrenia, paranoia, personality disorders, and psychological testing. Jeremy.ridenour@austenriggs.net

Sally E. Riggs, DClinPsy, is an ACT NY licensed Psychologist, Diplomate of the Academy of Cognitive Therapy. Founding Member and President of North American CBT for psychosis Network. Founder and Director of NYC CBTp, a private practice group providing cognitive behavior therapy for people with psychosis in New York City and training for mental health professionals nationwide. Dr. Riggs has previously worked in multiple inpatient settings in the UK and most recently in the US at NYC Health and Hospitals/Kings County in Brooklyn. sriggs@nyccbtp.com

Paul Saks, PhD, is a supervising psychologist at the Manhattan Psychiatric Center, New York, where he specializes in the treatment of psychotic disorders. He coordinates the Trauma Recovery Program, the Crossing the Bridge (community transition) Program, and Group Psychotherapy Training Program. He supervises psychological testing and individual psychotherapy for the intern and extern training programs and runs a poetry therapy group. In addition, Dr. Saks is an Adjunct Professor at Teachers College and has a private practice in New York City. paulsaksphd@yahoo.com. Paul.saks@omh.ny.gov

Shweta Sharma, PsyD, is an Assistant Professor of Psychiatry in the Menninger Department of Psychiatry and Behavioral Science at Baylor College of Medicine. She is a Senior Staff Psychologist at The Menninger Clinic, Houston, Texas, USA. ssharma@menninger.edu

Valerie Sims, PsyD, is a licensed Psychologist. At the time of writing her chapter, Dr. Sims was the Assistant Director of Internship Training at the Colorado Mental Health Institute at Fort Logan, Colorado, USA. Currently, Dr. Sims is a co-owner of Rocky Mountain Behavioral Medicine, a private practice focused on psychological and neuropsychological assessment. Dr. Sims continues to work with individuals with severe and persistent mental illness through the provision of comprehensive evaluations and engages in the training and supervision of doctoral level students. dr.sims@rmbehavioralmedicine.com

Malcolm W. Stewart, PhD, PGDipClinPsych, DipMgt FNZCCP, is a Clinical Psychologist at Thrive Psychology, Auckland, New Zealand. He was formerly Professional Leader – Psychology (Head Psychologist) for two District Health Boards in New Zealand and a Senior Lecturer in the School of Medical and Health Sciences, University of Auckland, New Zealand. He has worked as a Clinical Psychologist in both physical and mental health inpatient settings. thrivepsychology@mail.com

Peter Walker, MPsych (Clin), is a Clinical Psychologist. Principal Clinical Psychologist, Peter Walker and Associates. Senior Clinical Psychologist, The Kiloh Centre, Prince of Wales Hospital, NSW Australia (2000–2012). Visiting lecturer, University of New South Wales, University of Technology, Sydney. pete_w35@hotmail.com

About the editors

Meidan Turel, MA, is a licensed Clinical Psychologist and a licensed Supervisor in Psychotherapy and Psychodiagnostics. Mr. Turel has over 22 years' experience working within a psychiatric acute closed ward and as Director of Psychological Services in Sha'ar Menashe, a public mental health center in Israel. In his work, Meidan is engaged in leading the psychology department, treating and diagnosing inpatients, providing case consultancy services to staff, and teaching and supervising interns in psychiatry and clinical psychology. Mr. Turel has taught courses in psychopathology and psychotherapy in various academic and professional educational settings. He serves on the Board of Examiners for the Ministry of Health Certification Examination in Clinical Psychology. meidan.a.turel@gmail.com

Michael A. Siglag, PhD, is a licensed Psychologist, in New Jersey and Pennsylvania (USA). Dr. Siglag has over 30 years of experience working as a Psychologist in hospital settings with psychiatric and forensic populations. He received his PhD in Clinical Psychology from the University of Detroit. Dr. Siglag has provided clinical and forensic psychology services at New Jersey's Trenton Psychiatric Hospital and Ann Klein Forensic Center. In 2015, he was appointed to the New Jersey State Board of Psychological Examiners, where he served as the Government Representative. Additional previous experience includes Chairing the Psychology Department and Directing the APA-accredited Pre-doctoral Internship program at Trenton Psychiatric Hospital. Dr. Siglag has served as a Board member for professional organizations, served as an adjunct faculty member on doctoral dissertations, and has written and presented at local, national, and international conferences and symposia on topics such as group therapy, psychosocial rehabilitation, treatment approaches for individuals struggling with psychosis, trauma issues, and hospital systems. mikesiglag@comcast.net

Alexander Grinshpoon, MD, PhD, MHA, is a Specialist in Psychiatry and in Health Administration. Professor A. Grinshpoon is Director of Sha'ar Menashe Mental Health Center in Israel with over 35 years' experience in psychiatry. He currently heads the Department of Psychiatry in the Rappaport Faculty of Medicine, Technion, Israel Institute of Technology, Haifa, where he is also the Head of the CME courses in Forensic Psychiatry, and Addiction Disorders. Professor Grinshpoon is the former Director of Mental Health Services in the Israel Ministry of Health. Professor Grinshpoon is a certified psychotherapist. Alexandergrinshpoon@gmail.com

Introduction

The Practice of Clinical Psychology in the Mental Health Inpatient Setting

Meidan Turel and Michael Siglag

Clinical psychologists provide a variety of clinical services in mental health inpatient settings in many countries around the world. Yet, despite decades of such service, the unique role and contribution of psychologists' work in inpatient settings has not been presented in a dedicated volume. This book addresses that gap by bringing together a collection of authors who describe a wide variety of work, explicating the roles and functions performed by clinical psychologists in a range of internationally based mental health inpatient settings.

Clinical Psychologists began to work and become involved in psychiatric hospital treatment during the 1940s and early 1950s. This development went hand in hand with the advancement of the profession within the academic world as well as within community mental health services, and paralleled a growing social awareness of the need to improve the care given to the mentally distressed (Hetherington, 1956). During psychologists' early years of work in mental health inpatient settings, clinical psychologists' roles on the ward were both limited and vaguely defined. At that time, hospital staff lacked an understanding of the psychologist's abilities to constructively contribute to patient care and ward tasks. For example, Baker et al. (2012) described the lack of formally defined roles clinical psychologists encountered when first entering United States Department of Veterans Affairs (VA) psychiatric hospitals following World War Two. In the 1950s, Hetherington (1956) wrote about the inconsistency in roles and functions attributed to clinical psychologists working in psychiatric wards in the United Kingdom, and Sommer and Clancy (1958) described the ambiguities surrounding the psychologist's role within psychiatric hospitals in Canada. The clinical psychologist at that time was mainly recognized and identified in the hospital through the narrow role of psychometrician, appreciated for the contribution of assessment input to the psychiatric understanding of relevant cases.

Since that early period, much effort and hard work by clinical psychologists on psychiatric wards, along with significant advances within the profession itself, have contributed to the expansion and range of clinical psychologists' functions and roles as described and enumerated in this volume. Clinical psychologists provide individual and group therapy services, perform psychological assessment and psychodiagnostic evaluations, carry out diverse system oriented interventions, provide interdisciplinary training and consultation, and have become integral members of multidisciplinary teams in a variety of mental health inpatient settings.

Since the early years of psychologists' involvement in mental health inpatient settings, models of treatment have also developed in notable ways. For example, over several decades there has been growing recognition of early developmental factors, psychological trauma, and psychosocial factors in the etiology of severe mental distress and disturbance (Duhig et al., 2015; Varese et al., 2012). This recognition has influenced treatment approaches (Read & Bentall, 2012). There has also been an increased emphasis on empirically based psychotherapeutic treatments (Rosenbaum et al., 2012), and more concerted efforts to increase consumer participation in treatment planning (Foltz, 2009). Clinical psychologists have played an important role in driving these as well as other changes in the provision of inpatient treatment.,

Clinical psychologists' growing involvement within the mental health inpatient system has gone hand in hand with wider academic, scientific, and professional developments in the field of clinical psychology. Since the 1940s and 1950s, these developments have been substantial. Today, in many countries clinical psychology is a licensed profession with a regulated course of academic studies and practical training lasting many years. Increasing numbers of academic institutions now offer graduate and doctoral level programs in clinical psychology, in response to the growing demand for such studies, and reflecting the evolving need and appreciation within society for this profession (Shapiro, 2002).

Despite international variations in specific standards and procedures for academic studies, practicum and internship training, and professional licensure, three basic tenets of clinical psychology as a profession have become well established: (a) a rigorous academic and clinical training regimen (b) in-depth academic and applied training in psychological assessment and psychodiagnostic evaluation; and (c) the study and practice of psychotherapy. These tenets are universally recognized as identifying the features of the profession and have provided psychologists with the knowledge and skills enabling them to enter and flourish in an ever-widening scope of settings, including the mental health inpatient system. Notably, a fourth domain of the profession that has emerged is the application of wide-ranging systems-level interventions in psychiatric inpatient settings.

This volume is divided into four parts that represent these four domains of clinical psychologists' practice in the mental health inpatient setting:

1. Systemic multi-modes and levels of interventions on the wards.
2. Psychotherapeutic interventions.

3. Assessment and psychodiagnosis.
4. Clinical psychology internship and supervision.

Each part opens with an introduction by the editors, which describes the chapters in that part and provides an overview of the issues, challenges, and common themes encountered in the psychologists' work within the domain of the practice described. The book concludes with two chapters by the editors, in which they bring their perspectives and concluding thoughts.

Following is a brief description of these four parts:

Part 1: Systemic Multiple Modes and Levels of Intervention

The nine chapters in this part are organized into three thematic clusters. The first cluster consists of four chapters which provide an overview and description of the varied roles and functions that clinical psychologists perform in diverse mental health inpatient settings, and the unique issues and challenges that confront them. The second cluster is composed of three chapters which describe original and innovative systems-level interventions created and led by clinical psychologists in response to difficult and demanding situations encountered on the ward. Knowledge of these programs, as developed and implemented by the authors, can benefit professionals confronted with similar circumstances in their inpatient work. The third and concluding cluster of chapters in this part is comprised of two chapters that provide a more personalized narrative of their authors' experiences, challenges, and difficulties encountered in their mental health inpatient work.

Part 2: Psychotherapeutic Interventions in the Mental Health Inpatient Ward

The six chapters in this part describe a variety of psychotherapeutic strategies, interventions, tools, and techniques currently practiced by clinical psychologists, that are uniquely adapted for work in diverse mental health inpatient settings and with severe mental states. Chapters include case studies and vignettes that illustrate the text.

Part 3: Assessment and Psychodiagnosis in Mental Health Inpatient Settings

The three chapters in this part describe the significant benefit that clinical psychological assessment and psychodiagnostic work holds for understanding difficult issues in the patient's presentation. Through detailed examples, the chapters illustrate ways assessment work helps the psychologist provide input to the patient and multidisciplinary treatment team members in order to more effectively and efficiently plan and provide patient-specific interventions.

Part 4: Clinical Psychology Internship and Supervision in the Mental Health Inpatient Setting

The four chapters in this part describe the important and unique experience of clinical psychology internship training in inpatient settings. This part includes chapters in which interns describe their work and experiences, as well as chapters written by supervisors, presenting perspectives on internship training and supervision.

The contributing authors are clinical psychologists who work in a range of mental health inpatient settings, including public and private facilities, open units, closed acute units, and forensic wards. The contributors represent a broad international spectrum: the United States, United Kingdom, Australia, New Zealand, Czech Republic, and Israel. Despite this wide variation in settings, types of institutions, and countries represented, many common themes and challenges are evident in the work and experiences psychologists describe. These themes are woven through the book's chapters, tapping into what might be thought of as both unique and universal principles of the profession as practiced today in the mental health inpatient system.

While common themes, conceptualizations, and experiences of clinical psychologists appear throughout the chapters of this book, diverse theoretical orientations, treatment approaches, and personal perspectives are also presented. This diversity exemplifies the current and evolving state of the conceptualization and practice of clinical psychology in mental health inpatient settings today. One way this broad scope of perspectives is made evident is through varied terminologies used by authors throughout the book's chapters. For example, designations for persons receiving inpatient treatment include 'patients', 'inpatients', 'consumers', and 'service users'. The editors chose to keep this array of terms, in order to allow differing conceptualizations and thoughts to come through as intended by their authors.

One major theme recurring through many of the books' chapters centers on the challenges clinical psychologists face related to efforts to create space in the inpatient setting for the recognition and acceptance of a psychological perspective. This theme is manifest in many of the book's chapters, cutting across psychologists' theoretical and technical orientations (e.g., psychodynamic or cognitive behavior therapy), and levels and modes of interventions provided (e.g., systemic, group or individual patient interventions). A major quest and contribution of clinical psychologists in inpatient settings is creating space for psychological issues and making the underlying reality they represent visible while addressing their involvement and significance in patients' treatment.

Clinical psychologists, with their high level of professional expertise and training in human psychology and psychopathology, are uniquely prepared to discover and explore underlying psychological issues related to the patient's presentation and circumstances and to understand their impact on the multidisciplinary team and the systemic level of the work. Psychologists strive to articulate a psychological understanding of these underlying issues and integrate this understanding into the broader multidisciplinary treatment effort. Through that process, psychologists attempt to bring greater clarity and relevance to the therapeutic work at hand. This is a challenging task, and one not always possible or easy to achieve. However, when achieved, it contributes in an important way to the ward's therapeutic effort, helping the treatment team see the person in the patient, with all the human complexities and issues involved in the existing situation. Thus, the clinical psychologist contributes to the unfolding of a wider perspective of the patient, shifting from a more limited, two-dimensional, and phenomenological view of the patient, to a fuller three-dimensional and psychological view, creating mental space where meaning-making provides the context for therapeutic activity.

Suffering and disturbance presented by persons treated in mental health inpatient settings are conceptualized by many who apply the prevailing medical model of mental health inpatient care, as symptoms or disease entities that need to be remediated or removed. From a psychological perspective, these same mental and behavioral phenomena are viewed as 'entry points' that need to be understood in order to reach the inner workings of the patient's mind and help alleviate their suffering. Whether through CBTp,[1] psychodynamic, family-systems, or other psychologically based models, clinical psychologists seek to make contact with the thoughts and feelings, and the many facets shaping people's identities, motivations and behaviors, in order to build an individualized and unique understanding of the person and tailor the therapeutic work accordingly.

Bridging the seemingly divergent attitudes that characterize these medical vs. psychological perspectives, while managing the tension inherent to their disparity, is an ongoing challenge for clinical psychologists working within mental health inpatient settings. Rather than viewing the biological and psychological dimensions as opposite aspects of the person being treated, the clinical psychologist strives to promote and maintain an integrative perspective in which the many dimensions of human life interact in a complementary fashion to form the individual person.

The collection of chapters in this volume relates each authors' tale of difficulties, successes and at times failures encountered in meeting this and other challenges in these settings. The book offers a broad view of the profession as practiced in the early twenty-first century, and suggests future directions for clinical psychologists in mental health inpatient systems.

PSYCHIATRIST'S VIEW OF THE ROLE OF THE CLINICAL PSYCHOLOGIST IN THE PSYCHIATRIC HOSPITAL

Alexander Grinshpoon and Rena Kurs

According to the World Health Organization, one in four people in the world will be affected by mental or neurological disorders at some point in their lives. Around 450 million people currently suffer from such conditions, placing mental disorders among the leading causes of ill health and disability worldwide. However, there is only one psychiatrist per 100,000 people in over half the countries in the world, and 40% of countries have less than one hospital bed reserved for mental disorders per 10,000 people (World Health Organization, 2001). The distribution of mental disorders between developed and underdeveloped countries is similar.

Following the development of community-based mental health services during the past few decades, and the reduction of inpatient facilities, globally, in 2014, there were only 17.5 beds per 100,000 population in mental hospitals (World Health Organization, 2014). Considering the immense gap between the number of people with mental disorders and the number of available psychiatric beds, it is clear that only individuals with severe psychiatric disorders and those in crisis situations receive inpatient mental health care.

The field of psychiatry is unique in that it treats the person, not only the disease. Psychiatrists and psychologists are the largest groups of clinicians that provide mental health services. The integrative approach to psychiatry has become the norm. While psychiatry is a medical specialty, and psychiatrists may prescribe psychopharmacologic medications, monitor lab reports and brain imaging studies, psychology is an applied academic discipline that incorporates the systematic study of mental functions and human behavior. The therapeutic relationship with patients is based on the understanding of the individual's character and his/her adaptive mechanisms. Clinical psychologists are thus involved in understanding, preventing and relieving subjective distress or dysfunction in humans taking into account the biopsychosocial environment (Gbadebo-Goyea et al., 2012).

Thus, psychiatry is closely identified with clinical psychology. Indeed, Carl Jung, Otto F. Kernberg, and Heinz Kohut, fathers of psychoanalytic theories were world-renowned psychiatrists, and Aaron Beck, the founder of cognitive therapy, is a psychiatrist. Beyond receiving biological therapy, the psychiatric inpatient anticipates 'talk therapy' with the clinical psychologist. Interventions with the staff psychologist contribute to a better understanding of the patient. A deeper understanding of the patient in terms of personality and processes that the patient has undergone helps build trust between the patient and the multidisciplinary treatment team and contributes to engagement in therapy, including pharmacotherapy. A better understanding of the individual's defense mechanisms enable the staff, together with the patient, to choose the most appropriate treatment method, whether it be cognitive behavior therapy, supportive psychodynamic therapy, pharmacotherapy, or a combination of therapies.

Through the deeper understanding of the patient achieved with the expertise of the clinical psychologist, the patient can often enhance autonomy and participation in his/her treatment plan. Therapeutic alliances that are often established working with psychologists help build trust that can extend to the whole treatment team and serve as the basis for successful treatment. For example, a patient with schizophrenia, who has sporadic psychotic episodes that lead to hospitalization, might hesitate to take antipsychotic medications on a regular ongoing basis, because of the associated side effects that he has difficulties coping with. Prior to discharge, through the therapeutic relationship, the psychologist can help the patient identify the early signs of a psychotic episode, and owing to the mutual trust between the patient and the therapist, the patient will approach the clinic for appropriate treatment, when necessary. The building of patient autonomy and patient-specific care is the foundation for enabling discharged patients to re-integrate into the community.

Most inpatients are admitted at times of crisis or exacerbations of their mental disorders. Work in a psychiatric hospital is difficult, with most staff working on overload. Multidisciplinary staff work is the key to success. Teamwork of the multidisciplinary staff is the key to understanding the crisis and to preventing further deterioration. A team that works well together contributes to a better understanding of the patient and can promote the process of recovery. The presence of a clinical psychologist on the ward contributes significantly to the relationships among members and to the dynamics of the multidisciplinary team. Teamwork enables a broader perspective than that of the single therapist. While the psychiatrist often explains why certain treatments are necessary, the clinical psychologist is often perceived as a neutral person who succeeds in relating to the person. The clinical psychologist often initiates interventions and treatment plans and thus contributes unique input to the attending psychiatrist, the department, and the patient's treatment. Quality of care and patient satisfaction surveys routinely reflect the patients' appreciation of the input of the clinical psychologist and patients often request additional therapy sessions. In a survey of needs of mental health patients, the most salient patient reported need was communication (Grinshpoon & Ponizovsky, 2008). Psychiatry is based on talk therapy, and teamwork with the clinical psychologist ensures mutual contributions for the benefit of the patient.

The various chapters in this book bring to light the recognition of the importance of the interdisciplinary work of psychiatry and psychology in attaining the best possible therapeutic results in inpatient mental health care. We hope that this book will promote the understanding and practice of this approach in psychiatric hospital settings.

Note

1 Cognitive Behavior Therapy for psychoses

References

Baker, R. R., Goldstein, G., Gurel, L., & Stenger, C. (2012). Patient care by VA psychologists in the 1950s and 1960s. *Psychological Services*, *9*, 417–426.

Duhig, M., Patterson, S., Connell, M., Foley, S., Capra, C., Dark, F., & Scott, J. (2015). The Prevalence and correlates of childhood trauma in patients with early psychosis. *Australian and New Zealand Journal of Psychiatry*, *49*, 651–659.

Foltz, R. (2009). The experience of being medicated in schizophrenia: A subjective inquiry and implications for psychotherapy. In D. Garfield & D. Mackler (Eds.), *Beyond medication* (pp. 159–173). London & New York, NY: Routledge.

Gbadebo-Goyea, E. A., Akpudo, H., Jackson, C. D., Wassef, T., Barker, N. C., Cunningham-Burley, R., & Bailey R. K. (2012). Collaboration: The paradigm of practice approach between the forensic psychiatrist and the forensic psychologist. *Frontiers in Psychiatry*, *3*, 89.

Grinshpoon, A., & Ponizovsky, A. (2008). The relationships between need profiles, clinical symptoms, functioning and the wellbeing of inpatients with severe mental disorders. *Journal of Evaluation in Clinical Practice*, *14*, 218–225.

Hetherington, R. (1956). The clinical psychologist in the mental hospital. *British Medical Journal*, *2*(4994), 708–709.

Read, J., & Bentall, P. (2012). Negative childhood experiences and mental health: theoretical, clinical and primary prevention implications. *British Journal of Psychiatry*, *201*, 89–91.

Rosenbaum, B., Harder, S., Knudsen, P., Koster, A., Lajer. M., Lindhart, A., & Winther, G. (2012). Supportive psychodynamic psychotherapy versus treatment as usual for first-episode psychosis: Two-year outcome. *Psychiatry*, *75*, 331–341.

Shapiro, D. (2002). Renewing the scientist-practitioner model. *The Psychologist*, *15*, 232–234.

Sommer, R., & Clancy, I. (1958). Ambiguities in the role of clinical psychologist in a mental hospital. *Journal of Clinical Psychology*, *14*, 264–268.

Varese, F., Smeets, F., Drukker, M., Lieverse, R., Lataster, T., Veichtbauer, W., & Bentall, R. (2012). Childhood adversities increase the risk of psychosis: A meta-analysis of patient-control, prospective- and cross-sectional cohort studies. *Schizophrenia Bulletin*, *38*, 661–671.

World Health Organization. (2001). World Health Report: Mental disorders affect one in four people. Retrieved from www.who.int/whr/2001/media_centre/press_release/en/

World Health Organization. (2014). Global Health Observatory (GHO) data. Beds in general hospitals for mental health and beds in mental hospitals (per 100,000 population). Retrieved from www.who.int/gho/mental_health/care_delivery/beds_hospitals/en/

Part 1

Systemic Multiple Modes and Levels of Intervention

Introduction to Part 1

Meidan Turel and Michael Siglag

All of the work described in this book is carried out by clinical psychologists in systemically complex and challenging mental health inpatient settings. For clinical psychologists working in these settings, systemic work through multiple modes and levels of interventions forms a crucial and integral part of their practice. This dimension of their work provides psychologists with some of the most unique and challenging aspects of their practice there. Thus, this first and opening part of the book focuses on the systemic level of clinical psychologists' involvement and interventions in mental health inpatient settings.

The nine chapters in this part each describe interventions and perspectives informed by their author's understanding and attention to systemic aspects of the units and facilities in which they work. Settings include open units, community-oriented units, closed and acute care units, and forensic closed units in a variety of mental health facilities in various countries.

The term 'multiple modes and levels of interventions' refers to the wide and flexible range of possible systemic interventions uniquely available to the clinical psychologist in mental health inpatient units, beyond the foundational clinical interventions of psychotherapy and assessment, the backbone of the profession.

Such systemic multiple modes and levels of interventions include, among others:

- Leading unit group activities such as community meetings.
- Structured interventions involving multidisciplinary staff. These include consultations with team members individually and in group settings that concern patient treatment planning as well as unit management issues; leading staff in implementing systems-level interventions with patients (e.g., behavioral intervention programs with patients); training staff in acquiring therapeutic tools and programs; etc.
- Provisory interventions with both staff members and patients, spontaneously improvised or planned, in response to various situations and conditions as they arise on the unit. For example, leading debriefings following sentinel or other adverse events on the ward

(such as patient suicide or an injurious act of violence); creating an informal ad hoc consultation in the nurses' station on specifics of a patient's situation; etc.

A major challenge inherent to such systems-level interventions is the clinical psychologist's ongoing task of successfully translating psychological understanding of the issues at hand into language that can be heard on the unit and put to constructive use. Through the process of articulating issues so that they can be addressed in a shared language with all those involved and impacted, the clinical psychologist enhances the quality of the unit's therapeutic efforts, contributing to the evolution of a therapeutic approach more tailored and responsive to the specific needs and communications of the unit's patients.

The ability to achieve this mission is contingent on a myriad of factors active in the setting, not least of which is the person of the psychologist: his/her professional disposition, abilities, as well as previous experience in such work.

The systems-level dimension of the clinical psychologist's work is, therefore, to some extent, an open-ended venture. Beyond specific systems oriented interventions that might be structured into a given unit's program (e.g., scheduled staff debriefing group meetings), it is up to the clinical psychologist to flexibly and creatively find ways and means to fulfill this dimension of the work within the particulars and circumstances operating in the setting.

This aspect of the clinical psychologist's systems-level work is well represented in the nine chapters comprising this part of the book, in which authors describe their interventions in response to specific issues and challenges in their particular settings. The nine chapters fall into three thematic clusters and are grouped accordingly. Following is a brief description of these three clusters and the included chapters:

In the first thematic cluster (Chapters 1, 2, 3, and 4), authors present a broad perspective and overview of their roles and functions within their respective inpatient settings:

In the first of these (Chapter 1), Mark McFetridge describes his work of many years as a clinical psychologist within an open unit in an independent inpatient psychiatric facility in the United Kingdom. McFetridge highlights a variety of the psychologist's roles and functions, which extend beyond the confines of the consultation room and involve systemic and group work with patients and staff, all of which valuably contribute to an integrated and psychologically minded approach to the therapeutic work on the ward. McFetridge encouragingly concludes that although the work is challenging and at times daunting,

> clinical psychologist(s) … are perfectly placed and ideally trained to fulfill the range of roles outlined here, and through these have

a significant influence on the good work of the ward that extends well beyond the walls of the clinical room.

In the next chapter (Chapter 2), Marilyn Charles describes her psychoanalytically oriented systems-level work within a renowned psychoanalytically and psychotherapeutically oriented private psychiatric inpatient facility in the United States. Through her examples, the author describes the clinical psychologist's pivotal role in providing understanding and recognition of underlying dynamics at play around various treatment issues. Her description of the systemic model used in her facility highlights how multiple levels of dynamics play out in the hospital, allowing for more efficient and transformative therapeutic work to unfold between the staff and patients.

In Chapter 3, authors Peter Walker and Sophie Li describe the clinical psychologist's placement and position within the Australian mental health inpatient system. Relying on their own experience as well as on input they collected through a survey conducted with fellow colleagues, the authors paint a rather grim picture of the limited degree of clinical psychologists' involvement and latitude in providing quality clinical psychology services on closed wards in the public mental health inpatient system. They convey a perspective suggesting that overemphasis on a biologically-based medical treatment model, together with limited resources available for patient care and rehabilitation within the broader public mental health inpatient system, creates conditions in which infringements of patients' human rights may occur. Stemming from this perspective, they endorse and summarize a human rights advocacy stance that clinical psychologists can take to safeguard patients' rights. The authors describe the implementation of cognitive behavioral therapy-based interventions and techniques on both systemic and individual levels and argue that by their very nature such interventions can remediate some of the more harmful aspects of inpatient mental health care.

In this cluster's closing chapter (Chapter 4), Heidi Camerlengo discusses the ethical issues and challenges involved in clinical psychologists' work in mental health inpatient settings. The author describes a variety of ethical dilemmas and issues faced by psychologists; some derived from her own experiences and some from experiences recounted by colleagues in both public and private psychiatric hospitals in the United States. In her chapter, Camerlengo demonstrates how ethical dilemmas abound in clinical psychologists' work in these settings, and how their impact crosses over into several aspects of the psychologist's clinical and administrative work, and sometimes into personal aspects of their work and lives as well. While the ethical dilemmas discussed in the chapter are not exhaustive, they represent some of the more common situations that psychologists encounter when providing inpatient mental health treatment. The author shows how addressing ethical dilemmas and conflicts is an ever-challenging part of the inpatient psychologist's responsibilities.

The second thematic cluster of chapters in this part includes three chapters (Chapters 5, 6, and 7) that delineate specific, original, and innovative systems-level interventions, created and led by the clinical psychologists in response to situations and needs they identified within their units.

In the first of these, Jimmy Kim and Peter D'Amico (Chapter 5) describe their implementation of a positive behavioral support model within an acute care inpatient unit in a public psychiatric facility in New York. The authors describe how through the use of this model they develop patient-specific behavior plans that help the ward maximize clinical care, patient stabilization and reduction of aggressive behavior. The authors discuss how, as clinical psychologists cast in the role of behavioral consultants on the ward, they assist the multidisciplinary team, the patient, and family members to understand patient's disturbing behaviors as a form of communication. This, in turn, opens the way to address underlying needs generating such behaviors and facilitates change.

In the next chapter (Chapter 6), Amit Fachler describes three of the more implicit roles that may be undertaken by a clinical psychologist in an acute closed inpatient unit. Using composite case examples taken from such work in a public psychiatric hospital in Israel, the author describes a psychodynamically minded clinical psychologist functioning as (a) an interpreter of patients' and family members' communications, (b) an informal organizational consultant, and (c) as 'regulator' of the unit's social climate. The author shows how functioning in these roles provides the psychologist opportunities to enhance the team's benign and thoughtful stance when confronted with difficult and challenging situations in their work on the acute closed ward.

In Chapter 7, Enav Or-Gordon describes her work with a recovery-oriented behavioral tool, developed and implemented in a closed psychiatric forensic ward in a state hospital in Prague, Czech Republic. The author demonstrates how work with this tool (a personalized notebook allocated to participating patients), promotes integration of the varied interventions on the ward into a unified structure and contributes to a cohesive course of therapy, enhancing patient's self-agency and constructive involvement in shared hospitalization goals.

The last cluster of chapters in this part contains two chapters (Chapters 8 and 9) in which their authors address, through a more personal narrative, their first-hand experience of work within the mental health inpatient setting:

In Chapter 8, author Jim Geekie presents his personal, lived experience of work in a public mental health inpatient unit in the United Kingdom. The author explores some of the challenges encountered in attempting to reconcile personal and professional values while working in an institution dominated by medicalized approaches to understanding and relating to mental distress. Geekie considers from a personal perspective, if and how it may – or may not – be possible to work within such a system while remaining true to his values.

In this part's closing chapter, Michael Siglag (Chapter 9) describes his many years of work within public and forensic state psychiatric hospitals in New Jersey, USA. Michael describes many influences and challenges encountered through his career path, starting as a unit based psychologist and moving ahead to management positions such as director of the APA-accredited internship in the hospital, followed by chairing the hospital's psychology department. The author presents this personal narrative of his long-term experience within the public psychiatric inpatient facilities, seeing it as representing experiences and challenges faced by many clinical psychologists working in similar public settings.

This collection of nine chapters, each describing psychologists' systemic-level perspectives and interventions, demonstrates the unique and valuable contribution such work holds for the mental health inpatient service, its units, patients, and staff. For the clinical psychologist committed to this level of work, experiencing his or her contribution to the unit's ability to fulfill its patients' therapeutic needs is rewarding and satisfying. Continuously holding in mind the potential influence of systems-level interventions on the unit, the clinical psychologist can turn every excursion from the privacy of the consulting room to the unit's public arena, into an opportunity to promote the system's psychological mindedness for the better care of its patients.

1 Therapy Beyond Walls

The Clinical Psychologist's Multi-Level Work in the Psychiatric Ward

Mark Andrew McFetridge

Twenty-five years earlier, Michael's key nurse Dawn met me at the entrance of the Acute Psychiatric unit known as 'Derwent ward'. The river Derwent in the north of England is unusual in that it flows upstream (rather than Nature's design of downstream) into the tidal river Ouse; a Roman shortcut to York.

I noticed that Dawn seemed reluctant to facilitate my use of the ward's consulting room to meet with Michael for our seventh therapy session. 'How has Michael been since our therapy appointment last week?' I asked. 'He's cut his face again; it was the day after your session'. I thought privately that my nursing colleague just did not understand the importance of this crucial therapeutic work on Michael's experiences of childhood sexual abuse. Dawn privately thought this young clinical psychologist was misguided, causing Michael to become more disturbed and unnecessarily extending his admission to Derwent ward.

Having had a quarter of a century to consider this view (it is important to take a little time to reflect) I now consider Dawn to have been correct. There were key things I had yet to learn, including that any individual therapy on inpatient units needs to be fully integrated with the service and not undertaken by clinicians having little communication and shared formulation with the core inpatient team. I had yet to learn that clients who have histories of childhood abuse who self-harm must develop alternative ways of safely managing distress before addressing their traumatic memories in therapy. If not, the flow of the intrinsic emotional distress is inevitably against the self in a direction congruent with the invasion of their childhood.

Later in my career, I had the opportunity to work with, and learn from, a number of group analyst colleagues. I already had experience facilitating therapeutic groups for clients and training groups for staff; however, I was not aware of the therapeutic potential of the group within the inpatient setting for developing the sense of community, belonging, involvement and agency (Kennard & Haigh, 2009; Pearce & Haigh, 2017).

Over the next two decades, I had the privilege of being a staff member of the Acorn program, a DBT-informed Therapeutic Community at the

Retreat York, UK. Opening in 1796, the Retreat 'mental health project' and its founders rejected the inhumane treatments of the day (purging, burning, bleeding) and applied their Quaker values and practice to a new institution for the treatment of the insane that was to prove remarkably effective (Tuke, 1813). Samuel Tuke wrote of the importance of 'exciting the capability of the patient', implicitly acknowledging that the ward environment could have a powerfully enabling effect. The relevance of the Quakers original approach to contemporary mental healthcare is still apparent (Borthwick et al., 2001).

Too often, we presume that the problem is solely located within the patient, and the correct therapy will remedy this pathology. Comprehensive formulation of our patients' clinical presentations might still usefully take account of social, environmental, occupational, and spiritual factors, as did the Quakers. There was a reason this pioneering institution was built on an eminence, with beautiful grounds of sufficient size for animal husbandry (Tuke, 1813).

The importance (if not primacy) of attachment experiences and learning has been acknowledged as important for us all (Bowlby, 2005). Perhaps the nature of the anticipated interaction and the actual relationships between the patient and others might exceed the effect of any simple intervention. Wampold (2013) found 87% of outcome variance was due to client-related factors and other factors outside therapy. Only 13% could be attributed to the treatment itself, and of this the therapeutic alliance had by far the greatest contribution to the outcome, far greater than the therapeutic model (Green & Latchford, 2012). If this is correct, our therapeutic interventions need to extend beyond the walls of our therapy office in order to maximize effectiveness.

While the complexity of client presentation may be particularly challenging, the clinical psychologist is perfectly placed to make a valuable contribution to the care and treatment received during their psychiatric admission. The integration of theory, research, and practice is what differentiates the clinical psychologist from other professions. Skillful, collaborative formulation of the individual's mental health difficulties and strengths, in the context of their past/present relationships and life experiences, will effectively inform the inpatient team's considered interventions and care plans.

> Lucy was a 50-year-old teacher. She was admitted to the ward following a life-threatening overdose and now presented with depressed mood and marked intrusive thoughts about dangers befalling her family members. Lucy reported she was happily married to Rick, a train driver, and they had three adult sons together. When her youngest son Sam left the family home, as his brothers had, Lucy soon became unable to work as her mood deteriorated and her compulsive behaviors markedly increased. She began to

> self-harm by ligaturing, and subsequently took an overdose of prescribed and over the counter medications.

With Lucy, Michael, and Derwent ward in mind, let us consider a number of potential roles and contributions for the clinical psychologist within the complex system of a psychiatric ward.

The Individual Therapist

While this will be a familiar role to all clinical psychologists, the system in which this takes place requires additional attention. The level of possible direct clinical involvement with a client will clearly be influenced by the anticipated duration of admission to the psychiatric ward. In brief, a shared written formulation may be all that is possible; however, the potential benefit of this to the individual patient and to future treating clinicians should not be underestimated. The client has too often not encountered a clinician who is so actively and collaboratively curious about their difficulties and how these might 'make sense' through the lens of experiences, developmental learning, and current life context.

The clinical psychologist also brings a broader assessment and psychodiagnostic contribution to the inpatient unit. Screening measures (e.g., for Autism Spectrum Disorders) may be incorporated into initial assessment, alongside baseline clinical outcome measures. Following this, formal psychometric assessment may be undertaken to assess any cognitive or specific learning difficulties. If more clearly identified and delineated, any such difficulties will have implications for individualizing future interventions from the ward team.

In some cases the clinical psychologist may routinely undertake a full psychometric assessment on all new clients; this may be clearly indicated by the nature of the inpatient unit, e.g., neurobehavioral rehabilitation ward. In general, however, my own view is that while this is undoubtedly a specific skill of the clinical psychologist, it is also time-intensive for both the psychologist and client. If psychometric assessment is reserved for use as and when it is indicated by initial assessment or subsequent symptoms, this permits time for a broader contribution and involvement by the psychologist.

Following a series of assessment sessions with Lucy the following written formulation was shared with her:

> You were born a normal healthy baby to your parents Bill and Brenda; their first child. Brenda and Bill had planned to have a baby soon after Brenda's recent depression as they thought and were advised by family that it would help them through what had been a difficult time for everybody. You were a healthy and attentive baby girl and you were welcomed into the world but with heavy

expectations immediately placed on your little shoulders. What you could not be expected to understand as an infant was that your mother found being responsible for a child to be more difficult than she had expected, particularly as Bill was away from home, apparently working, for much of your childhood. She suspected he was seeing other women and felt frustrated at being unable to keep his attention as she had previously strived to do. As you made sense of how others related to you, and what you could come to expect from them, you learned to feel the source of difficulty for them and that your role was to make others feel better. Brenda very soon became pregnant again and lost this baby at birth; your mother became depressed and withdrawn and received medical care from community services.

You recall that by the time you started school you had difficulty making and keeping friends as you felt different from others; there was nobody at home able to help dress you like the other children in your class. You were teased by the other children, and you learned to avoid playtime by staying with the teacher after lessons had finished. You remember thinking it would be better if you died because people said nice things about dead people. You began thinking about things that might kill you, like your mother's tablets in the bathroom. You noticed that thinking about and visualizing this made you feel better.

This initial part of Lucy's formulation is not written in the language of a particular therapeutic model, but you may detect it draws from attachment, systemic, and cognitive-behavioral frameworks of understanding. It is more important to incorporate Lucy's own words and reported memories as closely as possible. Lucy found this a deeply validating, emotionally attuned and supportive intervention, which further facilitated collaborative work on the second stage of Lucy's formulation explicitly linking childhood experiential learning to her presenting problems and life context.

The clinician should, however, be cautious that we cannot be certain of the degree of accuracy of childhood memories; the British Psychological Society concluded that memories are records of people's experiences of events and are not a record of the events themselves (The British Psychological Society, 2010).

The longer admission permits a more comprehensive formulation and more active therapeutic engagement with the formulated issues. If a short admission, the client might take the formulation into their future therapy as an outpatient.

The space may be facilitated by the possibility that the clinical psychologist, unlike their psychiatrist colleague, may not be subject to the same degree of immediate transference. This has been my experience as a male clinician working closely with a male psychiatric colleague.

Alternatively, the more complex client may present and relate differently to members of the team due to a disorganized pattern of attachment (Liotti & Farina, 2016). The pattern of multiple relating should be understood as a whole so the individual can experience being held in mind by a benevolent, reliable team. To facilitate this, the clinical psychologist needs to be attuned to the involvement and responses of colleagues, and share details of their own work in the service of the client's therapy. To permit this, the boundary of confidentiality might be discussed with the client as existing around the therapy team rather than the individual clinicians. There may, however, be details of the client's history they may request the clinical psychologist to maintain on a 'need to know' basis. This would not include information about risk-related behavior of the patient, or information about imminent risk to others. Withholding other non-risk-related information from the wider team, while important in the careful management of information the patient may feel deeply ashamed of, needs to be used judiciously or risks perpetuating the client's disorganized and fragmented presentation. Many inpatients will have previously reported a history of traumatic events evident in their case notes (McFetridge, Milner, Gavin, & Levita, 2015) which may (but may not) manifest as a Complex PTSD presentation. In my experience, such clients have found this a validating framework for understanding their experience; several guidelines are available to assist clinicians in how to appropriately assess and safely undertake phase-based therapeutic interventions for patients with histories of traumatic experience (Cloitre et al., 2012; The United Kingdom Psychological Trauma Society, 2017).

Having worked in several inpatient and outpatient settings, my personal view is that when working within a skillful and well-managed inpatient team it is easier to sustain and contain the work than when carrying a caseload of complex clients as an independent clinician; risk is shared and potentially managed more therapeutically, and successes can be shared and acknowledged more effectively.

The Group Therapist/Facilitator

The novice clinical psychologist may have relatively less experience as a group facilitator, but appreciation of relational and systemic factors may assist in the assimilation of these skills. Many individuals with their difficulties conceptualized as a diagnosable personality disorder, or as Complex PTSD have been found to benefit from participation in a therapy group. There is evidence for the effectiveness of group therapy for adults with histories of childhood sexual abuse, regardless of whether these are trauma-focused or present-focused groups (Classen et al., 2011). More structured groups which include a 'safety and stabilization' phase have been found effective with adult survivors of childhood trauma. One recent variant, a 10-session group intervention called 'Survive and Thrive' has been developed with the aims of increasing stabilization, understanding links between past trauma and current symptoms, and preparing for trauma-focused therapy. Preliminary studies, including a controlled investigation, have demonstrated this may be an effective intervention for promoting stabilization (Karatzias et al., 2014). As a time-limited structured group this may also be suitable for inpatients with trauma histories.

Equally, there is evidence that patients without a reported trauma history benefit from participation in a residential Dialectical Behavioral Therapy (DBT)-informed therapeutic community (McFetridge, Milner, Gavin, & Levita, 2015). This model incorporates the therapeutic community as a method for delivering and enhancing the structured individual and group interventions. This facilitates therapy beyond the walls of the consulting room, and the clinical psychologist has the potential to play a valuable role in helping the client and staff colleagues to think about patterns of relating within groups.

> Following a period of my leave, a clinical colleague expressed concern about Michael's capacity to regulate his feelings and whether more specific work on this was needed. Michael had self-harmed during this time, and the staff team had felt concerned and confused as to why he was disturbed after quite a stable period. When I met with Michael as planned, we established he had indeed found it difficult not meeting for individual sessions as he believed he didn't have anywhere to take (his) feelings resulting from difficult conversations with his mother. I acknowledged that it was, of course, disruptive of his therapy for me to be on leave, however understandable and necessary this is. However, there were many other staff and fellow patients present during this time who may have been able and willing to offer support if Michael had been able to approach and seek such help. My absence had simultaneously highlighted both the therapeutic benefit of consistent appointments and the unintended negative consequences; Michael had not had to practice seeking support from peers or others as any difficult issues would be 'saved' and addressed with me within a session. We recognized that as an 'only child' he had, through no fault of his own, missed the opportunity to practice this key emotion regulation skill earlier in his life. We discussed the potential value of Michael joining a group on the ward to experience support seeking and giving with peers. Following participation in the group, Michael was more able to let others know when he was feeling distressed and at risk of self-harm,

and in turn experience the degree of emotional containment that can result from doing so.

Facilitator of a Psychologically Minded Team with Therapeutic Curiosity

If clients are to be helped, the staff team must be able to understand and digest the feelings they experience in their interactions with them. If this is overlooked or avoided there is a danger staff will become the unwitting (re-)enactors of the clients' life scripts. The capacity of the staff team to think will, in turn, be facilitated by organizational factors which promote this, including effective, consistent leadership and appropriate working conditions. If such organizational requirements are compromised or absent, the clinical psychologist should address this with higher management in a way that effectively alerts senior managers to the clinical and financial consequences of this.

The clinical psychologists, actively carrying their formulation skills and broad knowledge of psychological and clinical theory, can be key contributors to the 'psychological mindedness' or reflective capacity of the team. For this to be realized, I would argue, the clinical psychologist needs to be seen as a member of the ward team, even if this is not possible on a full-time basis.

Within the ward, a culture of curiosity combined with a shared model of understanding is fundamental. A regular 'staff supervision' (or alternatively named 'reflective care') group with a permissive expectation that all staff will attend regularly facilitates this. This opportunity for group processing enables the staff team to appreciate each other's perspectives, their differing experiences of the same client, and to diffuse and explore the feelings engendered by the team's shared work. An additional benefit of this arrangement is that there is a scheduled weekly meeting to address any serious incidents that would otherwise require a special meeting due to their impact. If services and resources permit, this might be facilitated by a clinical psychologist colleague from another unit, with a reciprocal arrangement. Such an arrangement allows the ward's clinical psychologist to actively and equally participate in the group supervision for their team, and through this to model openness to reflexive thinking.

Let us return to Lucy, who on the ward alternates between being 'the perfect patient' in supporting the staff and other clients, and occasions of angry denigration of staff members and acts of self-harm. The staff team is at a loss to understand this rapidly alternating presentation, and feel angry and critical of her in return as they know she can be so different. Lucy is aware that others are angry with her at these times. She feels troubled, and yet strangely reassured, by this. The supervision group was used to acknowledge the very real emotional demands of the teams' shared work, and to reintroduce aspects of the formulated understanding of Lucy's attachment patterns of interacting with others and responding to her own distress. As team members no longer felt as confused and frustrated by their subsequent interactions with Lucy, they were able to collaboratively problem-solve the day's emotional challenges with her.

Culture Carrier

Staff teams inevitably change over time as colleagues gain experience and career development elsewhere, and new members replace them, bringing fresh perspectives and valuable 'beginners' eyes'. This will also apply to the clinical psychologist, but it is equally important for there to be stability in the team (and career development within the organization to permit this) to allow the culture and norms of a service to become established. The clinical psychologist may then act in a culture-transmitting role, enabling new colleagues to observe, enquire, and then assimilate new ways of understanding and responding to patients within the inpatient unit. This will be of (at least) equal importance to any formalized training provided due to its timely provision when relevant and needed.

Researcher and Scientist Practitioner

The clinical psychologist is not only a therapist but also a scientist-practitioner. Many years before the advent of evidence-based practice and practice-based evidence, clinical psychologists were trained to continually evaluate and explore the effectiveness of their clinical (and other) interventions through appropriate measurement. This was later extended within the UK to a greater appreciation of mixed method and qualitative approaches following the development of methodologies such as IPA (Interpretive Phenomenological Analysis; Smith, Flowers, & Osborn, 1997) and Grounded Theory (Strauss & Corbin, 1997).

The psychiatric ward team and service first needs to be helped to clarify what it seeks to achieve through its work with clients; what are the aims of the service for its clients? Measures can then be identified to best assess these aims at intake, reviews, pre-discharge, and at subsequent post-discharge follow-up. A mixed method approach of quantitative and qualitative measures can be helpful in evaluating whether a service helps its clients to improve in specific ways and to examine the clients' personal experiences of these changes. Considering the example of 'the Acorn program for self-defeating behavior' at the Retreat, York UK, the primary aim was to help clients to reduce their self-harm and impulsivity. The primary measures of this were, therefore, the Multi-Impulsivity

Scale (MIS; Evans, Searle, & Dolan, 1998) and the patient reported outcomes and reflections of change on longer-term follow-up (McFetridge & Coakes, 2010).

The ongoing evaluation of clinical changes can also be useful for informing and influencing the clinical process. If multiple time points for all patients yield a data set for the developmental sequence of admission and post-discharge, the pattern becomes evident and useful in a range of ways. Within Michael's unit, Derwent ward, it was apparent from a representative sample of 56 previous patients, that measures of psychological distress improved during admission, worsened temporarily pre-discharge, and then improved again three months after leaving. This pattern made sense to the staff team as they recognized the anxieties, uncertainties, and loss that often accompanied their patients' discharge. It was also helpful for them to be made aware that this (generally) subsequently improved by three months post-discharge. This knowledge, in turn, facilitated more contained 'endings' between key nurses and Michael on his discharge and improved their ability to acknowledge Michael's emotional response to the discharge process. Supportively, Michael was also made aware that the data suggested that the period around discharge was difficult for people in general (not just for him) but that this did change for the better over the following year for his predecessors as they were perhaps able to put into practice what they had learned during their hospitalization.

As a service informed by clinical outcome data, the Derwent ward team were, in addition, able to think about additional support around discharge, introducing a weekly transitional group that clients were invited to attend as they approached discharge and could continue for the three months post-discharge. The service, assisted by the clinical psychologist, noted that readmission rates within three months of discharge significantly reduced following the introduction of this transitional group.

The nature and level of doctoral clinical psychology training also equips the clinical psychologist to design and implement primary research to extend the shared clinical knowledge base. Joint research with colleagues from the range of professions can, in addition, improve team morale, staff retention, and development, and further raise clinical standards. The successful dissemination of the research by publication and conference presentation may also serve to raise the internal and external profile of the service. While research is invariably the lowest day-to-day priority in the psychiatric ward, if successfully undertaken to completion, it can provide many positive benefits for the service. For example, a nursing colleague and I presented our clinical research at a national conference; we had examined the factors likely contributing to the remarkably positive clinical outcome of a small group of patients (McFetridge, Morton, & Berg, 2006). 'I am now a proper researcher', she said with evident pride on our return journey. She went on to develop a successful leadership role within the inpatient service.

Teacher, Trainer, (Skillful Team-Maker)

We have already noted the informal training opportunities the clinical psychologist can contribute to the inpatient team. It is equally important for us to be open to the opportunity to learn from others outside our profession as this can only complement and broaden our existing knowledge. However, the clinical psychology resource in a team will be utilized most effectively if more formal regular training opportunities are provided for colleagues. There is much to be addressed in the development and maintenance of a shared clinical model for the ward, whatever focus this takes. It is, however, in my experience, a more effective choice of model if this can enable those interacting most frequently with patients to know what to do in your absence. An overly complicated theoretical model that is experienced by the team as the province of more expert colleagues will have limited impact. To this end, clinical psychologists in Scotland have, in recent years, been actively involved in training and supervising nursing colleagues in Mentalization skills (Williams, Beedie, & Gumley, 2017). This is not the full Mentalization-based therapy training (MBT; Bateman & Fonagy, 2010), but an abridged version of the model focusing on the key skills that inpatient nurses can employ in their interactions with patients. A number of unexpected benefits have been found to follow from this training, commensurate with the teams having greater confidence to manage any difficult situation they may find themselves party to.

I recall my own experience of the unexpected non-specific benefit of undertaking Eye Movement Desensitization and Reprocessing (EMDR) level II training with Francine Shapiro in 1998. I predictably became more expert in this (then) new form of trauma processing therapy; however, the additional benefit was that I now felt able to approach the most appalling of traumatic memories with clients with a new found confidence and sense of containment. Clinical outcomes were impressive, but I continue to suspect this was disproportionately influenced by my new found palpable capacity to contain the clients' worst life-threatening moments; perhaps my own version of Dumbo's feather facilitating the belief he could fly (Walt Disney Productions, 1941). Like the author, inpatient team members need feathers too, and the clinical psychologist can engender these.

Leadership; Formal or Informal

The clinical psychologist may have a formalized leadership role within the inpatient ward, but more often this is an informal leadership born of the contribution to the team and service over time. I would advise any new clinical psychologist joining a team to go quietly yet confidently; your clinical knowledge and skills will become evident. Alternatively, a sales presentation of the many reasons you should be followed is likely to be (appropriately) poorly received and ultimately self-defeating. This is unnecessary and likely driven by anxiety on your part (May I offer a feather for your cap?); talk with your new colleagues about their patients' problems and notice what you bring to the developing shared understanding. The new setting in which you work may be unfamiliar as yet, but you will probably 'recognize' the clients discussed. Clinical psychologists in the main cannot help but be patient-focused, emotionally attuned, and supportive colleagues and soon become appreciated as such.

Container

Remembering the ward is a system within a system, there are important contributions to be made in ensuring others can enable these to function effectively. One important role is the supporting of the ward or clinical team manager. They are subject to all manners of displaced feelings and projections from both patients and staff members, coupled with unconscious (and occasionally conscious) 'attacks' from the parent organization. Often this will be prompted by fear of criticism, or actual criticism, of the unit from sources external to the organization. The effective management of anxiety at each level within a psychiatric institution is central to being able to sustain an effective service and is a key 'management' function.

Managing a psychiatric unit or hospital, however, brings inherent challenges and complexity, and this can be overlooked from a more detached managerial perspective and interpreted as evidence of a failing service. The pathological patterns of clients' past, of possible exploitation, deprivation, and abuse, can be 'pushed in' to the organization. The clinical psychologist, as a senior colleague, may often be in a position to offer the service manager personal support and informal systemic supervision 'as required'. The supported opportunity to appraise the validity of criticism (actual or perceived), hypothesize reasons for this, and interrupt otherwise impulsive responses may probably be both appreciated by your colleague and be of significant benefit to the service. Sometimes a staff member will have gone on to act inappropriately, and this needs to be dealt with by the manager and digested by their colleagues. The clinical psychologist's involvements already discussed can mitigate against this to a degree, but the emotional loads of this work should not be underestimated. This was formally recognized in the UK with certain enhanced employment conditions for those designated 'mental health officers' who spent the majority of time in face-to-face clinical contact with clients. Interestingly, this was removed for new staff two decades ago; could it be that the real impact of the work could no longer be heard, or had the systemic effects of working in mental health on managers and others perhaps never been equally recognized?

Conclusions

The river Ouse in York, UK, still floods with regularity, so much so that many visitors are unable to quench their thirst at 'the Kings Arms' public house due to the water climbing the doors and walls. Unlike riverside pubs, psychiatric institutions were purposely built on high ground to permit good drainage and sanitation, and therefore promote better physical health. Our forefathers realized this could contribute significantly to improving the mental health of patients within asylums, together with a culture of community, kindness, respect, and social responsibility (Tuke, 1813). In this way, they were not only addressing immediate distress but working 'upstream' from the presenting problems of their patients, and leaving the challenge for us to follow their lead.

I have suggested in this chapter that there are a number of roles and means by which the clinical psychologist might work upstream within the system of the psychiatric ward. A psychological formulation may not only help the patient, but also be of benefit to the team around them, and beyond the admission. In addition to the individual psychological therapy and facilitation of therapeutic groups, the clinical psychologist should contribute to the capacity of the inpatient team to reflect on their patients and interactions, and do this from a position of therapeutic curiosity. Bringing the formulation beyond the walls of the therapy room into the actively reflecting team will additionally assist with the containment of anxiety of the team during times of incident or uncertainty. As time and tide continue, new staff members need to be helped to understand and assimilate the culture of the service, and it is suggested the clinical psychologist can play a lead role here as a culture carrier. This forms part of a broader informal leadership role within the team, which takes shape during regular clinical discussion and other contributions to the teams' work. There is much informal training offered through this process, but the clinical psychologist might also usefully provide formal teaching input to the team. The support of those who manage and serve in formal leadership roles is crucial; the clinical psychologist can thus be both a good colleague and reduce anxiety-driven impulsive responses by managers. Rather than any implied criticism, this can be understood as an inherent effect of the work within a mental health system that Ballatt and Campling (2011) note may otherwise undermine the *intelligent kindness* within the organization. Last but far from least, the competency of the clinical psychologist as a scientist-practitioner and researcher can quality assure and further develop the work of the psychiatric ward, and contribute to the security of the service through demonstrating clinical and financial effectiveness. This latter role can be difficult to prioritize, but open to regret at your leisure. The good news is that as a clinical psychologist you are perfectly placed and ideally trained to fulfill the range of roles outlined here, and through these have a significant influence on the good work of the ward that extends well beyond the walls of the clinical room.

References

Ballatt, J., & Campling, P. (2011). *Intelligent kindness: Reforming the culture of healthcare*. London: RCPsych publications.

Bateman, A., & Fonagy, P. (2010). Mentalization based treatment for borderline personality disorder. *World Psychiatry*, 9(1), 11–15.

Borthwick, A., Holman, C., Kennard, D., McFetridge, M., Messruther, M., & Wilkes, J. (2001). The relevance of moral treatment to contemporary mental health care. *Journal of Mental Health*, *10*(4), 427–439.

Bowlby, J. (2005). *A secure base: Clinical applications of attachment theory*. (Vol. 393). London: Taylor & Francis.

Classen, C. C., Palesh, O. G., Cavanaugh, C. E., Koopman, C., Kaupp, J. W., Kraemer, H. C., & Spiegel, D. (2011). A comparison of trauma-focused and present-focused group therapy for survivors of childhood sexual abuse: A randomized controlled trial. *Psychological Trauma: Theory, Research, Practice, and Policy*, *3*(1), 84.

Cloitre, M., Courtois, C. A., Ford, J. D., Green, B. L., Alexander, P., Briere, J., & Van der Hart, O. (2012). The ISTSS expert consensus treatment guidelines for complex PTSD in adults. Retrieved from: www.istss.org

Evans, C. D. H., Searle, Y., & Dolan, B. M. (1998). Two new tools for the assessment of multi-impulsivity: The 'MIS'and the 'CAM'. *European Eating Disorders Review*, 6(1), 48–57.

Green, D., & Latchford, G. (2012). *Maximising the benefits of psychotherapy: A practice-based evidence approach*. West Sussex, UK: John Wiley & Sons.

Karatzias, T., Ferguson, S., Chouliara, Z., Gullone, A., Cosgrove, K., & Douglas, A. (2014). Effectiveness and acceptability of group psychoeducation for the management of mental health problems in survivors of child sexual abuse (CSA). *International Journal of Group Psychotherapy*, 64(4), 492–514.

Kennard, D., & Haigh, R. (2009). Therapeutic communities. In M. Gelder, N. Andreasen, J. Lopez-Ibor, & J. Geddes (Eds.) *The new Oxford textbook of psychiatry 2nd edition* (Section 6.3.9, pp. 1391–1398). Oxford: Oxford University Press.

Liotti, G., & Farina, B. (2016). Painful incoherence: The self in borderline personality disorder. In M. Kyrios, R. Moulding, G. Doron, S. S. Bhar, M. Nedeljkovic, & M. Mikulincer (Eds.) *The self in understanding and treating psychological disorders* (pp. 169–178). Cambridge: Cambridge University Press.

McFetridge, M., & Coakes, J. (2010). The longer-term clinical outcomes of a DBT-informed residential therapeutic community; an evaluation and reunion. *Therapeutic Communities: The International Journal of Therapeutic Communities*, *31*(4), 406–416.

McFetridge, M., Morton, C., & Berg, J. (2006). Traumatic memory; is it all in the mindfulness? *Therapeutic Communities: The International Journal of Therapeutic Communities*, *27*(2), 177–191.

McFetridge, M. A., Milner, R., Gavin, V., & Levita, L. (2015). Borderline personality disorder: Patterns of self-harm, reported childhood trauma and clinical outcome. *British Journal of Psychiatry Open*, *1*(1), 18–20.

Pearce, S., & Haigh R. (2017). *The theory and practice of democratic therapeutic community treatment*. London: Jessica Kingsley Publishers.

Smith, J. A., Flowers, P., & Osborn, M. (1997). Interpretative phenomenological analysis and the psychology of health and illness. In L. Yardley (Eds.) *Material discourses of health and illness* (pp. 68–91). Florence, KY: Taylor & Francis/ Routledge.

Strauss, A., & Corbin, J. M. (1997). *Grounded theory in practice*. Thousand Oaks, CA: Sage Publications, Inc.

The British Psychological Society. (2010). (Revised version) *Guidelines on memory and the law; Recommendations from the scientific study of human memory*. Retrieved from: www.academia.edu/2326108/Guidelines_On_Memory_And_The_Law_ Recommendations_From_The_Scientific_Study_Of_Human_Memory

The United Kingdom Psychological Trauma Society (UKPTS). (2017). *Guideline for the treatment and planning of services for complex post-traumatic stress disorder in adults*. Retrieved from: www.ukpts.co.uk/guidance_11_2920929231.pdf

Tuke, S. (1813). *Description of The Retreat, an institution near York, for insane persons of the Society of Friends*. York: Published by Isaac Pierce. Retrieved from: https:// archive.org/details/2575045R.nlm.nih.gov

Walt Disney Productions. (1941). *Dumbo*.

Wampold, B. E. (2013). *The great psychotherapy debate: Models, methods, and findings* (Chap. 9). New York, NY: Routledge.

Williams, A., Beedie, S., & Gumley, A. (2017). 'Tricky interactions': Exploring mental health staff responses to stressful interpersonal sequences following mentalizing skills training. Scientific paper presented to the British and Irish Group for the Study of Personality Disorders Annual Conference. Retrieved from: www.bigspd.org.uk/uploads/6/9/5/8/69584269/exploring_mental_health_ staff_responses_to_stressful_interpersonal_sequences_following_mentalizing_ skills_training__williams_beedie__gumley__.pdf

2 The Clinical Psychologist in an Open Inpatient Setting

A Psychoanalytic Perspective

Marilyn Charles

In this chapter, I use Psychoanalytic and Field Theory lenses as vertices through which to consider the role of the clinical psychologist in a hospital setting. These lenses help us to recognize the potential positive impact of the psychologist not only in his or her clinical roles but also, importantly, in relation to colleagues and to the institution as a whole. System perspectives help to mark the ways in which individual dynamics also play out in relation to the various structures within the hospital. Such recognition can help both therapists and patients to become better able to recognize various patterns and defenses at play in ways that may be transformative rather than merely repetitive. As someone whose expertise affords insight into the ways in which unconscious processes may play out in groups, the psychologist can offer formulations that enable other staff to perform their own roles more effectively. Examples will be given regarding the psychologist's role as part of the hospital treatment team, as a pivotal person who can help to allay anxiety and encourage greater understanding through recognition of the dynamics in play with a particular patient.

The Austen Riggs Center (ARC) is a psychoanalytically-informed psychiatric hospital. The four times weekly individual psychotherapy with patients there is augmented by a community program that offers patients ongoing opportunities to locate themselves in context and to recognize ways in which their behavior may undermine their conscious intentions, thereby also illuminating unconscious dynamics and motivations. Operating under the principle of *examined living*, all members of the community, including staff, are encouraged to speak from their own perspective such that the diversity of viewpoints can be considered. Being able to see a familiar problem across relationships helps to attenuate the tendency to personalize and attribute blame, and also highlights patterns so that we might recognize our own part. In this way, patients (and staff) encounter stumbling blocks they have experienced in other relationships but now with the opportunity to learn more directly about the roles they take on, patterns of reactivity, and the effects they have on others.

The Riggs treatment model is dynamically informed, with an appreciation for the ways in which the unconscious can play out in a group process, resulting in fixed ideas that can be projections rather than perceptions. These projective processes are amplified by the ways in which tensions can increase and discharge as groups become larger. Group relations concepts such as *task* and *role* help us to locate ourselves in relation to the larger whole, and to think about how to speak as a responsible member of the community, from whatever role we find ourselves in at that particular juncture, in relation to the task at hand (Obholzer & Roberts, 1994). These concepts are crucial to have in mind for the psychologist who plays diverse roles within the treatment setting.

Because there is an appreciation for ways in which meanings are nested and may become entrenched in idiosyncratic ways that can be hard to get hold of, we structure into our routine opportunities to talk with one another across staff/patient and guild-specific boundaries, to help us see beyond our blind spots. Our patients have all become waylaid in their lives to some extent, which often leaves them with entrenched ideas about authority, either deferring to or opposing it in ways that make it difficult for them to recognize and make use of their own legitimate authority in relation to their lives, well-being, and desires. To counter these tendencies, or at least make them more visible, we use ideas from Lacan (1977) regarding the analytic *Third*, the importance of having a third perspective through which to contextualize an understanding of the dyad (Muller, 2011); and also the *Subject caught by the desire of the Other*, the tendency to look for answers from an external authority rather than making use of and refining one's *own* internal sensibilities (Charles, 2012).

Our fundamental guiding principle is that the open setting affords people opportunities to take responsibility for their lives and well-being. There are no locks and no mandated treatments; rather, there is a continual negotiation between the individual and others within the institution regarding the extent to which that particular treatment is useful and viable. Entering Riggs requires making the choice to sign oneself in for a six-week period of intensive treatment and evaluation, and agreeing to keep oneself safe by asking for help when needed rather than moving directly into self-destructive actions. Developing relationships within which uncomfortable feelings can be talked about rather than acted on is the principle on which the open setting rests.

Riggs is unique in that it is a psychoanalytic treatment setting that is embedded within the context of a therapeutic community. In that way, there is an essential tension for the psychotherapist (who may be either a clinical psychologist or a psychiatrist), who is in a private, confidential psychotherapy relationship with his or her patients but who is also a citizen in the larger hospital community. Citizenship includes all center meetings, which include all staff and patients, as well as clinical staff/patient meetings that occur during alternate months. In these meetings, each community member is free to speak about any concerns they might have, from their dual roles with respect to their position in the hospital and as a human being within the community environment.

Although these tensions between roles can be difficult, they also serve as important reminders of the basic humanness that unites us all, and also the variety of roles we take up that incur particular obligations and responsibilities. Much as a staff member may have conflicting roles as person and therapist, for example, so, too, the patients take on diverse roles even within the Center, through the work program or by taking up roles in patient government. At Riggs, we are all part of the larger community, always at odds with the ways in which good intentions can go awry and the inevitable limits we come up against in our encounters with one another.

The psychologist at Riggs may take up various roles, including clinical and administrative functions in the therapeutic community, such as group consultation, psychological testing, supervision, and teaching of junior postdoctoral colleagues ('Fellows'), family therapy and the four times weekly psychoanalytic psychotherapy that forms the core of our treatment model.

The psychologist also participates in daily staff meetings, meeting first thing Monday morning to hear how patients have fared over the weekend, and then on Friday afternoon to lodge concerns as we head into the weekend. Twice weekly, we meet with the treatment teams that form an important part of our treatment offering. Each team is responsible for approximately one-fifth of the patients, around 15. These smaller groups help us to attend to each patient's needs and treatment as we sift through the material offered by each of the various representatives of that patient's treatment team. Psychotherapy, psychopharmacology, social work, nursing, substance abuse, and community staff are all available to share their particular perspectives on the work with a given patient. That diversity helps to widen each person's lens, thereby helping us engage more mindfully in our various roles. Discussions include both pragmatics and dynamic formulations, as we track the relationships between difficulties that arise and the underlying meanings, relational themes, and patterns that are being expressed and enacted.

The therapist plays a pivotal role in integrating the information from the various disciplines, through the lens of the evolving dynamic formulation that provides a synopsis of the individual and familial dynamics at play for each of his or her patients. That formulation provides a lens through which the patient's behavior can be understood within the context of the life and family histories through which he or she has evolved. Recognizing that identity is built in relation to life history, we try to understand the life narrative as it has evolved, as well as how it has gone awry.

Because our training is psychosocial and developmental rather than primarily biomedical, the psychologist plays a key role in these conversations and provides an important anchoring point. Psychologists recognize the basic human dilemmas at the core of most patients' problems, and ways in which a medical model can obscure those problems in living (Charles, 2015a). This grounding can be particularly important with patients who are difficult to engage with, or who have learned to think about themselves in relation to medical jargon and diagnoses rather than as human beings with needs and feelings. The role of patient can become another mask to hide behind.

Because the open setting rests on our ability to form relationships with each individual, patients who are difficult to reach and engage with generate anxiety and instability within the staff. From a psychoanalytic framework, we know that positive and negative aspects of the transference will be dispersed among members of the treatment team in ways that may be difficult for staff members to bear but must be borne if we are to come to an understanding of what the patient is working at and working toward (Janssen, 1994). The therapist tries to bring split-off aspects of the transference back into the consulting room so that they can be more actively reflected upon. Because this process takes time, other staff members may need interpretations by the therapist, seen through the lens of the dynamic formulation, in order to hold steady during periods of strain. Psychologists' awareness of transference/countertransference dynamics can help other staff members recognize their entanglement with a given patient as an enactment of family dynamics. Such awareness can help staff members be more sympathetic rather than anxious or angry. Much as the patients need conceptual anchors in order to better understand where they are caught, so do staff members.

As an example of the crucial role of the psychologist, consider one young woman who was extremely difficult to engage. Very bright and highly defended, she was experienced as contemptuous, deprecating, and hateful, inviting reactive hostility rather than empathy. In such situations, other staff members often assume that the therapist is sitting on the positive end of the split, and therefore cannot understand other staff members' feelings. However, I knew all too well what complicated feelings this young woman could engender. As the therapist, it was my job to hold in mind the dynamic formulation for team members. Through that vertex, I could invite nursing and community staff members into a more empathic recognition of the family dynamics that had left the patient suspicious of anyone who tried to offer care or support.

For this young woman, as for many of our patients, psychological difficulties could be traced to disruptions in development resulting from failures in mourning across the generations. As we see from the literature on disorganized attachment, the ways in which failures to work through loss result in preoccupied parents who are at times emotionally inaccessible to their children (Liotti, 1999; Main & Hesse, 1990). Those failures disrupt the development of self-regulation and identity, which are tied to parental attunement and sequences of disruption and repair (Beebe & Lachmann, 1994). Having an index of where the person is stuck developmentally can help us to recognize the 2-, 5-, or 12-year-old caught in an adult body, and to empathize with the difficulty of being both child and adult in moments of strain. A developmental perspective can help us to recognize the gap between the pretense of adulthood and the person's actual capacities, particularly under strain.

Psychotherapists have the benefit of the analytic field in the consulting room, through which to register subtle levels of meaning as they manifest in dreams, fantasies, and free associations. Over time, I came to imagine this young woman as a frightened kitten, snarling and batting away any extended hand. At a team meeting, I invited the nursing staff to imagine how young developmentally this woman must be, and to consider what it must be like to be a young adult functioning emotionally at the level of a 2-year-old. That type of interpretation, anchored in a dynamic formulation of the patient's problems, helps the nursing staff shift their view of the patient's behaviors and be more empathically connected to the child within the adult. That shift in perspective helped the young woman feel empathically engaged with by nursing staff, which was relieving on all sides, and also opened up more reflective space for the patient to consider her own behavior and its impact on others. Invoking a developmental framework has become a soothing move for staff members on our team, as we imagine where a given patient is stuck and how we might therefore most effectively and empathically intervene.

In order to keep track of comings and goings and new issues as they arise in relation to particular patients, we meet three times weekly as a full clinical staff. We try to reserve our mid-week meetings to reflect on the larger issues that may be bubbling up within the system, and what these issues might mean for and about us. Our awareness of group dynamics invites us to be proactive in our collective efforts to recognize problematic behaviors of individuals as possible symptoms of perturbations within the system that could use our attention. Wondering how trouble in the patient community reflects and speaks to trouble in the staff is an ongoing interpretive activity. Although moving toward *management of problems* may be important to consider (and tensions can certainly push toward management as either a relief from our distress or to more explicitly mark the frame and boundaries on which the open setting depends), we also try to remember that our patients will inevitably act out their troubles as a means toward obtaining recognition of nascent meanings that cannot yet be put into words, including commentaries on the community itself.

As part of our stance that a community needs access to each person's voice and perspective in order to best sustain itself, and recognizing that communication becomes more difficult as the size of the group increases, we also meet semi-monthly in medical staff, psychotherapy staff, and clinical staff meetings. These smaller meetings afford time and space to discuss how we are working together within each of these subgroups and to more explicitly discuss issues that are pressing and require joint reflection among staff members from our particular roles within this complex system.

Our treatment model is informed by the A.K. Rice/Tavistock tradition and the work of Menzies Lyth (1988) that highlights ways in which anxiety becomes mobilized and managed in hospital settings. That framework highlights that what might be termed *treatment-resistance* may be more usefully conceptualized in terms of alienation from treatments that are disrespectful and not useful (Shapiro, 2011). Such knowledge helps us counter the tendency to act on impulse rather than reflectively considering the impulse as useful information that might inform the treatment. The systems perspective also helps us to consider the role that a given individual may be fulfilling within the system, why that role has been mobilized at that particular time, and what purpose the individual may be fulfilling, for better and worse, for the system.

It is easy, for example, when anxiety begins to escalate, to find ourselves focusing on whoever is making the most 'noise,' particularly a rule-breaker whose behavior seems dangerous (whether patient or staff member!). Patients, too, can focus attention on the person who seems to be the 'problem' that we can get rid of by expelling that person from our midst. Often, that person is problematic, in part, because he or she confronts us with something we do not want to be confronted with. Consider for example the psychotic patient attending a process group who irritates other group members with her comment 'It's like eating popcorn without the butter.' Although the patients were utterly dismissive, certain that this was a 'crazy' statement, the group facilitator could recognize that the patient had come right to the point: the group was circling around and going nowhere because the patients were busy playing the role of 'good patients' and avoiding engaging with one another at a deeper level. Notably, a more senior patient was taking the lead in this particular group, acting as a facilitator rather than working at her troubles. Hearing about the incident helped staff members to wonder how we might be colluding with patients' desires to act as though they are functioning well rather than exploring more fully ways in which they are not.

Even more complicated for the psychologist is when staff behavior is implicated in the complaint. One experience that I found illuminating in this regard had to do with a patient who began to struggle explicitly with the pulls he was experiencing toward conformity within the system. One day he came into his session, sat down heavily, and said: 'Is it *1984* or *Brave New World* where they talked about "group-think"?'

'It's *1984*, *Brave New World*, and *Animal Farm*,' I replied, with empathy. So began for me the complex task of trying to use my own understanding of these pulls toward conformity without acting out a collusion between the reactive aspects of my patient and myself around shared issues concerning conformity and compliance. This meant a pretty steady internal consultation with how the other person was right when I was most convinced they were wrong. At Austen Riggs, there is the adage to *always listen for how the other person is right* (Shapiro & Carr, 1991). That reminder can be key at precisely those moments when we are most reluctant to attend to an alternate view.

I took the collapse of space that occurred when my patient's and my own views aligned too well to mean that there was likely another side I was not seeing. Pulling toward that other side often meant irritating my patient, as I insisted on there being more to the picture than what he described. In time, however, we were able to see how his tendency to split off conflicting aspects of the picture did not serve him in the long run. Affirming his need to grapple with difficulties, rather than merely discarding them, helped him to attain more complex representations of self and other instead of becoming mired in the good versus bad split that had precluded certain conversations and insights previously.

This type of engagement by the psychologist requires our ability to recognize aspects of transference as they play out at system as well as individual levels. In order to facilitate staff recognition of system dynamics that may feel personal but may also represent larger systemic tensions, all staff are encouraged to attend at least one of the group relations conferences offered nationally and internationally by the A.K. Rice Institute. The group relations setting helps to expose patterns of relating in which one's own character is inevitably implicated. Such a vantage point helps to offset the tendency to personalize conflicts and to make attributions that project blame rather than to take responsibility for one's own actions. Such a perspective also helps us to reflect on our own underlying feelings and motivations that may impact those around us, feelings that we otherwise may believe we are concealing, and thus to recognize ways in which hidden resentment, frustration, or other feelings may be tainting the work. Knowing that group dynamics may be at play helps each of us to pause so that we might reflect on our own participation in interpersonal tensions, and work on our own contributions. Trying to bring difficulties to the surface, where they might better be worked through, helps to ease tensions and frees us up to look together at the dynamic in relation to the particular patient–family dynamics that may be at play and also in relation to larger systemic issues. Being able to recognize ways in which patterns may play out at various levels within a system helps us make use of our insights rather than merely being oppressed by the patterns.

Because of our recognition of the importance of paying close attention to group dynamics, a weekly group consultation seminar is often offered for staff who wish to study group processes and organizational consultation more intensively. Participants learn to be more mindful of organizational dynamics, helping them to be more competent members of our particular system. In that way, they also do a service to their colleagues in refining their lenses and offering observations in staff meetings, as relevant. Process comments in group meetings from staff members during times of tension often help to open up a conversation that has become fixed and stuck.

In line with the A.K. Rice/Tavistock model (Colman & Bexton, 1975; Colman & Geller, 1985; Fraher, 2004), group work at ARC tends not to conform to a group psychotherapy model. Rather, psychologists consult groups as a way of highlighting interpersonal dynamics as they arise among group members. We look for patterns in relating. Weekly group supervision is offered for staff members who consult patient groups, both as a way of enhancing consultation skills and also as a way of trying to reflect together on how each group's process that week might inform our understanding of what is 'up' in the community, where the tensions are centered at that particular time. There is an ongoing dialectic between the pragmatic and meta-levels of understanding that can feel maddening, as we get caught between tolerating tensions versus the desire to solve or manage the *problem*. This tension rises most precipitously when we are concerned about patients' well-being. For example, we have noted that exclusive relationships between patients can be very destructive to their treatment and can even, at the extreme, lead to suicide. Knowledge of that history can invite staff members to try to control behavior rather than illuminating risks so that patients might make more adaptive choices. Moving toward reflection rather than impulsive reaction is a continual exercise for us all, particularly in moments of strain. Recognizing heightened affect as a sign of transference dynamics being played out helps to remind us of the utility of this *theater in the round* in which we all continuously participate. Trying to take a more reflective position precisely when we are feeling most defensive can afford useful insights that deepen our collective work with the patients.

Roles

As mentioned above, work in a psychiatric hospital can be likened to a theater in the round, in which patient's individual and family dynamics are always playing out in relation to staff, individual, and organizational dynamics, making self-reflectivity essential. The most important roles played by the therapist are to hold the dynamic formulation so that we can consider enactments in relation to the story being told, and learn to recognize patterns, countertransference reactions, and underlying meanings as they emerge, and thereby be more reflective and less reactive – and thus likely kinder – even when what is needed are firm limits. Team and staff meetings help the therapist to recognize bits of the transference that are being acted out so that she can try to bring the split-off bits back into the psychotherapy.

The psychologist also serves as the co-therapist, along with the patient's social worker, in family meetings and in family therapy. We distinguish between family meetings that have an express purpose that revolves around pragmatic concerns or information exchange, versus family therapy in which each family member must be willing to reflect on their own participation in the family dynamics and interactions. At Riggs, context is recognized as an essential aspect of meaning-making. A psychodynamic perspective recognizes that meanings are inevitably personal and that transference is ubiquitous. As Grotstein (2009) notes, perception is more accurately designated *apperception*, meanings colored by the social and cultural contexts through which they have been derived.

Recognizing the importance of context in understanding the individual, we gather as extensive a family history as possible, so that we can look for important patterns and themes across the generations. A troubled individual generally marks trouble in the family, in terms of negotiating developmental passages that have eluded family members (Ackerman, 1966). The family history helps to show ways in which transgenerational trauma infuses itself into an individual's life story, thereby inviting respect for each individual caught in her own way in that family dynamic. That respect provides a position from which the clinician can meet each individual's good intentions and invite collaboration with the task at hand. It also helps to recognize split-off aspects of the family history that have come to haunt family members because they are not consciously recognized sufficiently to be worked with (Charles, 2016).

Family work is an important part of the psychologist's clinical efforts. Working empathically with the family, while also recognizing limits and difficulties, can help family members to be less reactive and more accepting of self and other. Such acceptance puts them in a better position to work together in ways that feel more supportive and build greater understanding. Although participation in both individual psychotherapy and family meetings puts the psychologist in dual roles, those dual roles can be useful in modeling for the patient the negotiation between disparate roles.

Being able to engage empathically with the good intentions of family members can help to soften tensions and enable family members to more actively support the patient's work at the Center. Such efforts also tend to avoid exacerbation of the splits that can occur when the family becomes the *bad object* in relation to the therapist's role as *good object*.

Kleinian notions of splitting and projective identification (Klein, 1946) become useful tools in the psychologist's arsenal in family meetings to illuminate the relational entanglements that might otherwise be experienced as facts.

An initial family meeting through which the individual therapist and social worker can encounter and begin to name family dynamics is an important part of our evaluation and treatment process. Also important is a meeting following the case conference, in which the patient discusses with the family what he has been learning about his troubles. We work with families in teams, so that the roles of family contact and individual psychotherapist are balanced within the co-therapy team. Although it can be complicated to work with an individual patient and his or her family, it can also be extremely beneficial.

At Riggs, psychologists work collaboratively with the psychiatrist who prescribes for each of their patients. We try to hold to the adage that *the therapist is in charge of the case*, in terms of developing a dynamic formulation that helps the staff to hold the patient in mind. But prescribers are also mindful that the provision of medications has meanings for the patient. Working together helps us to more reflectively contain splits that might emerge, and to provide care that is more mindful. At times, our patients enter treatment on a regimen of medications that not only do not solve the problems but create further difficulties. Working with the psychopharmacologist toward understanding the patient's relationship to medications can be crucial.

The dynamic formulation provides reflective containment, a crucial holding function for both patients and staff, particularly important during times of high stress, when both staff and patients may feel pressure to discharge tensions through action rather than reflection. Trying to understand what is going on under the surface when such urgency hits can be incredibly difficult and even painful, as we try to look beyond the splitting, scapegoating, or other accusations or distrust that can so easily arise during moments of high tension and anxiety. It is in these moments that the ongoing work at collaborative engagement with fellow staff is pivotal in helping us to hold steady so that we might more effectively attempt to reflect on what is mobilizing us rather than merely reacting reflexively.

The culmination of the six-week evaluation and treatment period is the case conference. The psychologist as therapist plays a pivotal role in organizing the information that is offered to the clinical staff in the case abstract that summarizes the patient's difficulties, history, and treatment. The therapist compiles the life history and reports on the psychotherapy at the conference, inviting other staff members to offer reflections on important themes and possible transference and countertransference issues that might be useful to consider and integrate into the treatment. A detailed depiction of life and family histories afford insight into the contexts in which the troubles have arisen and in which they might be better understood. Reports from those team members working most closely with the patient help to chronicle aspects of the patient's engagements outside the therapy room. The therapist digests the feedback and then reports the findings and recommendations first to the patient and then to the family.

Psychologists also serve as faculty to our Fellows, mentoring, teaching, and supervising as part of our ACPE accredited psychoanalytic training program. Psychology Fellows, mentored by senior psychology staff, are responsible for the assessments that provide a crucial function in our evaluation process. Along with standardized intellectual testing, we use projective testing as a window into the patient's object relations, defenses, and underlying character structure. Testing results are offered at the case conference in relation to the therapist's questions that have guided the inquiry, to inform our understanding and guide treatment recommendations.[1]

Tensions Between Disparate Roles

Particular difficulties arise in relation to the disparate roles that psychologists take on within the institution. Confidentiality may be the most pressing issue facing psychologists, as they attempt to manage the at-times conflicting roles of psychotherapist and member of a treatment team. Countering the presumption that we will all share information in order to provide the best and most coherent care, for the psychologist confidentiality is critical to the psychotherapy. I find it important therefore to be clear with both my patients and my team regarding how I work with these conflicting obligations.

Confidentiality is an essential part of the therapy relationship. I want my patients to feel safe enough to vocalize unformulated experience and to share even their most shameful or painful secrets, to have an opportunity to put everything on the table and sort through it with someone whose job it is to assist them in that process. If there is no presumption of confidentiality, then it is as though the walls have ears. Much as occurs in work with adolescents and young adults whose parents are paying for the treatment, it may not be clear to what extent the patient is speaking toward their own self-discovery or to whomever is presumed to be listening.

As part of the hospital community, however, the psychologist has an obligation, not only to her own patients but also to the institution and to the other patients. In recognition of our embeddedness in a community, I encourage patients to recognize these complexities so that they can feel and be motivated by their own perceived tensions between needs of self and other. Grappling openly and honestly with these tensions requires a therapeutic space within which such dilemmas can be considered and worked through. As such, the assurance of confidentiality provides the safe space within which to reflectively consider possibilities for working through, *including* greater engagement with other members of the community. Pressures toward action tend to close down and preclude such reflective spaces. Psychodynamic and other insight-oriented therapies 'work,' in part, because they help to build the reflective capacities required for making mindful choices, and so it is important for the psychologist to trust the process and the person sufficiently to allow the work to proceed.

I find it important in the hospital setting to feel the multiple demands of self and other sufficiently that I can invite my patients to feel those tensions as well, so that they can be motivated to address difficulties that *they* encounter in the system. For example, I encourage them to work toward imagining how they might effectively address a secret another patient is holding that could be detrimental to that patient's treatment. Such action would require moving from the position of complicit child, not wanting to tell on one's friend, to seeing oneself as an adult who bears some responsibility for others' well-being. Once again, in the spirit of interpretation toward learning rather than moving toward management, I try to invite the patient to consider alternatives to any closed-down perspective they might hold, to consider how a defense might serve some needs while also foreclosing development.

Psychologists are also faced with challenges in managing tensions that arise for their patients in relation to other staff members. Much as with my *Animal Farm* patient, there are times when our patients' experiences too neatly collide with our own, making it crucial to recognize latent identifications with the patients. Reflecting on ways in which these identifications might be playing out can help us sort through complicated feelings so that we can better fulfill our roles. Because we are always trying to manage the level of tension and anxiety within the hospital, collegial relationships among staff are important. We depend on one another to support the work we are doing, which includes being able to challenge one another respectfully and usefully when differences arise. Our work on treatment teams helps us to get to know one another and to develop ways of engaging in productive discussions. Catching hold of the ways in which *we* may be splitting, as well, helps us to re-integrate the positive and negative aspects of our colleagues sufficiently to have them in mind in our work with our patients. That re-integration helps us to recognize the complications our patients encounter empathically and to believe that they can work through their difficulties, rather than further encouraging the splitting.

Because of these ever-present hazards, we work very hard to have in mind the dynamic formulation that might help us to recognize transferential aspects of an enactment and learn from our collective countertransferences rather than merely to be caught up in them. Feelings run high when there is a lot at stake, so the intensity of the affect itself becomes a signal that there is something further we need to understand. At these times, work on teams can be very helpful in trying to sort through the issues at hand so that we can bring that information back to the larger staff community.

For example, one young adult female patient invited intense reactivity from staff members. She was often working at the edge of some boundary within the Center, uncannily able to find any point of vulnerability within the system. At one point in time, her low weight had become an issue, which enraged her because, from her perspective, we were focused on the wrong problem, her weight rather than the underlying sources of her difficulties with food, nourishment, and her body more generally. Her apparent contempt for others' concerns had exacerbated those concerns, resulting in a weight plan that at a certain point outlived its usefulness. At that point, her unwillingness to work with us on a plan she had not truly signed on to kept the plan in place. We worked very hard as a team to recognize that we were 'into something' as a system that had more to do with inter-staff issues of power and authority than with the patient's well-being. Those efforts not only helped to ease the tangle with that particular patient but also helped us to work through system issues that had kept the problems in place. As we discussed this case as a full staff, we could recognize ways in which underlying staff fears over keeping our patients alive were driving us toward management rather than reflection.

Recognition of ways in which anxiety can usurp reflection helps to mark the anxiety as a problem in and of itself, inviting us back toward trying to understand the contexts within which the anxieties arise. The life and family histories that the therapist has in mind for each of her patients help us to recognize patterns of relating when they begin to play out in the community. It is always easier to view such dynamics from a distance, and so conflicts that arise between patients can be a useful index for making sense of similar dynamics as they play out in the staff. Our knowledge of group and organizational dynamics helps us to recognize our own patterns of relational reactivity as we get into them and provides reference points through which to regain our bearings during times of stress, knowing that even our good intentions may be experienced quite differently by others. Being able to step back from the tendency to personalize difficulties in ways that further divide us, and to recognize relational patterns together, are crucial efforts in this parallel process between working with our patients and their families, and working with one another.

Because of this parallel process always at play, ideas about reflective function provide a useful rubric for thinking about staff engagements (Lysaker et al., 2011). Knowledge of intra- and interpersonal dynamics helps us to recognize the intensity of our own affect as a flag signaling the need to downshift and reflect on the context rather than to merely act out from that reactive state. In this way, we actively work toward reducing tension levels and also model for one another and for our patients an allegiance to the type of reflective activity we believe will further development in us all.

When working with those who do not engage easily in relationships, reflecting on their dilemma provides a means for holding them in mind even when they resist our efforts to engage with them more directly. Being able to recognize ways in which the person gets caught and may experience sympathetic or empathic efforts as assaults or intrusions, helps us to persist in refining our attempts at engagements in ways that might be more accessible to that particular individual. Knowing the story can help us to have in mind idiosyncratic meanings we might otherwise stumble over. Recognizing, for example, that 'home' may signal danger rather than safety can be crucial in meeting the individual where he or she is, rather than trying to impose our own language and metaphors in ways that further close down the conversation.

On team, we try to keep an ear out for our own language that lodges the problem in the individual or suggests hopelessness, so that we can inquire into the dynamic at play. Attempts at management through medication, for example, often arise in relation to our work with individuals who are dysregulated and dysregulating. We have learned to provide patients with diverse opportunities for learning to manage dysregulation, so that people can better gain competence in managing their own affect and thereby have greater access to their intellects and other capacities. In this regard, psychologists can play a crucial role in didactic groups that teach interpersonal and coping skills as an adjunct to the other treatment offerings.

A further issue for psychologists is managing the pull between one's own ethical values in the work and opposing ideas within the staff or with external standards of 'care.' In this regard, it is important to keep in mind that various guilds are represented within a hospital setting, each with their own code of ethics and standards of care (Charles, 2011). Psychologists in the United States have a very different code of ethics, for example, than their psychiatry counterparts. Whereas the medical code of ethics is very specific in offering guidelines for quality of care in relation to specific diagnoses, the psychology code of ethics demands that the psychologist be informed as to the relevant parameters of treatment so that he can make informed decisions. In an era in which standards are becoming increasingly constricted and codified, the psychologist is still expected to make mindful decisions based on the available data. Being able to effectively advocate for one's treatment methods and goals, then, becomes an important offering to one's colleagues, so that they can either steer their efforts accordingly or engage in dialog regarding their different vision of good treatment.

Such efforts help to both illuminate and to soften tensions that arise in relation to staff conflicts over roles, relationships, visions, values, and ideas about treatment. Respectful listening is perhaps the essential key in managing such tensions. Willingness to listen to opposing or alternative points of view helps each member of the treatment team to place her concerns on the table, so that they can be reflected on collectively, thereby reducing the type of pressure that arises when worries cannot be adequately voiced and attended to. As mentioned, we try to keep in mind the adage to *always listen for how the other person is right* (Shapiro & Carr, 1991) to help us sustain our attention to other perspectives.

A Case Example

Healthy development depends upon a balance of sufficient attention and frustration in order for development to proceed, on parents who may falter in a given moment but who can be brought to attention when needed. Many of our patients have been waylaid by a particular type of trauma or neglect that can make even an otherwise good-enough (Winnicott, 1971) parent inaccessible to their children in moments of distress, leading to disorganized attachment and incoherence in autobiographical memory (Liotti, 1999). This trauma is a function of insufficient mourning in previous generations that results in moments of self-absorbed inaccessibility on the part of the parent (Main & Hesse, 1990). Never knowing whether one will encounter the present, receptive face or the absent, empty one is itself disorienting and dysregulating to the child. The psychoanalytically oriented psychologist is in a good position to recognize these developmental difficulties in ways that further understanding and learning for patients and also for other staff members.

For those whose stories have pushed them outside of the narrow margins of what is acceptable within the confines of the family story, truth and reality can be both precious and precarious, as one rendering of meaning seems to preclude another. For example, I worked with one young woman who had become increasingly dysregulated in relation to a story that could not be told because the early abuse was not held in conscious memory but rather lodged in bodily symptoms and cognitive disorganization that had never been effectively 'read.' Her attempts to make meaning had become so occluded that she was having trouble using her mind, having the experience that her mind was fractured and in pieces. Her mother was described as wonderful and loving, creating opportunities for enjoyment for her children but also, importantly, unable to tolerate information that might disturb that lovely family narrative. As a result, Virginia's attempts to obtain assistance from her parents were often met with a blind eye and a deaf ear, offered with a loving smile that invited her to stop 'creating' problems.

Virginia experienced a series of breakdowns in late adolescence and early adulthood. Although her parents tried to find assistance for her, by the time I met them, they clearly saw her as mad. As such, Virginia's earnest attempts to explain to them her troubles, from their perspective were read as a repetitive and relentless display that they could only register as assaultive, affording them further evidence of her madness. Family meetings enacted the impasse, helping us to confront these highly disparate meaning structures, and to recognize that the rendering of Virginia's speech as meaningless fed the repetition. Being able to hold in mind this variability of perspectives helped Virginia to put together a story in which her own experience could make sense even if it did not agree with that of others, and where others' experience could be reflected on as data points to be considered. These data points that marked the diversity of characters, vantage points, and experiences helped Virginia organize her thoughts and thereby build a more cogent life narrative through which she could better understand ways in which she had at times fallen through the cracks. Recognizing her own capacity to make and hold meaning helped Virginia recognize and accept limits in herself and others, which in turn helped her make more effective use of her own very considerable capacities.

There are truths that are as difficult to hear as they might be to tell. For Virginia's parents, it was difficult to face the possibility that their child might have been injured while under their care. Their lack of recognition of the source of her distress left Virginia unable to recognize her own distress until someone had marked her physiological symptoms as potential manifestations of early trauma. That recognition afforded the grounding that Virginia needed in order to begin to register and make sense of the symptoms she had been experiencing and to seek further assistance.

Virginia's nascent recognition of the sources of her distress helped her to make better choices in spite of her continuing disequilibrium. She was able to resist, for example, the diagnosis of schizophrenia that provided a *way* of *making sense* of her symptoms, but did *not* recognize the story *behind* the symptoms. A psychoanalytically informed psychological developmental perspective helped me to support Virginia in her efforts to make sense of what was and was not useful in what she was being offered, which in turn helped her to further stabilize and make better use of her cognitive capacities.

Reflective function depends on the ability to recognize and make use of one's internal experience in relation to others' minds that may be both similar and different (Lysaker et al., 2011). Virginia's ability to *oppose* the medicalized truth with the truth of her experience was an important stand she was able to take on her own behalf, insisting that the diagnosis did not make sense because it did not take into account her trauma history. That insistence helped Virginia to mark her own path in ways that enabled me, as her psychologist, to help others better understand the particularities of that path. For Virginia, the distinction between trauma and psychosis was meaningful because it helped to demarcate a story in which *something had happened to her* that impeded her development. Helping the treatment team to recognize these meanings helped them to better support her efforts. For Virginia, her abuse history did make a difference in terms of how her story was told and how one might proceed. Putting together the story of her abuse, and the ways in which her repression of that abuse had undermined her efforts to build a life, became the foundation on which her identity could more solidly be built.

Conclusion

Holding lightly to our theories while working with the metaphors as they emerge in the clinical work helps us provide a model for playful interaction that supports the development of reflective function in our sessions, as we *dream through* the sessions in the manner described by Bionian field theorists such as Ferro (2009) and Civitarese (2005). From that perspective, the goal of psychoanalytic work is to facilitate the patient's capacity to think, feel, and dream, those behaviors that we group collectively under the term *reflective functions*. Dreaming requires sufficient safety to allow ourselves that relaxation. Hospital settings where we work with people whose safety is at risk oppose the type of relaxation required for deep reflection. From a psychoanalytic perspective, the right interpretation at the right time helps us to downshift sufficiently to begin to allow our conscious and unconscious minds to do their work together. The psychologist can play a key role in this meaning-making de-escalation process, to the extent that she can take sufficient care of herself to enable her reflective capacities to function and also provide interpretive containment to her colleagues (Charles, 2015b).

Note

1 See Biedermann et al. (Chapter 16) in this volume on psychodiagnostic work carried by clinical psychologists at the Austen Riggs Center.

References

Ackerman, N. W. (1966). *Treating the troubled family*. New York, NY: Basic Books.

Beebe, B., & Lachmann, F. (1994). Representation and internalization in infancy: Three principles of salience. *Psychoanalytic Psychology*, *11*, 127–165.

Charles, M. (2011). System pressures, ethics, and autonomy. In: E. Plakun (Ed.), *Treatment resistance and patient authority: The Austen Riggs reader*, pp. 174–197. New York, NY: Norton.

Charles, M. (2012). *Working with trauma: Lessons from Bion and Lacan*. New York, NY: Jason Aronson.

Charles, M. (2015a). *Psychoanalysis and literature: The stories we live*. Lanham, MD: Rowman & Littlefield.

Charles, M. (2015b). Caring for the caregivers: Consulting with therapists in the trenches. Special Issue: M. Akhtar, Guest Editor, *Psychoanalytic Inquiry, 35*, 682–695.

Charles, M. (2016). Ashes of remembrance: Reconfiguring the phoenix. *Psychoanalytic Review, 103*, 41–67.

Civitarese, G. (2005). Fire at the theatre: (Un)reality of/in the transference and interpretation. *The International Journal of Psychoanalysis, 86*, 1299–1316.

Colman, A. D., & Bexton, W. H. (1975). *Group relation reader*. Sausalito, CA: A. K. Rice Institute.

Colman, A. D., & Geller, M. H. (1985). *Group relation reader 2*. Sausalito, CA: A. K. Rice Institute.

Ferro, A. (2009). Transformations in dreaming and characters in the psychoanalytic field. *The International Journal of Psychoanalysis, 90*, 209–230.

Fraher, A. L. (2004). *A history of group study and psychodynamic organizations*. London: Free Association Books.

Grotstein, J. S. (2009). *'But at the same time and on another level …': Psychoanalytic theory and technique in the Kleinian/Bionian mode. Volume I*. London: Karnac.

Janssen, P. (1994). *Psychoanalytic therapy in the hospital setting*. D. Cannell, Trans. London & New York, NY: Routledge.

Klein, M. (1946). Notes on some schizoid mechanisms. In: R. Money-Kyrle (Ed.), *The Writings of Melanie Klein Volume 3: Envy and gratitude and other works, 1946–1963*, pp. 1–24. London: Hogarth Press. 1975.

Lacan, J. (1977). *Écrits: A selection*. A. Sheridan (Trans.). New York, NY: W. W. Norton.

Liotti, G. (1999). Disorganization of attachment as a model for understanding dissociative psychopathology. In: J. Solomon, & C. George (Eds.), *Attachment disorganization*, pp. 291–317. New York, NY & London: Guilford Press.

Lysaker, P. H., Erickson, M., Ringer, J., Buck, K. D., Semerari, A., Carcione, A., & Dimaggio, G. (2011). Metacognition in schizophrenia: The relationship of mastery to coping, insight, self-esteem, social anxiety, and various facets of neurocognition. *British Journal of Clinical Psychology, 50*, 412–424.

Lyth, I. M. (1988). *Containing anxieties in institutions: Selected essays, Volume I*. London: Free Associations Books.

Main, M., & Hesse, E. (1990). Parent's unresolved traumatic experiences are related to infant disorganized/disoriented attachment status: Is frightened and/or frightening parental behavior the linking mechanism? In: M. Greenberg, D. Cicchetti, & E. M. Cummings (Eds.), *Attachment in the preschool years: Theory, research, and intervention*, pp. 161–182. Chicago, IL: University of Chicago Press.

Muller, J. (2011). Why the pair needs the third. In: E. Plakun (Ed.), *Treatment resistance and patient authority: The Austen Riggs reader*, pp. 97–120. New York, NY: Norton.

Obholzer, A., & Roberts, V. Z. (1994). *The unconscious at work: Individual and organizational stress in human services*. London: Routledge.
Shapiro, E. R. (2011). A psychodynamic treatment system for patients with treatment-resistant disorders. In: E. Plakun (Ed.), *Treatment resistance and patient authority: The Austen Riggs reader*, pp. 269–284. New York, NY: Norton.
Shapiro, E. R., & Carr, A. W. (1991). *Lost in familiar places: Creating new connections between the individual and society*. New Haven, CT and London: Yale University Press.
Winnicott, D. W. (1971). *Playing and reality*. New York, NY: Basic Books.

3 Clinical Psychologists in Australian Inpatient Mental Health Units

Enhancing Effectiveness and Relevance with a Human Rights Focus

Peter Walker and Sophie Li

Australia, a country of approximately 24 million people (Australian Bureau of Statistics, 2015), is a landmass that has been populated for at least 50,000 years by complex and diverse indigenous cultures. The native populations of Australia were largely decimated with the arrival of European settlers in the late eighteenth century, and with their arrival the psychological insights and therapies of that set of cultures were lost. In its wake, a medical system conceived of and developed in Europe was established (Kirkby, 1999).

The Australian mental health landscape has been rocked by the storm and stress of government intervention, social movements and clinical innovations. Shaped by similar processes occurring internationally, a focus on human rights in mental health settings was formally reviewed from the early 1980s. The findings were damning, describing the paucity of services for the mentally ill (Richmond, 1983). This process was repeated every 10 years, and each iteration revealed further deprivations (Burdekin, 1993; Mental Health Council of Australia, 2005).

In parallel, during the 1970s and 1980s, diverse social movements developed in a series of Western countries. Referred to variously as the "Consumer movement," "service-user movement" and "psychiatric survivor" movement, they sought to develop "strategies to change mental health consumers' status from powerless victims to agents of change" (Bassman, 1997). The movements shed light on the most oppressive elements of routine psychiatric treatment and led to some concrete beneficial changes.

As the consumer movements gained momentum and influence, an important development within academic psychology commenced as clinical researchers began studying the psychological processes underpinning psychotic symptoms (Bentall & Slade, 1988). From psychological models of delusions and hallucinations, sophisticated treatments were developed (Bellack, 1986; Chadwick, Birchwood, & Trower, 1996) referred to as CBT for psychosis (CBTp).

In addition, an evidence-based treatment for Borderline Personality Disorder (BPD) was developed – Dialectical Behavior Therapy (DBT). BPD is notoriously difficult to manage for health services, and as such the development of DBT has led a greater degree of optimism for psychologists. This context is a challenging but exciting one for Australian psychologists. The mental health landscape is chaotic and at times hostile, yet is actively being challenged by an inspiring social movement. At the same time, novel treatments are increasingly available that provide a key role for the clinical psychologist.

Clinical Psychologists in Australia

As of June 2016, there were 7481 psychologists with a clinical endorsement working in Australia (Psychology Board of Australia; Registrant Data, June 2016). The training involves the completion of a 4-year Honors Degree, which has no specific clinical content. To become endorsed as a clinical psychologist, one must complete either a Master's degree, Doctorate or combined PhD/Master's degree. These degrees consist of a combination of coursework, supervised clinical placements and an experimental research thesis. Once the formal clinical training is complete, clinicians become "clinical psychology registrars," and they are required to complete 2 years of weekly supervision of their practice with an endorsed clinical psychologist. For the most highly credentialed clinicians, the educational process can take 10 years.

University courses are accredited nationally, so there is a relative uniformity in the training process. The predominant treatment paradigm reflects the Cognitive Behavioral tradition, and most students leave university with basic skills in CBT (e.g., Cognitive Therapy, Exposure Therapy and Behavioral Activation among others) and the third-wave psychotherapies (Acceptance and Commitment Therapy (ACT), Dialectical Behavior Therapy (DBT), Mindfulness-based Cognitive Therapy and Schema Therapy).

There are no precise figures describing the numbers of clinical psychologists working in inpatient mental health units, the subject of this chapter. It is the authors' experience that there is no standard regarding the number of Full Time Equivalent (FTE) clinical psychologists on inpatient units. For other disciplines, most notably nursing, there are mandated ratios, nursing FTE to bed numbers that are legislated and protected. For clinical psychology, it appears that there is great variation. Where the clinical leaders (most often senior nurses and psychiatrists) value the unique role of clinical psychologists, the FTE numbers are relatively high. Where the clinical leaders were less valuing of clinical psychology, numbers are lower and at times clinical psychologists are absent.

Private versus Public Inpatient Units

Within the Australian mental health system, inpatient psychiatric care may be either publicly or privately funded. Public inpatient units are managed by the Department of Health and are free to the public as part of Medicare, the Australian universal health care system. Private units are mostly funded through private health insurance, with 56% of Australians privately insured in 2015. The different funding and governance models of the two systems have led to very different cultures, environments and treatment paradigms.

Public mental health units are often considered less desirable than private settings. Involuntary treatment almost always requires admission to the public system. A consumer who is at risk of self-harm in a private hospital will usually be transferred to a local public hospital. The acuity in public units tends to be higher, with psychotic disorders as the most common diagnosis. The population tends to be more socioeconomically impoverished, often living in government housing and unemployed. Both authors have worked exclusively in the public system and as a result the chapter provides more detail on this context and the consumers who tend to inhabit these wards.

The Role of Clinical Psychologists in Inpatient Facilities in Australia

There are a number of core competencies that are expected of clinical psychologists working in inpatient settings. Clinical Psychologists usually form part of a multi-disciplinary treatment team (MDT) along with consultant psychiatrists, registered nurses (often with a mental health specialization), occupational therapists and social workers. Clinical psychologists conduct psychological assessments of consumers, emphasizing the thoughts, behaviors and emotions that maintain a psychiatric condition. This leads to a psychological formulation and a related treatment plan. Clinical psychologists contribute to diagnostic discussions and influence the psychological aspects of treatment.

As a consequence of the training models provided by Australian universities, the majority of clinical psychologists (upwards of 65%) in the Australian mental health system align with the cognitive behavioral tradition (CBT) of psychotherapies (Byrne & Davenport, 2006) and implement these treatments in individual and group formats.

Consumers are commonly referred for mood management, the treatment of panic attacks, management of sleep problems, anger management and the management of emotion regulation problems that occur in those experiencing Borderline Personality Disorder. It is less common for consumers to be referred for psychotic symptoms.

The material in this chapter is influenced by the personal experiences of both authors working clinically within the Australian mental health system over the past 15 years. The settings from which experiences are drawn include that of a large, 50-bed public psychiatric unit, community health centers that offer rehabilitation, to private practice, where treatment is voluntary with a fee-for-service arrangement.

The authors were mindful of the possibility that their own experiences may not reflect those of other clinicians and thus a brief survey was constructed to prompt comment and opinion from clinical psychologists working in other inpatient psychiatric settings. This added informal input allowed for a richer description of the context.

Of the eight respondents who completed the survey, three worked in private settings and five in public. The descriptions from the clinicians working in private hospital settings were more positive in relation to their role, their value and their status. Clinicians working in public hospital settings reflected on the poor quality of the environment, felt less valued by their teams, but described a great deal of support from their psychologist colleagues. Further, public-based clinicians reported that they were able to expand their roles to include research and the implementation of novel treatments whereas privately-based clinicians had a far more circumscribed role.

Challenges Faced by Clinical Psychologists Working in Inpatient Psychiatric Contexts

Influence of Biological Psychiatry

It is the authors' experience that the overriding priority in inpatient care is biological treatment. The authors do not oppose biological treatment and see it as an important component of care. Their concern is that the bio-psycho-social model has become, as the previous American Psychiatric Association (APA) President Steven Sharfstein referred to it, the "bio-bio-bio" model (Read, 2005), where psychological interventions are seen as ancillary at best. A respondent to the clinician survey reflected "Some of them are on so much medication, like multiple antidepressants. I believe that as a result of all this medication, they appear quite disengaged ... I feel powerless to help."

The bio-psycho-social model is paid lip-service in inpatient settings, as practice affirms the centrality, if not exclusivity of biological conceptualization and treatment. Within public inpatient units, ward-based therapy programs are rare or very much ancillary. Consumers complain of boredom, and they are largely encouraged to wait aimlessly for medication to "kick in." When ward-based psycho-therapeutic groups do exist, consumers are regularly removed from them to see their doctor. This is often done respectfully and apologetically, yet clearly reinforces the priority of medical treatments.

Private psychiatric units in Australia tend to have functional multidisciplinary ward-programs. As care is largely funded by private health insurance, claims can be rejected if some aspect of treatment is not provided. Unfortunately, this can result in objectives of therapy groups not meaningfully targeting consumer's symptoms. This was reflected upon by a number of respondents to the clinician surveys who described very large groups, often with participants presenting psychological problems that bear no relation to the content addressed in the group, and little time for personalized application. When discussing their ability to work autonomously, a survey respondent wrote

> I feel my clinical judgment and decision-making is frequently overruled by visiting medical officers or my manager. Examples include having to accept persons into my group that do not meet criteria and who cause issues in group dynamics; accepting more patients into my group than should be.

The authors have observed a pervasive neglect of, and occasionally outright hostility to, social and psychological factors in mental health contexts, contributing to the perception that psychological approaches with these populations are futile. This runs counter to the scientific evidence which demonstrates that psychological and social factors contribute to the etiology and maintenance of major mental illness (Bentall & Fernyhough, 2008; Duhig et al., 2015). Here Loren Mosher's appeal to his psychiatric colleagues in his resignation letter from the American Psychiatric Association reflects our experience when he writes "No longer do we seek to understand whole persons in their social contexts – rather we are there to realign our patients' neurotransmitters" (cited in Read, 2005).

The initial promise of the several generations of anti-psychotic medication and advances in neuroscience gave rise to an expectation that clinical management of mental illness would lead to brief admissions and fast recovery. Within this context, psychological interventions are de-prioritized, and clinical psychologists are required to assert themselves to gain relevance and influence.

The experiences of survey respondents varied, however, in relation to the value placed on psychological interventions in their team. One respondent wrote

> Psychological therapy and its role in my organization depends on which unit is being considered. In some (alcohol and other drugs abuse and BPD) the role of therapy is considered vital. In others (e.g., depression) it is considered an afterthought.

Another stated that psychological intervention is "seen as more like the icing on the cake in my ward ... not absolutely essential."

The Nature of Multi-Disciplinary Teams (MDT)

As the name suggests, MDT's are composed of a range of mental health professionals who collaborate in order to maximize consumers' therapeutic outcomes. Despite minor variations, MDTs usually function hierarchically with a psychiatrist being the designated leader. It has been the authors' experience that psychiatrists usually act as the diagnostician and treatment planners. Most often the other members of the MDT are provided with the treatment plan and assigned specific tasks. As a supervisor, one author (SL) regularly faced this concern with new graduate supervisees. They were faced with a conflict between following the direction of a senior colleague or adhering to their own clinical opinion. Clinical psychologists refer to experiences in which they feel like "technicians" who are assigned "CBT" in a de-contextualized way without reference to a rationale or formulation. For instance, one author (PW) was regularly directed to provide breathing-retraining and distraction for consumers with panic attacks, despite this approach being considered obsolete and potentially counter-therapeutic. A survey respondent addressed this issue and presented a potential solution.

> There were superficial limits on autonomy owing to the fact that referrals often carried a prescriptive element (e.g., this person needs CBT for X). I would do as I would normally do as a clinical psychologist – thoroughly assess, arrive at my own formulation and deliver an intervention accordingly.

Many survey respondents described positive experiences on MDTs, although they noted the limitations. For example, this clinical psychologist described them as:

> Relatively team-focused with an opportunity to give your perspective and feel listened to; however, this became more difficult in areas where there was potential conflict between the perspectives of the clinical psychologist and consultant psychiatrist on matters such as diagnosis, treatment planning and discharge.

Encouragingly, despite challenges, a number of clinicians had developed flexible ways of asserting a psychological perspective. Another respondent stated,

> In my practice, I would generally approach the appropriate team member immediately to discuss a patient when necessary. It does not make sense to sit on information about a patient for a week before discussing it with the necessary team members.

We have also found that there is a perception by the wider team that certain psychological treatment approaches, most notably CBT and the related therapies, are simplistic and can be implemented effectively by those with little training or experience. Our perspective is that there are simplistic as well as highly complex aspects to these treatments; however, it requires a great deal of experience to work effectively with consumers whose conditions are serious enough to require hospitalization.[1]

When working with consumers suffering from psychotic disorders, personality disorders, bipolar affective disorder, and severe unipolar depression, psychological treatment processes are sophisticated and nuanced. Timing can be critical, and one has to learn to hold a consumer in a therapeutic relationship while engaging with their mental symptoms. We have found a number of effective ways of gaining a greater appreciation for the complexity of the work of clinical psychologists. We regularly present at case-reviews, outlining the assessment, our formulation and most critically, the tight-rope routine of intervention. Further, we often provide clinical supervision to other professionals who seek to gain experience in CBTp. We have found that professionals who seek practical experience in implementing these therapies often develop an appreciation for their complexity.

Pervasive Therapeutic Nihilism on Psychiatric Wards

Locked psychiatric wards can be bleak places. Consumers often cycle between the community and hospital, looking increasingly physically and mentally disabled with each admission. The majority of consumers are unemployed, funded through disability pensions and accommodated in social housing where violence, crime and drug use are pervasive. In this context, it is perhaps unsurprising that many hospital-based clinicians lose hope in the prospect of recovery from major mental illness.

We have observed a general pessimism that cuts across disciplines. The authors have witnessed senior staff refer to schizophrenia as "brain cancer." The enthusiasm and energy of junior staff gets worn down by the ward culture. One survey respondent described this phenomenon: "The psychiatrist who was leading the unit at the time was young and enthusiastic but was seen as idealistic and 'green' by the nursing staff, leading to a sense of cynicism within the team environment."

This can make the implementation of psychological intervention in this context difficult. Given the general pessimism, individual therapy is rarely encouraged, and group-based interventions not prioritized. We have found that clinical psychologists are called on when "all else has failed." When pharmacological intervention has had minimal effect, and there is a strong pressure to discharge, we have often been called on to implement CBTp, under crisis conditions. This runs contrary to the nature of CBTp which takes time and careful planning to implement effectively. This experience has been observed by others who state, "CBT can sit alongside the neuroleptics with a distinctive and complementary emphasis, rather than merely being brought on as a substitute in extra-time" (Birchwood & Trower, 2006).

Challenges of Working in Resource Depleted Services

Australia allocates a relatively small percentage of the health budget to mental health when compared to other Organisation for Economic Co-operation and Development (OECD) countries. OECD countries spend between 12 and 16% of their health budget on mental health services, and Australia spends just 8% (OECD, 2015). Hospitals run off lean budgets with frozen staffing levels and long waiting lists for services. The majority of public hospital admissions occur in the context of crisis. Consumers have had either an exacerbation of a psychotic illness, a manic episode or present as a suicide risk. This often occurs after consumers present to Emergency Departments (ED) or when they are brought directly to the psychiatric unit by police or ambulance. In order to remedy these structural problems hospitals have developed strategies to promote "bed flow." The unfortunate extension of this is an increasingly singular focus on discharge rates and shortening admission lengths by administrators. It is the authors' view that unrealistic expectations of admission times are set, hampering recovery. It is the consensual view of clinicians and caregivers (e.g., Mental Health Council of Australia [MHCA] "Not for Service," 2005) that consumers are often turned away when requiring admission and are commonly discharged too early. This crisis-driven process also interferes with psychosocial treatments, as consumers can be discharged suddenly without a plan for ongoing treatment in the community.

Establishing a meaningful role in this chaotic environment is challenging, yet many of the survey respondents described ways in which they are able to provide meaningful services. Some expand their role to include follow-up post-discharge. They focus on assessment and relationship building during admission and then assist in transition after hospital discharge. One respondent commented

> It may be the first contact with a clinical psychologist that a patient has, and it may determine whether they engage with one again. Admission is extremely stressful … processing, support and validation around all of this is extremely valuable. Discharge planning and the assumption that things can change quickly should be anticipated and discussed in the very first contact. Specific work around symptom relief is incredibly useful, when people are actively symptomatic and distressed they are often most motivated to try what you teach them. Be prepared to do/practice/

model strategies then and there as you might only see them a few times. Aim to see them multiple times a week while they are there (if you can).

Stigma and Hostility toward Specific Consumer Populations

In our experience, the Rogerian principle of "unconditional positive regard" has little influence within the Australian mental health system. The nature of the clinicians' attitude toward consumers often varies according to the diagnosis of the consumer. For psychotic disorders, neglect, disinterest and an attitude of hopelessness has been widely reported (MHCA "Not for Service," 2005). There is an assumption of wide-ranging disability that often results in consumers not being afforded opportunities for study or other meaningful occupation. Here, the assumption of disability often leads to disability. Perhaps more confronting is the quality of care afforded to those consumers who self-harm or suffer from Cluster B personality disorders. These consumers may experience hostility and often a refusal of service when encountering health services. Although inexcusable, it is likely driven by limited resources and poorly educated clinicians.

Clinical psychologists are often confronted by these behaviors and seek to address them. A number of survey respondents described hostility and the use of offensive language in relation to consumers suffering from Borderline Personality Disorder. At times, their attempts to humanize those with personality disorders have been viewed by other disciplines as naïve and evidence that the clinician is being "manipulated." We have also observed a "hardening of clinicians" and the development of stigma after a period working in an inpatient setting. For instance, clinical psychologists who had been otherwise respectful of consumers may start referring to those suffering personality disorders as "PD's," a pejorative term in the Australian context. Desensitization in these situations is not uncommon, and one challenge is to keep clinical psychologists sensitive to potential human rights violations that may occur in inpatient units. Our method of implementing this will be outlined later in the chapter.

Can Clinical Psychologists Work Ethically within a System that Violates the Human Rights of the Mentally Ill?

As can be seen from the description above, the inpatient mental health environment is complex in many ways. The clinical populations are diagnostically complex, with significant risks. Psychotic disorders, severe mood disorders and personality disorders, the main diagnostic categories of consumers treated in inpatient settings, are difficult to engage. When combined with an almost exclusive biological focus, depleted resources and shrinking admission periods, this context can be difficult to navigate for clinical psychologists. Perhaps more troubling are the human rights violations that have become routine in some settings. This is the factor that requires the clinical psychologist to consider whether they are able to operate in these settings while maintaining ethical standards. We do not claim that the mental health system necessarily intentionally harms, or that all consumers have a counter-therapeutic experience; however, clinical psychologists must consider their role in a system that is criticized in independent reviews of human rights (Burdekin, 1993; Richmond, 1983; Mental Health Council of Australia, 2005).

The authors argue that clinical psychologists can work ethically in inpatient settings, and are in fact, particularly well placed to confront and challenge human rights problems that arise. We have found over the last 15 years that a relatively standard model of care, Cognitive Behavioral Therapy for psychosis (CBTp) acts to directly counter some of the most troubling elements of the mental health system. Perhaps controversially, we argue that clinical psychologists should expand their role to encompass that of human rights advocates if we are to work with consumers effectively. The section that follows will describe this approach.

Cognitive Behavioral Therapy for Psychosis (CBTp)

The authors work within the Cognitive Behavioral Therapy (CBT) tradition. CBT is an active and directive treatment that was developed in the late 1970s and is ubiquitous today. It asserts that certain thinking styles and behavioral patterns precipitate and maintain emotional disturbance. Treatment aims to equip consumers with techniques to alter behavior and unhelpful beliefs in order to reduce distress.

The cognitive behavioral tradition has only recently turned its attention to major mental illness. We argue that CBTp can act to both manage distress associated with the experience of psychosis and in addition work to address and uphold human rights principles in the inpatient context. This approach will be outlined below.

A Sense of Being "Silenced"

We have reported elsewhere (Walker, Steel, & Shearsby, 2012) that consumers report feeling "silenced" when interacting with the mental health system. They complain that they have to wait for long periods before seeing their doctor who may then appear rushed. They report difficulties being able to access nursing staff, and that certain topics, namely details about their symptoms, are dismissed. The "Not for Service" (MHCA, 2005) report offered the following example, "I noticed that when I started talking he would reach for the prescription pad."

Given the compelling and distressing nature of delusions and hallucinations, consumers often report strong desires to discuss these experiences in detail. When engaging in CBTp, a thorough assessment of beliefs and behaviors that are associated with psychosis is conducted. In this act, the consumers are encouraged to express their distress and are reinforced for their elaboration. In order to treat effectively, clinical psychologists seek to understand the details of psychotic phenomena, how and when they occur, what meaning the consumer instills in it and how and when the psychosis developed. Consumers often reflect that they had not felt as valued and heard before engaging in this form of treatment. By providing the consumer with an experience of being listened to, and having their thoughts and emotions treated as meaningful, this CBT intervention directly confronts some of the more oppressive aspects of the mental health inpatient system.

Witnessing the Experience

Related to the experience of being silenced is the clinical psychologist's role in witnessing the experience of the consumer. This is rare for the consumer and is experienced as novel. Most consumers are guarded when they are encouraged to elaborate on their experience, the distress, their beliefs and consequences. For many, it is the first time that they have felt heard and had their experience taken seriously. This is not to say that the clinical psychologist colludes with the consumer, rather that they take the role of a "detached scientist." This role is made explicit to consumers, and it is explained that the clinician has no investment in any specific conclusion. Rather, the clinician aims to assist the consumer to test the beliefs they have dispassionately and draw conclusions from the resulting evidence. If the conclusions are flawed or unhelpful, they are abandoned; if the consumer's conclusion holds, then appropriate action is taken to manage their situation. The authors have found that regardless of how bizarre a belief, little good comes from stating this directly, and if collaboration can be maintained by a consumer believing they are taken seriously, much can be achieved.

Many consumers have expressed appreciation during the intervention because the clinical psychologist kept formal notes. Consumers suffering paranoia felt reassured that a "paper trail" was developing, so that justice may be pursued in the event of catastrophe. After a long period of treatment, one consumer explained that he had believed the clinical psychologist was "in-on" his conspiracy but was benevolent. Over time, he explained that the plausibility of their paranoid belief about the clinician's role reduced and the clinician had gently but consistently raised a series of inconsistencies that led to a reappraisal of his beliefs.

Trauma of Inpatient Psychiatric Admission

The experience of psychosis can be horrifying. This trauma can be compounded by interaction with emergency services, such as the ambulance service and police. Even if emergency services act with sensitivity, it can be a humiliating experience to be forcibly removed from the community and transported to hospital in a locked police-van. On arrival at an inpatient facility, a consumer will observe people in states of distress and disorganization and many report feeling unsafe.

The relationship between trauma and psychosis is complex. In a literature review, Morrison, Frame, and Larkin (2003) cited evidence for Post-Traumatic Stress Disorder (PTSD) arising from the experience of psychosis, trauma causing psychosis and PTSD in response to psychiatric admission. Clinical psychologists have an important role in assessing for trauma experienced by those admitted to psychiatric settings, a process that rarely occurs. Once identified, there are various alternatives that can be considered, including less-restrictive care or treatment of the traumatic reaction. Turkington (1998, cited in Morrison, Frame, & Larkin, 2003) published a case-study that applied imaginal-exposure and cognitive reappraisal successfully with a client with features of PTSD and psychosis.

Providing intervention for trauma resulting from admission can place the clinical psychologist at odds with other members of the MDT. This act identifies aspects of care as potentially harmful and can be interpreted as criticism. We would argue that identifying potentially traumatizing aspects of the mental health services is an ethical imperative for all professionals; however, we have found it more manageable to couch the trauma in terms of a reaction to the terror of psychosis. There is more evidence for this relationship (e.g., McGorry et al., 1991) and a study has found that the proportion of variance in PTSD scores accounted for by hospital experiences was much lower (6%) than that attributed to the psychotic experience (52%) (Frame & Morrison, 2001). The authors have found it most effective to treat the trauma when necessary and to work at changing the traumatizing aspect of the admission process through other channels (such as management meetings).

Social Isolation and Exclusion

Consumers are socially isolated and under-employed. A national survey (Jablensky et al., 1999) reported that 35% of those with mental illness had not had face-to-face contact with a close relative for over a year, 31% lived alone, and 72% had no regular employment.

Clinical psychologists work to address isolation and exclusion. Practical strategies that increase community participation and inclusion are often an early therapeutic target. They work against withdrawal when they attempt to engage consumers on the ward in conversation. With time, an avoidant consumer may be coaxed into a group where they may share their experience or express an opinion. This builds confidence and demonstrates the value of community. Links are made with community services and programs that work to activate and provide meaningful occupation for consumers. Clinical psychologists connect consumers to these services and work in parallel with them with a focus on social inclusion, training in living-skills or vocational rehabilitation.

Another important factor that reduces consumer's isolation is the development of the therapeutic relationship. Clinical psychologists are in a relatively unique position in relation to the depth of the human connection that forms across an admission. The frenetic nature of ward environments and the mechanization of assessment and treatment contribute to attrition of the sense of humanity in the consumer population. Consumers have become *risks to assess* and *symptoms to be treated*, rather than people with rich experiences and valuable lives. Intensive psychological intervention is at odds with these processes, and clinical psychologists are privileged to connect with those so often discarded. One author (PW) has lived in close proximity to the psychiatric hospital in which he had worked for many years. It is a source of pride to be greeted by consumers on the main street as he runs errands or buys his lunch. It is touching that those individuals considered outcasts by many in society go to great lengths to acknowledge him. In recognition of this relationship and acknowledgment of our shared humanity, their greeting is always returned.

Aggression on the Ward

Aggression on inpatient units in Australia is relatively rare but remains significant for staff and consumers (Barlow, Greyner, & Ilkiw-Lavalle, 2000). Techniques for dealing with aggression in Australia are in flux, influenced by a broader international movement. "Traditional" models such as physical restraint and seclusion are being phased out. These are usually combined with pharmacological sedation. The experience is described as aversive and at times traumatizing by consumers and is often seen as a mechanism of control (Duxbury, 2002). Although often viewed as unpopular by staff, there is also a perception that doing without these methods is naïve and unrealistic (Grigg, 2006). Regardless, a transition to the eradication of seclusion and restraint is underway in Australia.

The movement away from traditional methods of aggression management has opened up space for psychological intervention. This occurs at a systemic and individual level as described below.

Clinical psychologists provide expertise on the factors that contribute to consumer's distress, including anger, which gives rise to aggressive behavior. This enables them to intervene at the system level, facilitating organizational change to alter factors that contribute to agitation in the inpatient population. Consistency in the implementation of treatment, a respectful style in relating to consumers and harmony in the relationships between staff, are among factors that contribute to the potential for reducing consumers' frustration and anger (Cornaggia, Beghi, Pavone, & Barale, 2011) and can be readily manipulated.

MDT's regularly call on clinical psychologists to assist in developing behavior management plans to assist with consumer aggression.[2] These standardize the communication style of the team, allow for consistent consequences in response to specific behaviors and reward positive behavior in a consistent way. The experience of the authors is that on busy wards with high staff turnover, these plans were of limited effectiveness.

Perhaps more progress has occurred in the management of anger when it arises in the context of borderline personality styles. The survey of clinical psychologists revealed that private psychiatric units will often provide a consistent Dialectical Behavioral Therapy (DBT) model in which all staff are aligned and informs all aspects of practice. Clinicians report that the consistency for dealing with emotional lability improves effectiveness greatly.

Consumer aggression can also be treated individually, through assertiveness training, the challenging of the assumptions that are associated with anger (e.g., "I'm being disrespected") and by teaching mindfulness-meditation techniques to change a consumer's relationship to their context and emotion from resistance to acceptance. We have found that anger can be greatly reduced by engaging in meaningful, warm personal interactions, even brief ones. This may seem obvious, yet on a chaotic, fractured ward with pressure being maintained to treat and discharge, this simple expression of shared humanity can easily be lost. Taking the time to engage individually and doing so with the same respect and seriousness that would be paid to any other client helps to reduce arousal. This poses challenges for our discipline, as we are usually much smaller in number and as a result of the orientation described, the services can be in high demand.

The interventions described above, flow directly from the assumptions and style required to engage in CBTp. We argue that its very nature remediates some of the more harmful aspects of the inpatient mental health system in Australia.

Clinical Psychologist as Human Rights Advocate

Clinical psychologists inhabit an unusual space within the mental health inpatient context. We are part of a system that can often be experienced by consumers as oppressive and controlling. At the same time, the clinical psychologist is quickly identified by the consumer as distinct from other members of the treating team. Clinical psychologists do not medicate, they promote non-pharmacological treatments, and they employ strategies that require the consumer's distress to be elucidated at length and in detail. The authors exploit this ambiguity to engage consumers and implement various therapeutic interventions with the aim of assisting the consumer in achieving personally defined goals.

The authors argue, perhaps controversially, that in order to promote our relevance to consumers and provide the conditions for meaningful change, our role must expand beyond our traditional role. Whereas, in other settings, clinical psychologists' responsibility may be confined to assessing and treating psychological disturbance, we would argue that in the mental health inpatient system in Australia, the clinical psychologist's role should expand to encompass that of a human rights advocate.

This perspective evolved after many years of clinical work in inpatient psychiatry. As junior clinicians, we were left with a compelling sense that what we observed in relation to routine-care was unacceptable at various levels. We were confronted by ethical conflicts on a daily basis. Examples are listed below:

- At a ward round an adolescent consumer was encouraged to give up study to reduce stress.
- A senior clinician refers to a consumer as a "chronic schiz" (a highly offensive derogatory colloquial Australian term).
- A 30-year-old consumer's parents are called without permission to assess accommodation options despite many years of estrangement and evidence of abuse.
- A consumer yells at the team for "not listening." She is transferred to the higher acuity ward "to calm down," suggesting she is being punished with more restrictive care arrangements.
- A team-leader encourages discharging a consumer to a cave near a city beach as there is no other suitable accommodation.
- In a ward round, treatment is discussed prior to the consumer's attendance. Once the consumer attends, they are given limited information about treatment choices and protocol.

In the early 2000s we found that various ethical codes provided little guidance for the problems we were facing. Fortunately, after the turn of the century, the confluence between the consumer movement and CBTp had occurred, leading to tangible changes for those experiencing mental illness (Walker, Steel, & Shearsby, 2012).

Human rights are entities that have a long history but have become a particular focus since the middle of the twentieth century. The Universal Declaration of Human Rights (UDHR) was drafted in 1948 though it took until 2006 for the rights of the mentally ill to be protected with the ratification of the Convention on the Rights of Persons with Disabilities. Rights act as norms, entitlements and social practices that apply to everyone as a result of a shared humanity (Donnelly, 2003). They are established in order to promote the full and unimpeded expression of an individual's human potential (Dudley, Silove, & Gale, 2012) and are most often raised in relation to vulnerable groups, such as refugees, women and children. Given the vulnerability, social-exclusion and impoverishment that may be experienced by consumers admitted to inpatient facilities in Australia, the authors have used a human rights framework to enhance traditional psychological approaches.

For instance, we have used the following principles, derived from the UDHR and subsequent covenants, to guide clinical decision-making.

- highest attainable standard of health – right to health
- protection from arbitrary detention
- adequate standard of living
- self-determination
- social inclusion
- meaningful occupation – right to work and employment
- the right to information
- the right to choice of treatment
- the right to informed consent
- the right to freedom of association and contract
- the right to political membership of a community

We have found these principles useful in framing our responses to the kinds of ethical issues described above.

Using human rights as an organizing principle extends the role of clinical psychologists. The authors directly confront stigmatizing language when it is used by staff members; we provide information about consumer rights and we actively campaign for least-restrictive practices in managing mental health crises. We run ward groups where consumer rights are described and where consumers can report infringements and often work with peers to resolve such issues when raised. The resolution is at times simple (e.g., replacing a lock on a door). At other times, resolution can be more complex, requiring executive input and systemic change (e.g., reducing seclusion and restraint). We have observed wider change occurring as a result of taking these commonly neglected issues seriously.

The reader may wonder about the consequences for the clinical psychologist playing the role that has been described. To be frank, when the authors assumed this role, we feared direct conflict or ostracism. Although there have been instances of conflict, much more commonly we have found that our interventions have emboldened others to take similar action and for the standards, in relation to human rights principles, to improve.

Conclusions

The Australian mental health inpatient system is viewed by the chapter's authors as a complex and contradictory organism. The role of clinical psychologists within these settings had been neglected until this century. Since the 2000s, a number of changes within the broader international mental health system and academic clinical psychology have provided direction, increased relevance and momentum to the discipline. The consumer movement, developing alongside the development of novel psychological interventions such as CBTp and DBT has provided clinical direction, confidence and hope for consumer populations often viewed as most challenging for clinicians. The authors argue that the future direction of these interventions should be to more directly assess and incorporate human rights principles as they arise. It is only through addressing these issues, so commonly raised by consumers in inpatient settings, that clinical psychologists' relevance to consumers, caregivers and the wider mental health community will be realized and the human rights infringements that may occur in mental health settings be relegated to history.

Notes

1 See Chapter 10 by Parswani and Stewart, this volume, for a further discussion on differentiating levels of psychotherapeutic interventions by clinical psychologists and MDT members.
2 see Chapter 5 by Kim and D'Amacio, this volume, for discussion of aggression reducing behavioral support plans.

References

Australian Bureau of Statistics. (2015). Retrieved from: www.abs.gov.au/ausstats/abs@.nsf/lookup/3101.0Media%20Release1Dec%202015.

Barlow, K., Greyner, B., & Ilkiw-Lavalle, O. (2000). Prevalence and precipitants of aggression in psychiatric inpatient units. *Australian and New Zealand Journal of Psychiatry*, *34*, 967–974.

Bassman, R. (1997). The mental health system: Experiences from both sides of the locked door. *Professional Psychology: Research and Practice*, *28*, 238–242.

Bellack, A.S. (1986). Schizophrenia: Behavior therapy's forgotten child. *Behavior Therapy*, *17*, 199–214.

Bentall, R.P. & Fernyhough, C. (2008). Social predictors of psychotic experiences: Specificity and psychological mechanisms. *Schizophrenia Bulletin*, *34*, 1012–1020.

Bentall, R.P. & Slade, P.D. (1988). *Sensory deception: A scientific analysis of hallucination*. Baltimore, MD: John Hopkins University Press.

Birchwood, M. & Trower, P. (2006). The future of cognitive–behavioural therapy for psychosis: Not a quasi-neuroleptic. *British Journal of Psychiatry, 188*, 107–108.

Burdekin, B. (1993). *Human rights and mental illness: Report of the national inquiry into the human rights of people with a mental illness.* Canberra, ACT: Australian Government Publishing Service.

Byrne, D.G & Davenport, S.C. (2006). Contemporary profiles of clinical and health psychologists in Australia. *Australian Psychologist, 40*, 190–201.

Chadwick, P., Birchwood, M., & Trower, O. (1996). *Cognitive therapy for delusions, voices and paranoia.* Chichester, UK: Wiley.

Cornaggia C.M., Beghi M., Pavone F., & Barale F. (2011). Aggression in psychiatry wards: A systematic review. *Psychiatry Research, 189*, 10–20.

Donnelly, J. (2003). *Universal human rights in theory and practice.* 2nd ed. Ithaca, NY: Cornell University Press.

Dudley, M., Silove, D.M., & Gale, F. (2012). Mental health, human rights and their relationship: An introduction. In M. Dudley, D. Silove, & F. Gale (Eds.), *Human rights and mental health: Vision, praxis and courage* (pp. 1–49). Oxford: Oxford University Press.

Duhig, M., Patterson, S., Connell, M., Foley, S., Capra, C., Dark, F., Gordon, A., Singh, S., Hides, L., McGrath, J., & Scott, J. (2015). The prevalence and correlates of childhood trauma in patients with early psychosis. *Australian and New Zealand Journal of Psychiatry, 49*, 651–659.

Duxbury, J. (2002). An evaluation of staff and patient views of and strategies employed to manage inpatient aggression and violence on one mental health unit: A pluralistic design. *Journal of Psychiatric and Mental Health Nursing, 9*, 325–337.

Frame, L. & Morrison, A.P. (2001). Causes of PTSD in psychosis. *Archives of General Psychiatry, 58*, 305–306.

Grigg, M. (2006). Eliminating seclusion and restraint in Australia. *International Journal of Mental Health Nursing, 15*, 224–225.

Jablensky, A., McGrath, J., Herrman, H., Castle, D., Gureje, O., Morgan, V., & Korten, A. (1999). *People living with psychotic illness: An Australian study 1997–1998.* Canberra: Department of Health and Aged Care.

Kirkby, K. (1999). History of psychiatry in Australia, pre-1960. *History of Psychiatry, 10*, 191–204.

McGorry, P.D., Chanen, A., McCarthy, E., van Riel, R., McKenzie, D., & Singh, B.S. (1991). Post traumatic stress disorder following recent onset psychosis: An unrecognised postpsychotic syndrome. *Journal of Nervous and Mental Disease, 179*, 253–258.

Mental Health Council of Australia. (2005). Not for service: Experiences of injustice and despair in mental health care in Australia. Deakin, ACT: Mental Health Council of Australia. Retrieved from: www.humanrights.gov.au/sites/default/files/content/disability_rights/notforservice/documents/NFS_Finaldoc.pdf.

Morrison, A.P., Frame, L., & Larkin, W. (2003). Relationships between trauma and psychosis: A review and integration. *British Journal of Clinical Psychology, 42* (4), 331–353.

OECD. (2015). *Mental health and work: Australia.* Paris: OECD Publishing.

Psychology Board of Australia; Registrant data. (June 2016). Retrieved from: www.psychologyboard.gov.au/documents/default.aspx?record=WD16%2F21498.

Read, J. (2005). The bio-bio-bio model of madness. *The Psychologist*, *18*, 596–597.

Richmond, D. (1983). Inquiry into health services for the psychiatrically ill and developmentally disabled. Summary of recommendations. Sydney Health Commission NSW. Retrieved from: https://nswmentalhealthcommission.com.au/sites/default/files/Inquriy%20into%20Health%20Services%20for%20the%20Psychiatrically%20Ill%20and%20Developmentally%20Disabled%20-%20Richmond%20Report%20-%201983.pdf.

Walker, P., Steel, Z., & Shearsby, J. (2012). Can cognitive behavior therapy act as a human rights intervention for consumers experiencing severe mental disorder? In: M. Dudley, D. Silove, & F. Gale (Eds.), *Mental health and human rights: Vision, praxis, and courage* (pp. 623–634). Oxford: Oxford University Press.

4 Ethical Challenges for Psychologists Providing Inpatient Mental Health Care

Heidi Camerlengo

Clinical psychologists working in inpatient mental health settings encounter innumerable situations in which ethical decisions must be made. Often situations evolve in ways that provide the psychologist with sufficient time to recognize the dilemma unfolding and decide how to respond, or if a response is even necessary. Conversely, there are times when important ethical decisions need to be made on the spot. Psychologists working in the United States have a number of resources at their disposal to assist with ethical decision making including the *Ethical Principles of Psychologists and Code of Conduct* (American Psychological Association, 2017), the *Guidelines for Psychological Practice in Health Care Delivery Systems* (American Psychological Association, 2012a), and the *Specialty Guidelines for Forensic Psychology* (American Psychological Association, 2012b). Collectively, these documents establish enforceable standards of ethical conduct, suggest aspirational goals, and offer models for improving the quality and delivery of psychological services. Unfortunately, available guidelines often fall short in addressing explicit ways for resolving more complex ethical situations routinely encountered by psychologists engaged in inpatient mental health practice.

In this chapter, a variety of ethical dilemmas and issues faced by psychologists are described, some derived from the author's own experiences and some from the experiences recounted by colleagues with diverse backgrounds and varying years of practice in both public and private psychiatric hospitals in the United States. An attempt was made to categorize the issues into several distinct topic areas, but in reality, when ethical dilemmas and issues arise as they frequently do, their impact crosses over into several aspects of the psychologist's clinical and administrative work, and sometimes into personal aspects of their work and lives as well. While the ethical dilemmas discussed herein are not exhaustive, they represent some of the more common situations that psychologists encounter when providing inpatient mental health treatment. Balancing these overlapping and at times conflicting dilemmas is an ever-challenging part of the inpatient psychologist's responsibilities.

Clinically vs. Administratively and Legally-Driven Treatment

One of the more prevalent ethically challenging situations that inpatient psychologists experience is interference with treatment decisions by administrative and legal forces whose priorities may lead to decisions that diverge significantly from what is in the patient's best interest and in line with the clinician's ethical standards of practice. In the United States, the type and duration of psychological treatment offered and length of hospitalization is directly affected by patients' insurance coverage, institutional policies, oversight committees, the courts, and state commitment laws. The budget in many inpatient facilities is frequently a determining factor in service provision. If services are not reimbursed by insurance, then they are not offered, or they are only available on a limited basis irrespective of patient need. The impact of these issues on the provision of clinical care frequently results in decisions about important aspects of treatment being made in response to factors outside of the treating psychologist's control. While state and federal inpatient facilities have more flexibility than private-for-profit entities in offering mental health services to uninsured or indigent patients, there are still limitations that adversely influence treatment availability and continuity, and place psychologists in positions where organizational and other standards of care are at odds with ethical practice.

Psychologists employed in private inpatient settings lament the negative impact that insurance coverage has on the ethical provision of patient care due to coverage limits on clinically indicated services. "Every treatment decision is based on how many days insurance providers approve patients' stay and what therapeutic modalities they will reimburse." A psychologist working in a private psychiatric hospital discussed his dismay when the insurance of one of his more unstable patients ran out, and he was instructed by his administrator to prepare her for transitioning to outpatient treatment.

> I couldn't imagine how this woman was considered stable by insurance and no longer eligible for inpatient services. She was still talking about suicide although she contracted for safety. I didn't feel I knew her well enough after two days to say that she was credible and would be safe outside of the hospital, but I had to discharge her. I've tried contacting insurance companies myself and advocating for patients, but my efforts are often ignored.

Interference with psychological services also occur from authorities within institutions, at times challenging inpatient psychologists to ethically terminate therapeutic relationships in order to minimize harm to patients. A former colleague commented that her institution's administration thinks nothing of abruptly transferring patients when bed space is needed, without consulting the treatment team or providing the team with appropriate notice so that termination issues can be addressed. She recounted one case where a severely depressed and paranoid patient who had only recently begun to talk to the team after two months of hospitalization was moved from her unit to make room for a new admission. When the team reconvened the following day, they were informed of the transfer and immediately attempted to address their concerns with the administrator and other executive staff. Not surprisingly, their concerns were dismissed while the "efficient functioning" of the hospital's admission's process was given precedence. The displaced patient subsequently had a near-lethal suicide attempt shortly after the transfer.

In order to achieve an ethical resolution to this conflict between the ethics code (American Psychological Association, 2017) and organizational practices, the psychologist consulted with her supervisor, then she, along with her treatment team, sent a dissenting email detailing the event to all levels of hospital administration. She also visited the unit where her patient had been transferred, met with the new treatment team and her patient to have closure, and wrote a note in the patient's chart expressing clinically supported opposition to this unethical management decision. The psychologist commented on her reaction to the situation, "I had to do something to cope with feeling so powerless because this type of thing happens all the time and can be traumatic for everyone involved."

The seemingly random and unforeseen transfer of patients among inpatient units and the possibility of sudden court-ordered discharges directly influence psychologists' decisions whether to initiate clinically indicated individual and/or group therapies and perform assessment batteries. Furthermore, these circumstances also affect the assignment of interns to cases since institutions are contractually and ethically responsible for providing opportunities that facilitate interns meeting their training goals. Psychologists are obligated professionally and ethically to execute appropriate termination of therapy and provide patients with feedback regarding the results of testing. When patients are abruptly removed from psychological care, therapies are interrupted, testing may be incomplete, and psychologists may not fulfill their ethical obligation to enact appropriate termination or explain test results. It can be frustrating for psychologists and interns alike, as well as harmful to patients, when patients who are engaged in clinical services unexpectedly leave the unit.

The sudden voluntary or involuntary administrative transfer of psychologists to different hospital units can be destabilizing for patients and disruptive to psychologists working with these patients in treatment. A psychologist who formerly worked in a state psychiatric hospital commented that in his 27 years of service, he was transferred among units nine times, mostly due to the institution's need for psychological coverage in a particular area.

> There were times when I had only one day to prepare my patients and ward for my transfer. It was extremely difficult to have proper termination with my patients and co-workers. I also left knowing that the ward would be without consistent psychological coverage until a new person was hired or one of my peers wanted to work there.

Another disruption in patient care that poses ethical, as well as professional challenges to psychologists, are court-ordered discharges of patients against the psychologist's and team's recommendations. Some of the patients discharged in this manner have been evaluated as still dangerous and in need of inpatient treatment in order to ensure theirs' and others' safety. Involuntary commitment laws in many states cite either "foreseeable" or "imminent" risk of dangerousness to self, others, or property as reasons to mandate psychiatric hospitalization. Attorneys defending involuntarily committed patients may not appreciate the clinical evaluation of risk and often use patients' "recent" behavior as a guide for legally determining dangerousness. Defense attorneys have successfully argued in court that their clients "have not exhibited any aggressive or violent behavior in two weeks and therefore should be discharged." Furthermore, it is usually the psychiatrist who is called upon to provide testimony concerning a patient's need for continued inpatient care, not the psychologist who frequently has more contact with patients and knowledge about their clinical stability including readiness for discharge. While many psychiatrists seek input from psychologists and other team members before making such decisions, some offer their opinion to the court without obtaining this important information. In these situations, psychologists have a professional and ethical responsibility to present their clinical opinions to the court, even when they may differ from other professionals' opinions and could have treatment or judicial implications for patients.

One inpatient psychologist's approach to ethically managing the commitment hearing process is to work with her team's psychiatrist and provide him with a summary of patients' progress in treatment and any findings obtained from psychological testing that support a particular course of action. The psychiatrist incorporates these summaries into his commitment hearing reports for consideration by the court. Another psychologist routinely accompanies his psychiatrist to commitment hearings and will testify whenever he is concerned that patients whom he has evaluated as still at risk may be discharged by the court. In both of these cases, the psychologists note their careful attention to providing informed consent to clarify how information

obtained through psychological interventions could be used within the legal system to either support or oppose patients' preferences regarding their mental health care.

Involuntary commitment laws also impact patients' ability to independently choose mental health treatment, subsequently creating another ethical dilemma impacting psychologists; how does one respect patients' rights to self-determination when treatment is legally mandated? Patients who are involuntarily committed to a psychiatric institution are often resentful of their loss of control over this decision and frequently lack insight into their behaviors that have caused others concern. Some have no interest in participating in treatment and refuse to cooperate with required psychological assessments or interventions, while others can become quite hostile. It can be a difficult balancing act between supporting patients' wishes and rights to make autonomous treatment decisions including treatment refusal and providing ethical and clinically appropriate psychological services within the involuntary setting where it is expected that all patients will receive some type of mental health services.

A clinical psychologist working in a state psychiatric hospital discussed what it was like being "forced" by administrative oversight committees to provide services to involuntarily committed patients after they determined that the patients posed a high risk of engaging in violent behavior and required psychological intervention. These management decisions were made irrespective of patients' willingness to accept treatment or the psychologist's clinical assessment of their readiness to benefit from services.

> I really resent non-clinicians telling me what to do with my patients and how to manage their treatment needs. How can I possibly attempt to engage patients in treatment who are threatening to harm me or even kill me if I come near them? When my clinical evaluation of a patient is in opposition to administrative directives, I write a detailed progress note in the patient's chart documenting all of the reasons why psychological treatment is contraindicated at that time and my plans for future attempts to offer services if/when the situation changes. I am not always popular with hospital administration, but I feel my responsibility is to my patients first, not to mention my own safety. I also want to set an example for colleagues by asserting my commitment to ethical, clinically-sound practice despite pressures to behave otherwise.

In my inpatient work, I have found it useful to directly address involuntary commitment and treatment issues with patients and empathize with their position in order to facilitate cooperation. Patients are more likely to work productively with me if they feel that I understand their views regarding forced mental health care and am doing what I can within the institutions' legal and administrative constraints to give them a voice and make their desires known. When patients object to involuntary mental health treatment, I believe it is beneficial to contact defense counsel, not only to discuss plans for upcoming commitment hearings, but also to provide a model for patients of how to navigate the legal system and assert oneself appropriately, whether or not I agree with their opinions. Such contact is always made with my patients' consent and usually with their participation. I also encourage patients to discuss with their attorney the pros/cons of refusing to cooperate with recommended psychological assessments, therapy, and other clinically indicated treatment as well as the possible impact that their choices may have on the court's decisions regarding future treatment and discharge. In this way, I feel that I have demonstrated respect for my patients' dignity and right to choose participation in psychological services by offering an avenue for them to assert their wishes irrespective of my clinical opinion.

Providing involuntary mental health care becomes more complicated when my patients and I have to "agree to disagree" on a particular treatment plan, and I am unable to clinically support their preferred course of action. The ethical dilemma subsequently becomes magnified and I have to decide when, if at all, and under what circumstances, my professional decisions can override patients' beliefs about what constitutes their own "best interest" and thus potentially place constraints on their right to voluntarily choose mental health treatment. What factors should psychologists consider when deciding to move forward with clinically indicated interventions that may not represent what patients' request, and how important are patients' rights to self-determination when their treatment preferences could place themselves and others at risk?

A clinical indicator commonly considered by psychologists when evaluating the need for involuntary mental health care is a patient's level of insight into their mental illness and how likely they will be to follow through with recommended treatment once discharged from the hospital. The high re-hospitalization rate of patients who psychiatrically decompensate due to noncompliance with prescribed medications and aftercare is a well-known challenge in inpatient mental health care. Some psychologists argue that the trauma associated with ongoing episodes of involuntary hospitalization is itself a consideration for asserting a treatment agenda with uncooperative patients in an effort to mitigate harm resulting from such unsettling disruptions in their lives.

What options do psychologists have when institutional practices and laws negatively influence ethical aspects of treatment by affecting their ability to initiate clinically informed psychological interventions? The majority of private inpatient mental health treatment facilities and many public psychiatric hospitals operate on short-term, medically-based treatment models that emphasize crisis stabilization, psychopharmacology, and brief therapeutic interventions. How does one determine if a particular treatment intervention or assessment battery is appropriate when patients can be abruptly removed from our care by termination of insurance coverage, administrative practices, or court-ordered discharges? Psychologists are consequently charged with developing a multitude of approaches to treatment and providing therapeutic interventions that fit the needs of both their patients and their particular inpatient setting.

A senior psychologist said that his approach to ethically managing administrative interference in psychological treatment that contributes to unexpected interruptions in therapy is to make the most of every encounter:

> I treat each session with my patients as if it's the only one I'll have with them. Together, we set goals that can be accomplished quickly and discuss what issues they would like to explore with a mental health professional once settled in the community. I am always cognizant of avoiding harm to my patients by refraining from initiating therapeutic work that I won't have time to address or terminate properly. I want patients to have a good therapeutic experience with a psychologist to increase the likelihood that they will seek assistance in the future if needed.

Ethical Challenges Related to Treatment Team Functioning

Administrative and legal interferences in mental health treatment are not the only factors to consider when attempting to provide clinically relevant and ethical psychological services to psychiatrically hospitalized patients. Clinical psychologists who practice in the inpatient mental health setting also need to consider ethical issues that arise as part of their participation in a multidisciplinary treatment team. Along with the psychologist, treatment teams generally consist of a psychiatrist, a social worker, an administrative coordinator, and nursing staff including direct care workers. Ancillary team members may include physicians, addiction counselors, physical therapists, dieticians, chaplains, and rehabilitation staff. These professionals and paraprofessionals work together to address the biopsychosocial needs of each patient under their care. Their organized efforts are formalized in the creation of individualized treatment plans for patients that specify the services that each team member will provide. Ideally, each discipline would function in a consistent, singular relationship with patients that is defined by clear role expectations and boundaries; frequently this is not the case.

The very nature of the inpatient treatment team presents numerous situations where members find themselves required to perform a variety of duties in order to fulfill team and discipline-specific responsibilities. Such duties frequently place team members in multiple relationships with patients and challenge efforts to establish good treatment boundaries and maintain patient confidentiality. There was a time when I was the only psychologist assigned to an inpatient unit with 40 patients who had differing treatment needs and legal situations. Minimally, my responsibilities included treatment planning, psychodiagnostic testing, violence risk assessment, individual and group psychotherapy, crisis intervention, family therapy, and evaluating eligibility for Social Security benefits for every patient on my unit, as clinically indicated. I was also required to serve as a witness when patients were accused of involvement in dangerous incidents during their hospitalization.

These varying and often overlapping responsibilities lead to unintended, yet predictable multiple relationships with patients. The growing role of psychologists in court-related functions (i.e., court-ordered patient evaluations and testimony) presents additional challenges to maintaining appropriate boundaries within the psychologist–patient relationship and taxes adherence to ethical standards of conduct as they pertain to multiple relationships and patient confidentiality. A psychologist working in a federal inpatient psychiatric hospital said,

> Right from the start, I tell my patients that even though my title says clinical psychologist, at any given time I could wear a number of different hats. I try and preface my patient contact with an explanation of whom I represent at that moment, but it always overlaps.

Consider a situation in which a psychologist is required to assess risk for violence recidivism and provide group psychotherapy to a patient who is court-ordered to the hospital for treatment after she was arrested for burglary and found to be psychiatrically unstable. Upon the patient's admission, the psychologist is simultaneously placed in the roles of a team member, evaluator, and group therapist with the added potential for serving as a fact or expert witness in court due to the patient's legal situation. Each of these roles has different responsibilities and requirements with implications for informed consent including limits on confidentiality.

Over many years of work in the inpatient psychiatric setting, I have learned that it is good practice to try to anticipate the potential role(s) I may assume with my patients from the time of our initial encounter along with the possible uses of information acquired through psychological interventions. I convey these possibilities to patients as soon as feasible, both verbally and in writing, through the use of a separate consent form. In addition, I document my efforts regarding informed consent by composing a team or discipline-specific note in their charts whenever this topic is discussed. I also routinely check in with all of my patients to assess their understanding of confidentiality limits prior to conducting testing or therapy and provide ongoing reminders.

It is also important for psychologists to clarify their various roles, job responsibilities, and area(s) of proficiency as well as limitations in clinical experience with fellow team members to avoid practicing outside of their boundaries of competence. Psychologists are often perceived by team members as global experts in psychology and as such are presumed to possess the requisite knowledge and skills needed to evaluate and treat most issues that patients may present. Such unrealistic expectations of their abilities can create pressure for psychologists to offer opinions on clinical issues or provide evaluation and treatment without having appropriate training and supervised experience. A newly hired psychologist recounted a situation when the team's dietician asked for her opinion on how to manage an anorexic patient's meals. Apparently, this psychologist's predecessor had extensive experience treating eating disordered patients, and team members expected that she too was knowledgeable about these issues. The psychologist subsequently felt inadequate because of her limited training in this area.

> I wanted to be perceived as helpful by my new team. It was uncomfortable having to tell members that I wasn't sure how to proceed with this patient and would need to consult with someone in order to be of assistance.

Another challenge for psychologists working on a multidisciplinary team can be asserting one's position within the hierarchy and possessing the ability to independently evaluate patients and implement treatment plans that meet professional and ethical standards of psychological practice. The majority of inpatient mental health facilities in the United States operate on the medical model and as such place the psychiatrist in a position of power on the treatment team. In general, psychiatrists choose and prescribe psychotropic medications, write orders for privileges/behavioral precautions, evaluate for guardianship, and testify in court regarding a patient's need for continued commitment or readiness for discharge. They, as well as each discipline, have their own treatment priorities and ethics code that may or may not be consistent with the priorities and ethical responsibilities of other members. Many treatment teams successfully establish mutually respectful, egalitarian relationships among members that acknowledge each member's clinical opinion and incorporate discipline specific services into overall patient care. Difficulties ensue when members feel that their opinions are ignored, or they feel forced to behave in ways that are counter to clinically and ethically responsible practice.

A colleague recalled the first time he was involved in a team conflict regarding whether a patient who was occasionally uncooperative with taking prescribed medication should be permitted to have home visits. His opposing argument to the visits was primarily based on safety; if

this patient was not willing to accept medication administered by a nurse in the hospital, how likely would he be to take it without supervision? The team was divided on the issue, but ultimately the patient was allowed a visit home. In response to this decision, the psychologist wrote a dissenting team note explaining his opposition to home visits at that time, which he justified clinically. The note was not well received, particularly by the psychiatrist who had written the order and held the position that it was her license, not the psychologist's at stake if anything problematic occurred. It was initially uncomfortable for him to discuss his decision with the discordant team members, and he was later informed that his actions were perceived as a betrayal. Fortunately, the patient's visit was successful, and the event stimulated a dialog regarding strategies for handling future team disagreements in ways that promoted an attitude of cooperation among all members and respect for clinically and ethically appropriate interventions.

A related ethical issue involves the misuse of psychological reports and test results by team members to justify a particular course of action for patients. Psychologists have a professional and ethical responsibility to ensure that patient evaluations, and other data acquired through psychological interventions are used accurately and for the intended purpose. There are times when other disciplines may take assessment information out of context and use it to support their own agenda. During group supervision, a psychology intern discussed how a team member selected quotes from her supervisor's report and used them inappropriately to justify referring a patient to once weekly outpatient groups while the patient required significantly more support in order to remain psychiatrically stable. Another psychologist complained how her organization's clinical oversight committee misinterpreted psychological test results and labeled a patient as being at high risk for violence; thus the committee would not approve the patient's preferred discharge plan to an independent apartment. The psychiatrist was subsequently mandated by the committee to discharge the patient to a group home against the recommendations of the social worker and psychologist.

It can be extremely frustrating and potentially contentious for psychologists to rectify misuse of their work when addressing the issue with fellow team members. Even if psychologists make a concerted effort to develop and maintain positive professional relationships with their team and model respectful, collegial discussions, attempts to clarify misstatements of psychological data may contribute to treatment team members feeling disrespected, thus negatively impacting smooth team functioning. A clinical psychologist discussed what it was like confronting the team psychiatrist after he not only plagiarized a section of her report but also misrepresented her conclusions concerning recommendations for discharge.

> I thought the psychiatrist and I had a mutually respectful relationship that precluded such improper use of my work. The patient in question was difficult to deal with, and the psychiatrist's actions were an attempt to get this patient discharged, which in itself represents unethical behavior. When I confronted him about these issues, he took responsibility for his actions, apologized, and wrote an addendum to his report explaining his error and changed his recommendations to accurately reflect the assessment results.

Not every team dispute over the unethical misuse of psychological data resolves so positively. Another psychologist was concerned that her team social worker ignored a portion of her neurological assessment indicating that the patient was in need of a structured living situation and instead referred the patient for placement in an apartment with minimal supports. When the psychologist attempted to discuss the situation, the social worker justified his actions by explaining that he was unable to locate housing that met the psychologist's recommendations. In addition, he was feeling pressure from his administrator to effect a discharge and intended to follow through with his plans. "The social worker basically admitted that he succumbed to administrative force and accepted the first available placement for this cognitively impaired patient." When the psychologist's efforts to resolve this disagreement were unable to be rectified informally with the social worker, she was ethically obligated to take her concerns to the next level of administration since in her clinical opinion the patient could sustain substantial harm if left unsupervised.

Reporting unethical behavior on the part of team members has the power to divide teams and irreparably damage relationships. Psychologists have a clear ethical and at times legal responsibility to report unethical behavior on the part of their colleagues when attempts at informal resolution are unsuccessful or contraindicated due to the severity of the misconduct. A clinical psychologist discussed her experience with reporting a team member who used abusive language when speaking with an argumentative patient.

> I had tried several times to address this issue directly with the nurse, yet she continued to behave in an improper manner that eventually crossed the line into verbal abuse. I was required to file an incident report, and she was subsequently suspended. After her suspension, I felt team members and unit staff viewed me differently. It was as if they didn't trust me and were cautious in their communications with patients when I was around. I was also uncomfortable and had to work hard to regain their trust and respect.

Hospital/Accrediting Body Policies in Conflict with Psychologists' Ethics Code

An ongoing challenge for clinical psychologists who practice in inpatient mental health settings is the clash between ethical standards of psychological practice and institutional policies that are in part based on accrediting body standards. Many mental health institutions have administratively driven policies that require psychologists to complete evaluations of psychiatrically unstable patients and render treatment (i.e., suicide risk assessment; group therapy) within very short time-limits. Frequently, critical background and legal information is not readily available for use in completing required assessments within the timeframes outlined in these policies. It is equally concerning that often times newly admitted patients are unable to provide appropriate informed consent/assent to treatment due to their mental state. Acutely psychotic patients and those experiencing severe mood episodes usually require time to benefit from psychotropic medications and milieu therapy before they can fully appreciate and understand team functioning and limitations on confidentiality. These types of policies tax psychologists' ability to provide clinically and ethically appropriate services.

A psychologist employed by a state psychiatric institution described how psychologists in her department were expected to complete a comprehensive sex offender risk assessment within eight days of their patients' admission whether or not the patient was stable and regardless of their access to necessary legal and background information needed to perform the assessment. When her director attempted to inform hospital administration that such a requirement was unethical, he was essentially told, "It's a legal decision that is now policy, and we need to follow it." Her department's response was to email the institution's chain of command including the Board of Trustees to begin formally documenting their concerns and outline what they felt was a reasonable approach to addressing all parties' needs while protecting their patients' rights. Although her department was unsuccessful in changing their institution's formal policy regarding assessment timeframes, they did sensitize hospital administration to the various issues psychologists face when mandated to perform certain evaluations without required legal and other collateral information and successfully negotiated some exceptions that allowed additional time to collect this information prior to completing the assessment. Their approach to this ethical dilemma of maintaining professional standards of practice in the face of institutional pressure to bypass such standards supported a collaborative relationship with the administration while making clear the department's commitment to ethical practice. Senior psychologists agree that it is usually better to engender a spirit of cooperation and mutual respect with the administrative staff if one desires to have their concerns taken seriously and addressed in a manner in line with ethical and professional standards of care.

A senior colleague said that his approach to addressing ethical obligations to patients who are too psychiatrically decompensated or cognitively impaired to appreciate their circumstance and give informed consent/assent, yet are mandated for treatment, is to refrain from asking detailed, personal questions that are unrelated to the required task. Instead, he suggested exploring only those areas that can answer the specific referral question. For example, "Is this patient in imminent danger of harming himself or others?" He also developed a therapy group for patients whose mental state precludes them from fully understanding their situation. The focus of this group is to assist members in becoming oriented to their surroundings and adapting to the hospital environment. If called upon to testify in court regarding his patients' treatment, he makes a point of explaining the nature of their participation and their compromised ability to provide informed consent/assent before answering questions about their case. His psychological documentation similarly reflects patients' inability to give consent/assent and directs the reader to consider this factor when using information contained in their medical record.

Another colleague who works on an admissions unit described her approach to treatment with acutely ill patients who lack the ability to appreciate informed consent as "supportive," with the overall goal of rendering the least invasive form of psychological intervention that protects her patients' rights yet satisfies institutional and/or court requirements.

> I regularly spend about half of my workday asking patients basic orientation questions and offering information as tolerated. More importantly, I make a point of being the "friendly face" on the unit, which facilitates forming and establishing helpful treatment relationships.

This psychologist also remains cognizant of the possibility that her patients may be in need of a guardian, and she readily takes the necessary steps to expedite the process so one can be appointed as early in their hospitalization as possible.

An ongoing ethical matter for psychologists in many institutions concerns the ability of psychiatrically unstable patients and patients with intellectual disabilities and dementia to understand and appreciate informed consent to treatment and how their Protected Health Information (PHI) will be used. In the United States, PHI refers to any information about health status, provision of health care, or payment for healthcare that is part of a patient's medical record. Are these patients capable of giving consent/assent or is it necessary to pursue guardianship? Often psychologists are at the forefront of identifying deficits that could prompt a referral for further evaluation. Although all hospitals have policies in place for evaluating patients' needs for legal guardianship, their understanding and efficiency in completing the process vary considerably. A psychologist working in a state facility said, "Our guardianship process can take several weeks to complete; meanwhile, I'm being asked to sign as a witness to consent for medication when many of these patients clearly do not understand."

A former intern commented that very few psychologists and psychiatrists on staff at her public psychiatric hospital were clear how the guardianship process worked including who was responsible for performing the evaluations. As a result, evaluations were not being completed, and psychiatrically unstable patients and patients with suspected cognitive deficits were asked to sign consent for treatment including medications, financial agreements, aftercare plans, and other legal documents without fully understanding their meaning or potential implications. This practice did not sit well with the psychologist who was part of the treatment team and therefore an unwilling participant in this unethical treatment of cognitively compromised patients. Additionally, one of her more fragile patients was denied care at a local medical hospital when staff there questioned the patient's competency and sent him back to the psychiatric hospital for evaluation.

> I recognized the potential ethical and legal violations inherent in the institution's apparent disregard for pursuing guardianship, but I felt that I was too new and therefore unsure how to proceed in addressing the situation. I decided to consult with my former internship supervisor and a current colleague who shared my concerns and was willing to collaborate with me and take the issue forward. We initiated a discussion at a psychology department meeting and solicited our colleagues' and director's support in addressing the guardianship process with administrative staff and the institution's Board of Trustees.

Because of their actions, they were appointed to lead a state-wide task force to review current guardianship policies and draft a uniform process for ensuring that every patient undergoes evaluation in a timely manner if their ability to give legally informed consent is in question. "It's a work in progress, but we feel strongly that to ignore this issue is an egregious violation of patients' rights and does not support ethical practice."

A related concern is ascertaining whether patients have appointed a power of attorney (POA) who has the legal authority to provide consent on their behalf. Sometimes treatment teams are not aware of a patient's legal status as it relates to POA or guardianship until later during the course of hospitalization. There have been a number of times when patients admitted to my unit did not disclose this information and no documents were on file; thus we proceeded with treatment. Upon learning about the existence of a guardian or POA, we have found it helpful to immediately arrange a team meeting with this person and the patient so that each discipline has an opportunity to explain their particular role and the potential uses of PHI and answer any questions. By taking a proactive stance, we are usually successful in enlisting the guardian/POA in supporting the recommended treatment and engaging them in the treatment process.

Ethical Challenges to Protecting Confidentiality

Maintaining the confidentiality of patients' PHI is an ongoing challenge for psychologists employed in the inpatient mental health treatment setting. Many people from various disciplines, both inside and outside of these institutions, have access to information contained in patients' charts including information regarding patients' involvement in psychological services. While such information sharing among disciplines facilitates the development of comprehensive treatment planning, it also necessitates that psychologists establish a balance between protecting patients' confidential psychological information, and deciding what is professionally or ethically appropriate to share with team members and other clinical staff for their benefit.

I have found it extremely helpful for patients to understand my responsibilities when making decisions about protecting their confidentiality or exposing information acquired through their participation in psychological services. As part of my informed consent, patients are told from our first encounter that I am a part of the team and will provide members with ongoing updates of their progress in treatment and results of any assessments that I perform in order to provide the most beneficial interventions possible. I try, however, never to reveal personal information that is unrelated to the specific treatment issues without patients' consent. If I am bound by professional and ethical obligations to divulge PHI, I encourage patients to participate in sharing this information with me during a team meeting. Empowering patients to take responsibility for themselves and actively participate in their treatment not only reflects the intent behind the American Psychological Association's General Principles of Respect for People's Rights and Dignity, and Fidelity and Responsibility (American Psychological Association, 2017); it can also be therapeutic. Patients are less likely to have their trust compromised by releases of information if they are informed of the limits of confidentiality at the outset of treatment and have an active role in the team disclosures. Although I spend a good amount of time explaining my policy and ensuring that patients understand, this method has not always been successful in supporting their confidence in our relationship.

Another challenge that psychologists face in protecting patients' confidentiality concerns their legal status. Any time that psychologists are charged with treating legally involved patients, there is always the potential to be ordered to write reports for the court on patients' progress or be subpoenaed to testify regarding various aspects of their care. Psychologists may be legally bound to provide clinical information to the court either with or without patient consent. When court-ordered to release PHI, I find it a useful practice to first meet with patients and discuss the information that has been requested. Another colleague of mine encourages his patients to contact their public defender or a private attorney to discuss the request and explore what options might be available if they object to disclosing certain parts of their medical record. For example, will the court accept a summary of the patient's participation and progress in therapy rather than specific treatment notes? Once he is clear on the extent of information that must be released to the court, he reviews it with his patients and documents their discussions in the chart. He asks them to sign the consent to release the agreed upon information despite the mandated nature of this dissemination. Such practice provides psychologists with an additional layer of protection against perceived breaches of confidentiality and offers patients a sense of autonomy and control over their PHI.

Ethically protecting patients' confidentiality is sometimes challenged by institutional policies on PHI disclosures. While all hospitals in the United States must conform to the Health Insurance Portability and Accountability Act of 1996 standards (HIPAA, 1996) that in part establishes policies and procedures for maintaining the privacy and security of PHI, the manner in which psychiatric hospitals apply these standards to actual practice can vary. Psychologists may not have control over the release of psychological reports, risk assessments, or psychotherapy notes. Hospital policy may direct nursing or social work staff to have patients sign a general authorization that permits the hospital to share all information contained in their medical record with any agency/provider that has a role in their ongoing treatment or supervision. These could include case management services, partial care programs, residential facilities, substance abuse programs, probation, the legal system, private practitioners, medical facilities, specialists, and insurance companies. When such broad access is authorized, we may not know or fully understand how psychological records will be used and if such use is for the intended purpose(s).

In order to prevent the unnecessary release or misuse of our work, psychologists need to be proactive. If the unit's social worker is responsible for executing patients' authorizations to release PHI, then I meet with this person as soon as possible upon assignment to the unit. I make sure to understand the actual process of how psychological information contained in my patients' charts physically moves from that chart to the receiving entities. I ask to be notified when PHI is requested so that I can evaluate the appropriateness of the request and clarify any misunderstandings immediately with the receiving agency. If I believe the release of specific psychological records could be harmful to my patients, I have the ability to intervene and perhaps provide documentation that more appropriately addresses the potential clinical/legal issue(s) in question in order to protect my patients' rights. Awareness of this process also gives me an opportunity to discuss the release of psychological information with my patients and address any questions or concerns that they may have because of these disclosures.

One experienced psychologist obtains her own authorization from patients whenever psychological information is requested by an outside entity in order to exercise some control over its dissemination and to maintain an accurate record of locations where it has been released. Patients have a legal right under HIPAA to an accounting of all release of records. She supports the ethical management of her patients' PHI by taking this extra step. Despite her best efforts, unintended releases of PHI can and do occur. On several occasions, this psychologist found her assessments and other medical records in a centrally located copier accessible to any staff member of the institution as well as individuals from outside agencies. Apparently, clinicians from community programs were on site reviewing charts and copying materials without notifying team members.

The psychologist who encountered this violation of confidentiality immediately informed her treatment team of the incident and sent an email to her director with copies going to higher-level administration to make them aware of the incident. To the extent possible, she also attempted to manage any potential harm that could have resulted from such disclosures including helping patients to understand and process feelings they had regarding the breach. When the mistaken release involves psychological records, she immediately contacts the recipient(s) of the materials and requests that they are destroyed. As always, she carefully documents her attempts to address the problem in the patient's chart along with progress made or any barriers encountered.

Ethical Issues for Administrators

Psychology directors are usually the first line of hospital administration that are called on to assist and support unit psychologists in resolving ethical dilemmas encountered in the inpatient mental health treatment setting. Staff present myriad ethical concerns related to their work to administrators of psychology with the expectation that action will be taken, and problems resolved in a manner consistent with the ethics code. This might not always be the case since department heads are limited in their recourse to ethical issues by the same administrative policies and laws that affect psychological service provision as a whole. What are some strategies that seasoned directors of psychology have found helpful in addressing ethical dilemmas that occur in systems where practices may be entrenched and resistant to change? How does one increase the likelihood that such strategies will be perceived as helpful and engender a spirit of cooperation with governing bodies?

An experienced director of psychology with 25 years of service in state psychiatric hospitals suggested that having knowledge of the institution's by-laws is crucial to understanding the scope of psychologists' practice and where the profession fits within the organizational structure.

> I have worked in institutions where psychology was not recognized as an autonomous discipline, and therefore psychologists were unable to make independent treatment decisions for their patients. The differences in ethical standards among professions were at times in conflict and thus made it more difficult to resolve disagreements in ways that satisfied everyone's ethical responsibilities.

This director found that involving department members in hospital-wide committees gave psychologists opportunities to get to know administrators on a more personal level so that they were not just names and titles to one another. In addition, psychologists were able to educate administrators about ethical psychological practices and include such standards when developing policies and procedures governing clinical work.

A retired director of psychology with over 30 years of inpatient psychiatric experience was involved in many committees that developed hospital-wide policies and procedures. He said that whenever he had the opportunity, he would volunteer to draft policies that influenced psychological services in order to define the psychologist's role in ways that were consistent with professional and ethical practice. He maintained that if psychologists did not take the initiative to define their job responsibilities and policies affecting ethical practice, then someone without their knowledge and expertise would define it for them. This psychologist said that hospital managers would rarely challenge him on his policies because he always had data available to support his position and a pragmatic and accommodating way of delivering the information.

Conclusion

Practicing clinical psychology in the inpatient mental health setting is a rewarding experience for many psychologists despite the ongoing challenges they face to providing ethical patient care. Many of the ethical issues that arise for psychologists in these settings overlap with professional issues; the two are frequently inseparable. These issues are rooted in our professional and personal values, formal ethical guidelines, and our clinical training. The origin of many of the ethical and professional dilemmas psychologists encounter while performing inpatient work involves their experiences of being pulled in multiple directions as they attempt to balance their roles as employees of the hospital and professional members of the larger mental health system while making known their commitment to their patients and good, ethical treatment.

It can be overwhelming for psychologists at any stage in their career to successfully address the multitude of ethical dilemmas commonly encountered in inpatient mental health settings. There will always be obstacles to providing ethical treatment; however, while unethical practices continue to occur, sensitivity to such issues is growing, largely through the efforts of psychologists and other clinicians charged with providing professional and ethical services within these facilities. The ability of psychologists to openly discuss ethical issues and participate in scholarly work also increases awareness and helps to sustain attention to the matter and ongoing dialog. Institutions are responding appropriately to these concerns by formally addressing ethical standards of care through changes in policies and procedures. A retired administrator of psychology with many decades of state service believes that ethical practice is the goal of every setting and begins with psychologists taking responsibility for their own ethical conduct. "I always tried to advocate and influence my peers and colleagues to act in accordance with good, ethical treatment. I worked to establish a collaborative experience with everyone toward the provision of best care." His philosophy resonates with many psychologists engaged in inpatient mental health treatment who continually strive to find innovative and creative ways to work cooperatively with their institutions to uphold and model ethical standards in their practice.

References

American Psychological Association. (2012a). Guidelines for psychological practice in health care delivery systems. *American Psychologist*, 68(1), 1–6.

American Psychological Association. (2012b). Specialty guidelines for forensic psychology. *American Psychologist*, 68(1), 7–19.

American Psychological Association. (2017). *Ethical principles of psychologists and code of conduct*. Retrieved from: https://apa.org/ethics/code/ethics-code-2017.pdf.

Health Insurance Portability and Accountability Act of 1996 (HIPAA). Pub. L. No. 104–191, 110 Stat. 1936 (1996).

5 The Benefit of Behavior Support Plans in Psychiatric Inpatient Settings

Jimmy I. Kim and Peter J. D'Amico

Psychologists by training are well suited for the provision of behavioral consultation in interdisciplinary inpatient psychiatry teams (APA, 2013). As a professional discipline, psychology has accepted the mantle of behavioral assessment, planning, and intervention in all settings where there is a need for such services. Psychology is most often the "holder" or "bearer" of the technology, and so the psychologist often has a central role in providing formal and informal consultation about facilitating positive behavioral supports in clinical settings.

Most research on behavioral consultation has been on school systems with an emphasis on individuals with developmental disabilities, with less attention given to inpatient psychiatric settings (Moravecek, 2015). However, behavioral consultation is well suited, and one could even argue that it is especially necessary today for inpatient psychiatric settings, given the shorter stays, which require a quick study of the patients. Patients also now often present with higher levels of distress and disturbances in behavior. Bernstein and Saladino (2007) discuss positive psychotic symptoms as common triggers for aggression risk on inpatient units including hostility, persecutory delusion, hallucinatory behavior, grandiosity, and excitement. Sailas, Keski-Valkama, and Wahlbeck (2008) propose careful functional analysis to individually identify the purpose of behavior in an effort to modify the stimuli and consequences associated with escalations in incidents of aggressive behavior. The model of behavioral consultation offers important stages of problem behavior identification, behavioral plan construction, and implementation and intervention evaluation (Kratochwill & Bergan, 1990). The model facilitates behavior change by emphasizing the "discovery" of objective detailed knowledge about the patient's problem behavior (i.e., a functional assessment), and engaging others in problem-solving strategies to facilitate a more adaptive approach for the patient to secure their needs. Both patient and staff behaviors are thereby targeted by the consultation process which when effective leads to positive behavioral changes in the patient and staff. The emphasis on viewing other disciplines as equal partners in this process is helpful in all stages including identification of problem behaviors, data gathering, writing of behavior plans, implementing the behavior plans and, finally, assessing the success of the behavior plans. The trick is to establish an effective working model of behavioral consultation that meets the quickened pace of the modern inpatient psychiatric unit while preserving treatment integrity (Sanetti & Kratochwill, 2008).

Working on an acute inpatient psychiatric service is not for the faint of heart. It is difficult, time intensive, at times chaotic and emotionally intensive with (seemingly) little tangible rewards. There is also the real possibility of physical danger to patients and staff. The fast pace of the unit, rapid admission and discharge of patients, staff turnovers as well as staff that is under increasing pressure to "do-more-with-less" creates a crisis mode environment that is a direct challenge to best clinical care. Time to get to know the patient in an empathic manner and to create a therapeutic alliance is almost antithetical to this fast-paced setting. Time is a phenomenon that is much desired but often in rare commodity. Yet, we deal with people who come to us at what could quite conceivably be the worst moment of their lives. Those who walk through our doors are often unable to tend to their most basic hygiene needs, are unable to sleep for days on end, or have become so tormented by the torrent of delusions and hallucinations that they will do almost anything to stop them, including ending their own lives. That is the bad news. However, the task of the inpatient staff is not to find "the cure" or "the magic pill"; it is about finding a way to stabilize and help the patient get back up on their feet as quickly as possible. Even this very practical short-term goal is not an easy task given the brief inpatient stays.

Here is the good news. There may be no better time to truly make a lasting impact or at the very least set an optimistic or positive tone for all future interventions for the patients. During those moments of desperation and hopelessness, we can do truly great work. Nurses greet the patients that come through the unit's doors for the umpteenth time and comfort them like a long-lost relative who has had a bad stretch of luck. mental health workers (MHWs) literally help patients back onto their feet and whisper words of encouragement during those dark hours. Attending psychiatrists and nurse practitioners listen to the stories that patients share while working hard to find the best medication with the optimal dosage. Psychiatric rehabilitation therapists teach adaptive coping skills and relapse prevention so that patients have a fighting chance once they are back on their feet. Social workers work tirelessly to find discharge resources so that the patient can continue to make progress in their treatments in an outpatient setting and have a more successful transition to the real world.

And then, there are the psychologists who will listen, validate, challenge, and encourage patients in their own treatment. Psychologists who will observe and record behavior, and gather and weave together all the information to make sense of all the pieces in the puzzle that is the patient. The psychologist who will use translation of behavior as a tool to communicate with the patient, family, and team, and facilitate change. In this chapter, we will be talking about our challenges and successes and our pursuit to do even better.

The challenges are many. During one psychology group session about mental illness psychoeducation, one of the patients blurted out, "I just wish I had a broken arm instead." When asked to explain, it made more sense. What happens when you break your arm? In this simpler world, you go to the emergency room, get an x-ray, have your arm placed in a cast, four to six weeks later get the cast removed, and then receive physical therapy if necessary. The arm, once healed, does not need anything more. When we are physically ill, we take medicine until we feel better. Once we feel better, we can stop taking medications. Treatment of mental illness follows a very different model. For some patients, medications become a lifelong constant. Stopping prescribed psychotropics can lead to relapse or worse. For many patients, medications, while necessary, are not sufficient to correct the problem. Behaviors need to change. Skills need to be learned. Environmental supports need to be identified. Learning and maintaining healthy behaviors can often be a lifelong endeavor.

In the New York metro area, a particular challenge is a patient who is visiting or has recently moved to the area, speaks little English, and/or has no available support system in close proximity. The prospect of making any progress in treatment is daunting, to say the least. However, we here at the Zucker Hillside Hospital are very fortunate indeed in this respect. Our hospital is located on the eastern edge of Queens County, which is considered to be one of the most multiculturally diverse areas in the United States. The chances of finding a staff member that speaks the particular dialect from one of the Caribbean islands or knows someone who knows someone from a particular neighborhood is actually quite high. Thus, our staff often becomes the first real resource for the patient. You do not need to imagine the look of relief when you see a patient who is able to converse with someone from the same island that they are from. Or the mute patient who is able to verbalize his first words after being hospitalized for multiple weeks – his yearning for a particular food from his native country – and to have it satisfied when a staff member brings the very food back to the unit after buying it during their break using their own money. There are many challenges on the inpatient service; however, staff often rise to the occasion.

The ERASE Model as a Behavior Support Plan

Staff on the acute care adult inpatient service will usually approach and ask the psychologist to "please make that patient stop doing *x behavior*." This can be a sign that the staff are struggling with setting limits on the problematic behavior (Lowe, Wellman, & Taylor, 2003). The very manner in which the statement is posed highlights a human tendency to focus on reducing negative behavior as a direct goal and immediate need. It is our observation that this tendency to inhibit or punish the problem behavior can derail the efforts to understand the behavior and find adaptive replacement behaviors. This tendency is especially likely in cases of patient aggression risk. This is often the context in which the behavioral consultation takes place, and the psychologist must have a model that offers a firm grounding in positive behavioral supports with accompanying tools that are effective and easy to use. Our experience with one such model based on sound functional assessment is adapted from the work of Terrance M. Scott, Ph.D., of the University of Louisville. The ERASE model (Scott, 2003) has been instrumental in assisting our patients in learning how to utilize adaptive coping skills in a secure setting. We adopted this model as part of a strategic aggression reduction initiative in our inpatient psychiatric hospital, which includes both adolescent and adult patients across 10 programs. The goal was to offer a standardized, user-friendly tool around which our psychologists could consult and train staff in positive behavioral practices. The implementation of ERASE provided both concrete written plans for tough patient situations, as well as a mechanism for staff education and gradual culture change. In our efforts (D'Amico, Kim, & Kumar, 2016), we found that behavioral consultation on the inpatient unit, involving implementation of the ERASE model, led to reduced scores on a measure of patient aggression risk (DASA, Ogloff & Daffern, 2004). Observations indicated these perceptible changes in aggression risk led to reduced staff anxiety and fear (which result in defensive displays) with concomitant increases in proactive/confident approaches by staff toward the patient.

The first step of the ERASE model is to (E)xplain or specify the behavior that you wish to change. The challenge here is to define the behavior in a way that it can be recorded reliably. For example, we are often told by staff that the patient is "agitated." We will ask the question – what does the patient's "agitation" look like? Once we can describe or define the behavior objectively, we can quantify the behavior by measuring the intensity and frequency of the behavior. We can also note details of this behavior (e.g., What time did it occur? What happened before?). An important aspect of this detective work is to identify possible triggers or something that has the potential to set off a series of events. Can the environment be modified to avoid the triggers? What are some of the early warning signs in the patient's behavior (e.g., clenching teeth, shortness of breath, etc.) that serve as a cue or signal that the behavior is about to present itself?

The second step in the ERASE model, (R)eason is seeking why this behavior works for the patient. Why does the patient exhibit this particular problem behavior? Because it works! Even though it probably works badly. So we need to ask what function does this behavior serve? There are usually only a few reasons why one engages in these behaviors. Usually, it is to gain attention from others, avoid demands, escape from situations, obtain an object or a privilege, or self-stimulation. Finding the motivation and reason why someone engages in the problem behavior is critical in developing an individualized plan that can meet the need and thereby truly help the patient.

To meet the need, the next challenge in the ERASE model is identifying the (A)ppropriate replacement behavior that is more adaptive for the patient to perform instead of the problem behavior. We will often use the example of nicotine replacement therapy (NRT) when teaching staff and patients about this stage. Quitting smoking is difficult enough but doing so "cold turkey" (without any aids) makes the experience quite unpleasant and often too difficult. NRTs will help address the physical cravings of nicotine, while therapy and counseling helps to address the behavioral components that are often paired with smoking (i.e., smoking with the morning coffee, smoking while driving, etc.). The behavior plan aims to substitute adaptive coping mechanisms to replace the maladaptive ones. Everyone works better when there is a safety net.

When identifying the appropriate replacement behavior, it is important to ask if the patient is capable of performing the behavior. For example, if we ask a patient to maintain the identified appropriate replacement behavior for 24 hours and they are unable to do so, we can reduce the time required to ensure success. If 24 hours does not work, we ask for 12 hours. Often, it is better to start in smaller steps – start with an hour or two – particularly if the appropriate replacement behavior is new or difficult. Once the patient is able to maintain the appropriate replacement behavior for the time requirement, we raise the bar by incrementally increasing the time in order to gain the reward. Soon after, we can then change the positive reinforcement schedule from a Fixed Interval (i.e., receiving a reward every time at the chosen time interval) to a Variable Ratio Interval (i.e., receiving a reward at changing time intervals). This becomes an important component of the behavior plan because the Variable Ratio Interval resembles "real life." As much as we would like it to happen, we are often not rewarded for every good deed we do. Over time, we become content with secondary gains (i.e., feeling good when helping others, the joy of seeing someone else benefit from our deed, etc.) so that it becomes the reward itself. The Variable Ratio Interval prepares us and our patients for the real world at large.

The next question in applying the ERASE model is how we can best (S)upport the desired behavior? What positive reinforcers can we offer to make the behavior occur more often? In other words, we try to find the "carrot" – the "something" that motivates the patient to execute the behavior we are asking of them. This is no easy task. As noted earlier, patients who are admitted to our acute care service often come to us during the most distressing periods of their lives. Whether it be during a psychotic break because they did not take medications or the loss of a loved one, patients arrive at our doorstep, often unwillingly. It is during this time that we have to ask them to stop a problem behavior that has "worked for them." It is for this reason that an encouraging word, a kind expression, a compassionate action without any expectation for return can be powerful. We remind our staff that in doing so, we are planting seeds with the patients we work with even though we often never see the fruit grow. However, by planting the seed, we give our patient the chance to approach the same situation with a fresh and more adaptive perspective as well as new skills and new behaviors. By finding what motivates the patient to try the appropriate replacement behavior, we improve their odds for success and change the trajectory for the patient when they are discharged.

The following is one account of our work. "Joshua" was a 26-year-old morbidly obese patient with moderate intellectual disability who was hospitalized due to aggression toward the staff at his residence. The team asked us to consult on Joshua's tendency to take his pants off in public spaces on the unit. When observing Joshua, we saw him playing games appropriately in his room and then become bored and move into the open area of the community room. Once there, he hooked his thumbs on the waistband of his sweatpants, and in slow motion, pulled down his pants. The women on the unit screamed, and the staff ran toward him trying to cover him up. What was Joshua doing? He had a big grin from ear to ear, and he seemed to enjoy the overwhelming attention he was receiving for his behavior. Joshua clearly wanted attention. Attention was the identified "carrot." We consulted with the staff and recommended that a male staff respond in these situations by giving Joshua a curt response and covering him up quickly without fanfare. At the same time, Joshua was given positive attention when he engaged in the most appropriate replacement behavior (i.e., "keeping his pants on") or other general positive behaviors such as brushing his teeth, playing with toys, or joining groups. The behavior plan was highly successful as Joshua responded to the praise he received from the staff, and he was able to eliminate the problem behavior and maintain the appropriate replacement behaviors. He was discharged soon thereafter to a residential program because he was able to follow the structured programming of the unit; he was also able to keep his pants on in public areas.

The final step in the ERASE model is to ask how we (E)valuate this newly created behavior plan? Does it work? When consistently applied and religiously followed – yes, it does. Does it happen immediately? No, it does not – but it will. There is a "buy in" which is critical, and this "buy in" needs to take place with all staff on all shifts. This "buy in" can be accomplished if staff help to formulate the behavior plan. Once the plan starts to take off, the staff realizes that their input has helped the patient make progress in their treatment and, fortuitously, make the unit an easier and safer place to work. All it takes is one; one person who is willing to try what you are proposing. One staff member who is willing to try anything else because everything else to date has failed. Put simply, when the staff does not "buy in," the plan fails. From a behavioral perspective, the staff is not being reinforced for their efforts. At every level, reinforcement principles are operating. However, when a behavior plan is put into motion that is targeted, concrete, and simple to follow, success becomes tangible. Considering the truly dangerous nature of the work, we remain ever vigilant about contributing to a culture of staff recognition and praise for the daily courage that we witness.

Implementing ERASE on the Inpatient Unit

So how and when is the ERASE model implemented? When patients are first admitted to our hospital, the nursing staff will ask a series of questions to ascertain if there is a risk or history of aggression – this is part of our inpatient individual safety plan. The rationale for gathering this kind of information is akin to preparing a "Go Bag" (a bag of items that include a first aid kit, supplies, etc. to take with you "on-the-go") in the event of an emergency *before* the crisis occurs. Dean, Duke, George, and Scott (2007), discuss the importance of collecting information from patients and families upon admission concerning triggers for aggression and methods used at home to manage challenging behaviors. Removal of potential or known triggers is an important factor to consider in managing behavior (Bisconer, Green, Mallon-Czajka, & Johnson, 2006). By assessing for triggers early on in one of the first interactions with the patient, the team is setting the tone and opening the discussion about behaviors that can play a major role in their treatment and during their stay. Safety of the team is also enhanced because information about possible triggers and warning signs are available from the patients themselves. Some of the relevant questions are:

- Triggers associated with feeling upset, frustrated, angry.
- Early warning signs: what behaviors does a patient identify engaging in when feeling upset, frustrated, or angry?
- Strategies identified that help patients feel calm, safe, and in control.
- Strategies identified to regain control after an incident of aggression.
- If PRN medication is required, preferred route of medication (oral or intramuscular).

The inpatient individual safety plan then becomes a tremendous resource that helps us to begin formulating our behavior plan, especially for helping to find (A)ppropriate replacement behaviors and finding the best way to (S)upport the desired behaviors.

Our inpatient psychiatric unit typically has a census of 30 patients served by three teams (Red, Green, or Blue). Each team consisting of an attending psychiatrist (or psychiatric nurse practitioner), team nurse, psychologist, and social worker is responsible for about 10 patients. The team nurse is responsible for administering the prescribed medications as well as tracking and informing the team about the progress of the patients in their care. The team nurse often provides invaluable input in the development of the behavior plan, but it is the feedback of the staff at the front line that is critical in the early stages.

The mental health workers (also known as patient care associates or mental health therapy aides, depending on the psychiatric/institutional setting) are part of the nursing department staff who work most closely with the patients during their time on the inpatient units. MHWs will often check vital signs, administer finger sticks, and assist patients in completing their activities of daily living scale (ADLs), as well as many other routine tasks that help us track the progress of the patient. MHWs are the eyes and ears on the unit as they inform the rest of the treatment team if the patient is eating, sleeping, interacting with others, and whether engaging in adaptive or maladaptive behaviors. The MHW is invaluable in telling us the day-to-day movements of any of our 30+ individual patients on the unit down to the smallest details. Given the MHW's role, we will often first approach them and preface by saying, "this is the genius behavior plan that we have written for this patient – tell us how it's not going to work." And they will tell us (often with more brutal honesty than we were looking for). They will tell us about the lunch being served at the time the intervention is to be delivered, the staff's shift change that we did not anticipate, or the sleep schedule of this particular patient that the behavior plan did not consider.

We informally refer to patient engagement specialists (PES) as "super MHWs." They are staff who have demonstrated an uncanny ability to engage in verbal dialog with our most difficult patients. We modeled the PES after meeting with the inpatient team at Bellevue Hospital Center's behavior health associates (BHAs) in New York City, who were kind enough to spend several hours explaining their role and the many benefits to the inpatient units. The PES are paired together and float onto each of the inpatient units of the hospital, touching base proactively with those patients who were noted by the staff as being at risk for aggression. Our PES are paged the moment a patient is noted to be in distress, wherever they might be in the hospital. The success of the PES in becoming the liaison between the unit treatment team and the patient comes from their time and talk with the patient; the more time the PES have to talk with the patient, the greater their success. As key players, the PES are involved in developing the behavior plan, and they help the patient learn and follow the behavior plan.

Another key player on the treatment team comes from an unexpected resource: Housekeeping. Our housekeeper knows every single inch of our unit. More important, he is also able to tell us which patients do not come out of their rooms or even get up out of bed. He lets us know who hoards their food and those who have a difficult time attending to their ADLs. With our ever-present-and-observant housekeeper, he is able to bring to our attention the needs of the quiet patients who do not stir up trouble on the unit.

Our unit is also staffed by psychology trainees. We are invested in the training of our trainees, nicknaming them the "baby birds" of the hospital. During orientation, we often instruct the trainees to "bow to the milieu" and "plug themselves in" each time they enter the milieu, making them accountable. The trainee cannot come onto the unit, ignore the staff, meet with their patient for "island therapy" and then leave without informing staff of what happened during the session. The trainee is called upon to engage with the treatment team – to inform the staff of what transpired during the session (e.g., something new they learned about the patient) in an effort to assist the team in going forward in the care of the patient. The role of the trainee is to help maintain the treatment flow on the unit. By doing so, the trainee becomes one of the team.

ERASE as a Communication Tool

There are also some practical considerations. The behavior plan must be written in the simplest terms. It is important to convey clarity and conciseness. As such, the length of our behavior plans is typically one page. Any longer and it becomes impractical as a tool for the staff. Going further, we underline the "best parts," which are the most important and helpful parts of the plan that all team members must know and understand. The behavior plan becomes a guide, a resource to refer to when there are questions in dealing with the patient. It is not a one size fits all or a cookie cutter template, nor is it a static or one-time event. Instead, the behavior plan is a living, dynamic tool that needs to be reassessed, modified, and sculpted during the entire length of the individual patient's stay so that it becomes a best fit for that patient for that period. After writing more than several hundred ERASE behavior plans, it is still true that no plan is the same. Each behavior plan is individually tailored for each patient. Even for the same patient with multiple hospitalizations, the behavior plans often differ for each hospitalization. The final hope for a well-written behavior plan is that it should generalize to the outside world so that the patient is best prepared for his/her imminent discharge.

After incorporating the feedback from key team members, the psychologist now asks one or more staff to join in engaging the patient in a discussion about the behavior plan. When patients are able – cognitively and psychologically – we verbally go over the reason for the behavior plan and explain its finer points. Yes, there are times when the patient becomes upset, crumples the behavior plan, and throws it into the garbage can. It is our job to allow them some cool off time and find ways to re-engage at a later point. It is important for the patient to feel a sense of inclusion and better yet an ownership of the behavior plan. It is also important to convey the message to the patient that the team is working together to help him/her make progress in treatment. "The team is here to help you when there are difficulties." "The Team is prepared to help you make progress in your treatment." "The team ..." You get the idea.

We find that one of the many roles of the psychologist on the inpatient service is lending a voice to positive behavioral supports and making themselves heard in the multidisciplinary team (MDT). However, it is also important to not have an "ego" about it. There have been many times when we have made recommendations to the treatment team only to have our concerns not heeded (and yes, in honesty, we have had many "I-Told-You-So" moments too). It is important to state that your role is to make the best recommendation at the time – and understand there may not be team consensus for many reasons (i.e., length of stay issues, restrictions in the patient's insurance, etc.). It is not personal, so do not take it that way – it just *feels* that way.

This might also be a good time to note the type of authority a psychologist has on the inpatient service. In 1959, the social psychologists John French and Bertram Raven determined that there were five forms of power in leadership authority. These include reward, coercive, legitimate, referent, and expert (French & Raven, 1959). The psychologists on the units are often referent and expert authority figures. If we are doing our job correctly, staff have observed what we have done in the past, and we have earned their trust and respect. They value our expertise, skill, and experience in understanding difficult patient behaviors in acute situations. They look to us to be objective, fair, and at times creative in coming up with solutions to benefit the patient and maintain the safety and harmony on the unit.

In addition to the use of ERASE as a communication tool, our health system has adopted team STEPPS (Strategies and Tools to Enhance Performance and Patient Safety), a program designed to facilitate communication and teamwork skills among health professionals. In this model, the treatment team meets twice a day during "briefs" when we review the patients on the unit with high aggression risk or display of some other noteworthy behavior. Usually, at 9:15am, we have our morning brief. This allows us to inform all the team members of possible challenges we may face that particular day but also sets the tone for the remainder of the shift.

This is usually followed up by our team meeting, when the three MDTs gather sequentially to discuss each patient's progress (or lack thereof) while planning for future interventions as well as discharge. We have our afternoon brief at 3:30pm, which allows us to review the progress of the day as well as inform the evening shift of any possible difficulties they might encounter in the hours ahead. Briefs are a crucial time to notify staff across all three shifts of the individualized behavior plan for each patient. It is also an opportunity to get real-time feedback about the utility of the behavior plans and suggestions for changes that would enhance success. Problems with specific patients are addressed during "huddles," which are special times carved out with specific treatment team members to address the particular patient and issue at hand.

Our standardized approach toward patients who are having a difficult time on the unit is verbal intervention first with a healthy respect of personal space. The power of an empathic stance and a kind word are often underestimated, but it can truly make a world of difference. Approaching with a sense of calm and serenity, while conveying respect and empathy in our nonverbal body language, can be a good starting point for many potentially volatile situations. When the patient is ready to speak with you, they will. We stand in anticipation for that moment; when it arrives, the first words we speak are ones that resonate with the patient – choose those words carefully. Never, ever cite a rule (or the patient's breaking of that rule) – as that will often end your conversation abruptly (and quite possibly, violently). Instead, in the gentlest of tones, try validating the patient's experience without condoning it. Whichever words you choose, convey that you stand in support of them (and not in judgment of them). The next obvious reference is the patient's specific behavior plan. The value of the behavior plan in anchoring the staff in a crisis when emotions can get out of hand cannot be overstated.

ERASE as a Teaching and Therapeutic Tool

Since the psychologist is intimately familiar with the behavior plan, he or she can also use the behavior plan as a teaching tool. Sometimes the immediate reaction of the staff when a patient does something wrong is to punish them – "take away their dessert," or "send them to their room." In the heat of the moment, the psychologist can provide a teaching moment not just for the patient. For example, the psychologist can stop a patient from taking an impulsive action by engaging directly with the patient thereby distracting both the patient and staff from an inevitable conflict. We can then help redirect the patient from the problem behavior, and engage in appropriate replacement behavior to meet their needs. By modeling implementation of the proposed behavior plan, staff can learn by example and carry it into their future interactions with the patient. The greatest success in implementing a behavior plan is having it applied consistently across staff and all shifts. The key to this success is constant vigilance about the target behaviors and consistency in applying the interventions the right way and at the right time; the process to achieve it is exhausting. All staff have to "buy in," and the staff at the front line need the most support because they have the most face-to-face contact with the patient and his or her difficult or unsafe behavior.

Spoiler alert/Please note: Behavior plans are not always written to address a patient's behaviors. More times than not, the behavior plan is actually written for the staff. It becomes a step-by-step guide to help staff in their engagement of a particularly difficult patient. Our staff here at the hospital are an incredible group of dedicated professionals who have spent their careers taking care of the severely emotionally and behaviorally disturbed population and do so with a compassion that is unparalleled. However, the staff are increasingly challenged in this reality of high psychiatric disturbance/short stays that we live in, and the chronic stress of this work can upend many good intentions.

It goes without saying that the behavior plan must be written in a manner that is tailored to a specific patient because ultimately it is an individualized therapeutic tool. We end this chapter by sharing a final anecdote. One of our psychologists entered a team meeting with a patient who, the night before, had punched his roommate for turning on the light. The team members were gently reprimanding the patient for injuring the roommate as the patient sat sullenly in his chair, avoiding any direct eye contact with the room full of people. The psychologist as the behavioral consultant, always thinking functional assessment, learned that the patient had arrived early in the morning, coming slowly down from a manic state and verbalized his request to get some sleep. As the patient tried to rest, his roommate, upon exiting the room, would turn on the lights. A verbal request by the patient to keep the light off was met with an apology by the roommate, and yet the roommate again turned the light on. Another verbal request was made; another apology was promptly made and again the light was turned on. When the roommate tried to exit and turn on the light the third time, patient clocked him right in the face.

In an effort to steer the team toward being good behavior detectives and not just the police, the psychologist attempted validation with humor with the hope of getting patient "buy in" for a plan to engage in nonviolent alternatives and still get his needs met. The psychologist shared with the team that he found it hard to understand why the patient didn't clock the roommate sooner. For the first time since the event, the patient made eye contact. The psychologist then noted that while the release of frustration and anger in the moment may have been highly rewarding, there were probably a few other steps that could have been taken prior to any physical solution; for example, telling staff or requesting a room change. Patient nodded his head but remained silent for the rest of the meeting. Later that day, loud noises were heard from the patient's room. The psychologist was the first staff member to approach the room as the door swung wildly open, the patient exiting with a part of the desk leg in hand wielding it like a major league baseball player. The loud noise was the patient breaking his wooden desk and removing one of its legs. As the patient was about to swing, the psychologist, with hands open in supplication, gently called the patient by name. The patient made eye contact with the psychologist for the second time that day, nodded his head, and dropped the desk leg to the floor as he walked away.

As fortune would have it, patient and psychologist would cross paths again 7 years later. When the psychologist approached the patient who was engaged in a conflict with yet another patient, the patient stated very clearly that he was not ready to speak with the psychologist. The patient, however, took the time to say that he respected this psychologist and remembered how he looked after the patient during his last stay. He also noted that he could have hurt the psychologist the last time but did not do so because of how the psychologist didn't "dis-(respect)" him. The patient asked for some space and then later approached the psychologist to speak about what had been bothering him, a beautiful two-step behavior plan. It is difficult to ignore the powerful impact of kindness and respect that resonates even years later. As behavioral consultants, psychologists should remember that positive behavioral supports are compatible with these values. Again, seeds planted and, once in a while, something good grows.

References

American Psychological Association (2013). Guidelines for psychological practice in health care delivery systems. *American Psychologist*, 68, 1–6.

Bernstein, K.S., & Saladino, J.P. (2007). Clinical assessment and management of psychiatric patients' violent and aggressive behaviors in a general hospital. *Medsurg Nursing*, 16(5), 301–332.

Bisconer, S.W., Green, M., Mallon-Czajka, J., & Johnson, J.S. (2006). Managing aggression in a psychiatric hospital using a behavior plan: A case study. *Journal of Psychiatric and Mental Health Nursing*, 13, 515–521.

D'Amico, P.J., Kim, J.I., & Kumar, A., (2016). Implementation of the E.R.A.S.E. Model of behavioral of consultation and aggression reduction in an inpatient psychiatric hospital. Poster presented at the annual convention of the Association of Behavioral and Cognitive Therapies, New York, NY.

Dean, A.J., Duke, S.G., George, M., & Scott, J. (2007). Behavioral management leads to reduction in aggression in a child and adolescent psychiatric inpatient unit. *Journal of the American Academy of Child and Adolescent Psychiatry*, 46, 6.

French Jr., J.R.P., & Raven, B. (1959). The bases of social power. In D. Cartwright (Ed.) *The studies in social power* (pp. 150–167). Ann Arbour, MI: University of Michigan.

Kratochwill, T.R., & Bergan, J.R. (1990). *Behavioral consultation in applied settings*. New York, NY: Plenum.

Lowe, T., Wellman, N., & Taylor, R. (2003). Limit-setting and decision-making in the management of aggression. *Journal of Advanced Nursing, 41*(2), 154–161.

Moravecek, M.J. (2015). Behavioral consultation within a psychiatric hospital setting. *The Behavior Therapist, 38*(8), 256–258.

Ogloff, J., & Daffern, M. (2004). *The dynamic appraisal of situational aggression: Inpatient version-adult*. Melbourne, Australia: Center for Forensic Behavioral Science, Monash University.

Sailas, E., Keski-Valkama, A., & Wahlbeck, K. (2008). Inpatient agitation and aggression. In F. Ovsiew & R.L. Munich (Eds.) *Principles of inpatient psychiatry* (pp. 221–233). Philadelphia, PA: Wolters Kluwer Health: Lippincott, Williams & Wilkins.

Sanetti, L.M.H., & Kratochwill, T.R. (2008). Treatment integrity in behavioral consultation: Measurement, promotion, and outcomes. *International Journal of Behavioral Consultation and Therapy*, 4, 95–114.

Scott, T.M. (2003). Preparing for an FBA meeting: What should I bring? *Positive Behavior Interventions and Supports Newsletter, 2*(3), retrieved from www.pbis.org/common/cms/files/Newsletter/Volume2%20Issue3.pdf

6 Three Dynamic Roles of the Clinical Psychologist on the Acute Closed Psychiatric Ward

Amit Fachler

Was there a shield or spear seen?

Judges 5:8

It was 8am and the psychiatric ward staff were about to begin their daily report meeting. Everyone had a printout list of current inpatients and Dr. Rachel, the ward's clinical psychologist, was surprised to see a patient she had discharged the previous day, still on the list. Had he been readmitted in the past 16 hours? "No," said Dr. Wolf, the ward's head and Dr. Rachel's boss. His name should definitely not be on the list of ongoing hospitalizations. "Perhaps', suggested Dr. Wolf, 'Dr. Rachel was too preoccupied yesterday to check her patient out on the computer.' 'No,' retorted Dr. Rachel, she definitely checked him out the moment he left the building – as the computer would clearly show. Maybe the ward secretary, Ms. Dahan, who was supposed to confirm the checkout, forgot to do so." After a few moments of tense silence, Dr. Wolf called the secretary to join the meeting. Ms. Dahan appears at the door. "How come Mr. Aniston is still on the current inpatient list?" asked Dr. Wolf. "Em," said Ms. Dahan, "whose patient was he?" "Mine," said Dr. Rachel angrily. "Oh," said Ms. Dahan, "the thing is ... well, I ... it's a mistake." "You see?" said Dr. Rachel to Dr. Wolf, and to everyone else in the room. "Yes, but ..." continued Ms. Dahan, "it's because I got it into my head that Dr. Rachel comes in early in the morning and logs on to my computer and tampers with the data." "WHAT?" asked a bewildered Dr. Rachel. "Forget it," said Ms. Dahan, "I know it sounds stupid." With a sheepish smile, she left the room. "Right," said Dr. Wolf, avoiding Dr. Rachel's furious gaze, "now that that's settled, let's get on with the report."

This episode, based on true events, may convey an aspect of the dynamics at work in a psychiatric ward: the potential for paranoid ideation among staff members, in this case directed at the ward's psychologist. The psychologist's role here is an implicit one: to serve as an object for paranoid projections. However, it is not a role she had chosen. In this chapter, I will address the psychologist's dynamic roles in the acute closed psychiatric ward and ways the psychologist may work with these constructively.

To paraphrase the old catchphrase, "What is a nice girl like you doing in a place like this?" What is the thinking behind having a clinical psychologist in an acute psychiatric ward (see Silver, 2014). Curiously, while this question may frequently be raised by members of the ward team, it is never asked by the patients. The patients crave having someone listen to them. The psychiatric residents are too busy giving physical checks, prescribing drugs, writing reports; the nurses' hands are full taking vital signs, giving medication, changing sheets, etc. The occupational therapists help the inpatients improve their various skills; the social worker is engrossed in devising and implementing rehabilitation plans. Often, the question might be raised, what is the clinical psychologist's contribution to this beehive? Is she not a disturbance, getting in the way of the other mental health professionals, whose functions on the closed ward are specific, clear, and purposeful?

The focus of this chapter is on the more implicit, unofficial roles of the clinical psychologist on the closed acute psychiatric ward, and as such, not necessarily recognized and acknowledged by other staff members. Each ward environment differs, and the underlying psychological issues and themes on specific wards vary. While it is not always the psychologist who plays all the roles described in this chapter, psychologists' training makes them more prepared than most other professionals to detect psychologically driven dynamics on the ward. Psychologists' training related to psychological phenomena and dynamics can help sensitize them to projections and other distortions when they occur on the ward. This can increase the likelihood of their awareness of these phenomena when they occur, and can help them to consciously respond in ways that are productive to staff and patients, rather than to fall into patterns of re-enactments or repetition of disturbed patterns of interactions among staff.

Dr. Rachel, the clinical psychologist in this ward, has a unique status among her co-workers: she is, in a phrase coined by Harry Stack Sullivan (1956), a *participant observer*. She is an *observer* inasmuch as she witnesses certain phenomena, occurrences, and interactions. Being psychodynamically minded, she is motivated to reflect on her observations. This, in turn, involves interpreting to herself what *actually* is going on around her, in terms of the interplay of the psychodynamic forces and their resultant manifestations. She is a *participant* inasmuch as she takes part in, affects the emotional atmosphere of, and is affected by, the daily chores of the ward staff. A similar concept that is relevant in this context is the ward psychologist's role as *observing ego*. Coined by Richard Sterba (1938), the observing ego is that function of the personality which maintains perspective on the ebbs and flows of one's experience, as opposed to the *experiencing ego*, which is taking a full part in the action. Thus, if the ward is akin to a collective personality, it is the psychologist's function to keep an eye on what is going on, in order to facilitate awareness and insight among the ward members.

In this chapter, I focus on three roles of the (psychodynamically-informed) clinical psychologist as a staff member on an acute closed psychiatric ward, that stem from her functioning as the ward's "observing ego":

1. Psychodynamic interpreter of patients' and family members' communications.
2. Organizational consultant.
3. Regulator of the ward's social climate.

In my experience, some key aspects of this triple role remain unnoticed by staff members and the clinical psychologist alike, because of the hectic atmosphere in the department, and the psychologist's function as case-manager, busy running the day-to-day chores of inpatient care.

Psychodynamic Interpreter

Understanding Inpatients' Communications

We live in times of medically-informed psychiatry. In an acute closed ward, this means that the doctors seek rapid diagnoses in order to quickly prescribe psychotropic drugs. The standard psychiatric interview: the "Structured clinical interview for the diagnostic and statistical manual" (SCID), is based on closed-ended questions revolving around overt symptoms. Much relevant information can be lost when this is the dominant approach for obtaining knowledge, with the patient becoming an amalgam of symptoms with a "neat" psychiatric label (see Williams, 2010).

Psychodynamically-informed therapists like the British clinical head of nursing, Marcus Evans, offer a contrasting approach. Evans argued that

> the diagnosis and active interventions employed by psychiatry need to be accompanied by a receptive psychological approach to treatment and care. Mental health professionals need to be interested in the *meaning* of their patient's symptoms together with verbal and physical communications, which convey important information about the patient's *internal world* and *underlying conflicts*.
>
> (Evans, 2016, italics added)

The search for covert meanings and hidden communications cannot be taken for granted in a concrete-thinking milieu. Ronald Laing is one of the pioneers in applying psychodynamic listening to psychotic inpatients' discourse. In an oft-quoted vignette, Laing demonstrated how the fragmented monologue of a psychotic patient, interviewed in public by Emil Kraepelin and diagnosed as showing "'signs' of catatonic excitement" (Laing, 1960, p. 30), actually made sense in light of the immediate and exposed situation in which the patient found himself.

The patient wants to be heard. It is the ward psychologist's professional responsibility to use her expertise to help give voice to the patient's feelings and implicit preoccupations, in order to understand his behavior more fully and engage with him more effectively. For example, an inpatient diagnosed with bipolar disorder was admitted to the ward due to delusions of grandeur, including a belief he could talk to God. When Dr. Wolf, the chief psychiatrist, asked the patient, "Can you speak to God now?" the patient replied "Yes." "Who is God?" asked Dr. Wolf. "You are," answered the patient. Metaphorically speaking, the patient is correct: within the confines of the ward, the chief psychiatrist is the one who controls the freedom of the ward's residents.

In another example, Dr. Rachel heard an inpatient telling the resident during the grand round that he liked to watch TV. Dr. Rachel inquired about his favorite programs. When he answered that he enjoyed the National Geographic Channel, she encouraged him to say more. He replied that he was intrigued by a special about rhinos, and was also interested in the special about anteaters. By this stage, Dr. Rachel had achieved two goals: she enhanced genuine interest in the patient as a person, and she constructed a hypothesis about the patient's preoccupation with his sexual functioning. Dr. Rachel saw the horn of the rhino and the nose of the anteater as graphically representing the male organ. During the weekly staff meeting, Dr. Wolf expressed his reaction to Dr. Rachel's thoughts on this matter: "You psychologists – always thinking sex, sex, sex." This should not deter Dr. Rachel from maintaining her hypothesis, especially as the patient's case manager later reported that the patient was worried that his medication was making him impotent.

> Reuben, a 20-year-old soldier, was admitted due to repeated suicide threats. During the initial intake, it emerged that he threatened to kill himself with his rifle every time a quarrel broke out among his fellow soldiers. Dr. Rachel listened silently while the patient answered the SCID interview questions. When the interviewer invited other staff members to ask further questions, Dr. Rachel said quietly, "Hello Reuben, my name is Dr. Rachel, and I am the ward psychologist. Tell me please, do your parents live together?" "No," came the answer, "they divorced when I was

> 14." "And before they separated," continued Dr. Rachel, "did they use to quarrel?" "Oh, all the time!" said Reuben, "it was a living hell. Thank God they broke up." "Thank you," said Dr. Rachel. When the staff met later to discuss Reuben's case, Dr. Rachel said she was convinced that Reuben had fantasies that unless he killed himself, his parents might kill one another quarreling. That is why he cannot bear witnessing loud conflicts between people surrounding him.

This, again, was a mere hypothesis on Dr. Rachel's part, a psychodynamic formulation. But it was a hypothesis that broadened the team's picture of Reuben's mind. It held a piece of potentially valuable insight about what made this particular patient, this particular person, tick. Reuben's case is an example of how the ward clinical psychologist pays attention to life's adversities in the inpatient's story. Following Searles' seminal paper, "Schizophrenia and the inevitability of death" (Searles, 1961), it is wise to consider the impact of death, loss, grief, separation, abandonment, and other traumatic events, as triggers for the patient's current crisis. As Ann-Louise Silver (2014) has shown, if the patient himself does not mention such events, it might be fruitful to ask him directly about his thoughts around death. Either way, Dr. Rachel is alert to the possibility of delayed reactions triggered by similar situations (e.g., two soldiers fighting/two parents quarreling). Thus, the psychologist functions in a way that enhances the patient's subjectivity; this, in turn, enables the latter to regain some of his dignity and sense of agency – both rare commodities for a patient confined, wearing pajamas, to a closed acute ward.

Meeting the Parents: Understanding Inpatients' Family Members' Communications

> Marty, a 24-year-old student, was hospitalized under compulsory admission. This followed a psychotic breakdown during which he stopped sleeping, called the police to report he had been abducted by two imposters who pretended to be his parents, talked obscenely to his father, and later threatened to kill him. After a brief interview in the psychiatric ER, Marty's parents came into the department and asked to meet with the head of the ward. Dr. Wolf was not available. Marty's case manager was dealing with an emergency in another department. Carmen, the head nurse, greeted Marty's parents and offered to meet them herself until Dr. Wolf was available. To tell the truth, Carmen said later in the staff meeting that she felt overwhelmed by Marty's parents' questions: What is his diagnosis? How can we set limits to his behavior? How often should we come to visit

during hospitalization? Should we tell extended family members and friends about his shameful condition? Should we withhold from Marty information regarding his sister's engagement? Who will take care of him after we're gone? How can we get him to cooperate with the treatment plan? As she was describing this interaction to her co-workers, Carmen gave an exasperated sigh. "It's the same questions every time. The mother keeps fidgeting; the father seems to be on the brink of a nervous breakdown himself. How come I end up feeling guilty for their son's condition?"

It is my belief that the psychodynamically-informed clinical psychologist's expertise in such situations is invaluable. Society in general, and mental health professionals in particular, tend to focus on the explicit complaints of service users. In so doing, they fail to address messages conveyed in the subtext. Like the pilot in St. Exupery's book *The Little Prince* (1943), we automatically draw a concrete sheep instead of focusing on creating a proper box for containing the stressful emotions that arise in the present moment. The wish to know Marty's specific diagnosis (the "sheep") actually masks the parents' horror. The parents' plea for a diagnosis of a non-chronic mental state and their question regarding limit-setting (another "sheep"), camouflages other things: It could be parental guilt over their handling of Marty's behavior ever since he was a small child. Marty's parent's ultimate question, "the $64,000 question" as his mom called it, i.e., how to get Marty to cooperate, might hide strong ambivalence in the parents' ability to accept his mental illness.

Dr. Rachel's task in this context is to recognize these underlying themes and to contain (create "a box") the intense emotions attached to them. Returning to Carmen's account of her conversation with Marty's parents, the psychologist should recognize and address the head nurse's difficulties in containing the parents' plight. And what of Dr. Wolf? Parents kept asking to meet him. He seldom seemed to find the time for them, because the work in the ward was so intense and time-consuming. Psychiatrists on a closed ward work under the most demanding conditions: the ward is under-staffed; the missions are challenging and draining; it is only natural that the head psychiatrist is experienced by inpatients' family members as unavailable. Dr. Rachel would be wise to help Dr. Wolf by meeting with parents – and other inpatients' family members – herself. By handling and containing their ever-present experiences of guilt, shame, exasperation, anger, and helplessness, she reduces some of Dr. Wolf's burden. The clinical psychologist's role as someone who helps reduce the head psychiatrist's *emotional* burden leads to the next unofficial role of the ward's clinical psychologist: the boss's covert "right-hand (wo)man."

Organizational Consultant

Director, manager, administrator, executive, chief, chairman, and president are synonyms for the person running the company, the institute, the organization (see Adizes, 2016), or, in our case, the inpatient unit. Likewise: coach, corporate consultant, organizational psychologist, chief advisor, and consigliere are all synonyms for persons who support and stand by the manager. Their job is to advise the manager on to how to run the business or organization more effectively, how to reach organizational goals and how to manage crises.

In dynamic terms, one of the consultant's roles is to assuage the manager's loneliness. As Shakespeare's Henry IV tells us, "Lonely is the head that wears the crown." I will focus on the ward's clinical psychologist's role as organizational consultant. For example, let us suppose that the head of the ward, Dr. Wolf, is in conflict with the head nurse, Carmen, who is "working to rule," i.e., she is performing no more than the minimum official requirements of her job. Exasperated, Dr. Wolf shares his distress with the ward's psychologist, Dr. Rachel, asking for her insights. How should she intervene? If she is on good terms with the head nurse, she might mediate between the two. If, on the other hand, the head nurse's protest is because she feels devalued by her boss and by the para-medical sectors (including the psychologist), Dr. Rachel's role of psychologist might be a hindrance in itself. However, the very fact that the head of the ward wants to share such delicate matters with her could potentially relieve some of the head's stress, which in turn could have a positive effect on his functioning in the crisis, allowing him space to think and reflect: enhancing his "observing ego" capacities.

However, unlike an organizational consultant who is officially hired as such, the psychologist in the psychiatric ward is not officially assigned to aid the ward head in such a capacity. She is subjected to the same everyday demands as her co-workers: case management, meeting patients, attending ward meetings, writing and sending clinical reports, and more. She has to answer to the ward head and is not considered an official advisor on ward matters. As a participant, the clinical psychologist is also part of the web of ward politics (see below). Unlike the situation that would exist with an official consultant, if the ward clinical psychologist becomes involved in ward problem-solving, she might threaten the ward head's own sense of authority. That is why she might find herself only implicitly acting as consultant to the ward head.

> From the outset, it was clear that Doris would not cooperate with a formal intake. She was admitted by her parents after she had taken an overdose of sleeping pills and wrote a suicide note. In the

ward, she introduced herself using several different names, male and female. She refused a medical examination and insisted that the intake should take place in her room on the ward while she was in bed. The staff gathered around her bed, and Dr. Wolf started the interview. Why did you try to kill yourself? I was bored and depressed. How long have you felt this way? All my life. Did you have reasons for feeling depressed? Doris did not answer. Don't you care that you have caused such distress to your parents? Doris looked Dr. Wolf in the eye. "Are you here to judge me, like all the rest of them? Have you ever been depressed yourself, doctor?" For a moment, Dr. Wolf was speechless. Regaining his composure, he announced that the interview was over, adding, "You better behave yourself while you're here." As Dr. Wolf and his staff turned to leave the room, Doris suddenly started making strange noises. She began twitching in her bed, her eyes shut, mumbling "No, no, please stop, you're hurting me ... stop, I beg you ..." All stopped and returned to her room. Dr. Wolf asked, "Doris, can you hear me?" but she kept moving as if in a trance. Later, back in his office, Dr. Wolf said to Dr. Rachel: "Will you be able to prepare for tomorrow a presentation for the staff on treating Dissociative Identity Disorders?" Dr. Rachel invested a couple of hours in preparing a PowerPoint presentation that combined historical and theoretical perspectives, adding psychodynamic insights into the dynamics of DID and its effects on caregivers. She described the ongoing debate surrounding the viability of Multiple Personality diagnosis and emphasized the traumatic events that might ignite self-fragmentation. Dr. Rachel highlighted the expected split on the ward: male staff tagging Doris as "a typical Borderline" claiming she was putting on a show to receive attention; the women empathizing with her. Dr. Rachel pointed to the way that dissociation may be contagious, and she gave recommendations for how staff members could watch out for such effects. She added how the nurses were most invaluable in this regard, as they were at the forefront in dealing with such patients.

Dr. Rachel recognized Dr. Wolf's bewilderment when Doris asked him whether he ever felt depressed. By combining psycho-education with descriptions of dynamics, Dr. Rachel helped ease some of Dr. Wolf's tension. After the presentation, he called an urgent meeting with Carmen and asked her to prepare a list of what the nursing staff needed in order to handle the situation with Doris.

The above example illustrates how the involvement and input of the clinical psychologist helped focus the staff on the ward toward better, more effective treatment.

Climate Regulator

The ward clinical psychologist is trained and experienced in group processes. In addition to her role as dynamic interpreter and implicit consultant to the manager, she can use her professional intuition, perceptions and interpersonal skills to monitor changes in the ward atmosphere and to intervene accordingly. In this final section, I will describe three dynamics that are likely to occur in the psychiatric ward. I call these dynamics: pinball paranoia; the Iago effect; and the mysterious somatic symptom.

Paranoia Pinball

Paranoia is a state of mind characterized by delusions of persecution. Melanie Klein and her followers showed that every human being may, at times of stress and primitive anxiety, return (or regress) to paranoid-schizoid positions. That is, modes of relating to our inner and outer reality via unconscious mechanisms of splitting, denial, projection, projective identification, accompanied by experiences of hyper-vigilance and heightened suspiciousness (Segal, 1979). Behind the closed doors of the psychiatric ward, where a large proportion of admitted patients are prone to suffer from paranoid ideation and action, it is expected that an atmosphere of paranoia will prevail (see Sharfstein, 2009). Searles (1979c) addresses this phenomenon in his paper "Paranoid processes among members of the therapeutic team." In the opening vignette of this chapter, the secretary expressed some paranoid ideas in relation to Dr. Rachel, whom she accused of logging on to her computer and tampering with the data. In practice, however, people usually tend to ward off such feelings by activating them in others through the mechanism of projective identification (Segal, 1979).

I propose a specific dynamic that characterizes the ward's climate when these processes appear, which I term *paranoia pinball*. Pinball, of course, is the arcade game where the player must manipulate a steel ball inside a glass-covered cabinet, scoring points as the ball hits various targets, but preventing it from falling down the drain for as long as possible by flipping plastic bats (flippers) on both sides of the drain. Whenever the ball approaches the drain, the player presses buttons on both sides of the machine that control the flippers, striking the ball back into the cabinet space. Each time the ball hits a target, the pinball machine emits sparkling lights, loud bleeps, electric sounds, and musical motifs. To apply this simile to the dynamics of the closed ward, paranoia pinball refers to certain "players," i.e., members of staff, who cope with stressful events by flipping away their own emotions of guilt, shame, and horror, and stirring these emotions in their colleagues. This is a specific case of contagious affects (see Mitchell & Black, 1995), or of projective identification within the sphere of the group. Professionals may "flip" their own anxieties, amplifying those very anxieties among the professionals around them.

As is usually the case with projective identification, where unwanted feelings are unconsciously split and shoved into someone else, to be contained and processed by that someone, the pinball action is performed in such a way that the object of the projection is prevented from pointing to the projecting person's aggressive intentions. Searles provides a vivid example that is very common in medical institutes:

> When, for example, a charge nurse dutifully reported, concerning a psychotic physician-patient, Dr. Ryan, "'Searles is a shit,' observed Dr. Ryan calmly", I clearly heard the message from both of them.
>
> (Searles, 1979c, p. 104)

The charge nurse is stating what the patient said, and she does so matter-of-factly. But what she is really doing is expressing some unfinished business between herself and Searles. She is also making sure that the patient's negative focus is on Searles and not on her. To sum up, paranoia pinball is a special type of group dynamic, common to psychiatric inpatient teams, whereby the persecutory anxieties flip between its various members in order to prevent those anxieties from "falling into one's own void," and from remaining within a given person. Some people are more prone than others to stir paranoia in their co-workers. The next section discusses such processes on the ward.

The Iago Effect

Almost every group of people has at least one member who, whether consciously or not, is strongly motivated to create splits and who succeeds in causing mistrust and suspicion among their fellows. The character of Iago in Shakespeare's play Othello (Shakespeare, 1987) is a well-known literary prototype of such a person. In the play, Iago, Othello's ensign, is a paranoid person. He manages to maneuver his superiors and his peers to turn against one another, with tragic consequences for all concerned. How does he do that? There is a famous dialog in Act 3, Scene 2: Iago had previously arranged for his commander, Cassio, to be seen together with Othello's wife, Desdemona. As soon as Cassio exits, Iago kindles the sparks of jealousy in Othello.

Iago: Ha! I like not that.
Othello: What dost thou say?
Iago: Nothing my lord. Or if, I know not what.
Othello: Was not that Cassio parted from my wife?

Iago: Cassio, my lord? No, sure, I cannot think it, that he would steal away so guilty-like seeing your coming.

(Shakespeare, 1988, p. 834)

By using negation as a tactic ("Nothing my lord"; "I cannot think it") and planting the malevolent seeds in Othello's mind ("steal"; "guilty-like"), Iago is touching Othello's paranoid nucleus. Every office has its own Iago, someone who, in the bard's words, practices upon their mates' "peace and quiet even to madness." "Tis here, but yet confused, knavery's plain face is never seen till used" (ibid, p. 830). In an acute closed ward, where madness prevails by definition, it is all the easier for such types of spinning, to spread rumors, and to sow webs of conspiracies – real and imagined. What is the ward clinical psychologist's role when facing paranoia pinball and the Iago effect? The following extended vignette brings together several aspects of these dynamics and discusses how the clinical psychologist copes with them.

> Emanuel Cooper was 37 when admitted to the ward following a suicide attempt through overdosing. He was admitted to the acute closed ward from the general hospital where he had his stomach pumped. On the ward, Emanuel was assigned to the case management of Dr. Young, a clinical psychology intern. Emanuel was also placed under special watch. Round the clock, a team of nurses watched him wherever he went, including while he slept. During the grand round, Dr. Wolf assessed Emanuel's potential danger to himself. Emanuel was much more talkative than he had been when he entered the ward. He showed the staff a red string he wore around his wrist ("like Madonna," he said with a smile), explaining that it was an omen to keep his mind focused and his spirit intact. When he asked if he was allowed to wear his own pajamas, Dr. Wolf replied that he would consider it once the danger of Emanuel killing himself had passed. "Oh, but it has passed, Doctor," replied Emanuel. "We'll see about that," answered Dr. Wolf. Later, during the ward staff meeting, Carmen the head nurse said that Emanuel seemed fine to her, and there was no reason to continue the special watch, which was draining her team. Dr. Wolf was reluctant. He said that Emanuel seemed to be dissimulating suicidal contents and hinting at some nihilistic thoughts. Carmen retorted that Dr. Wolf was being over-careful, and was prejudiced against spiritual beliefs. Dr. Wolf sighed, and agreed to consider canceling the watch before the nurses' evening shift began at 3pm. He and Carmen saw Emanuel once more at 14:30, and Emanuel told them of his plans once he was discharged: he would spend more time with his son and daughter and would resume his job as journalist, saying:

> "no one in his right mind, who has children, could ever seriously ponder killing themselves." "See?" said Carmen as they exited the patient's room. Dr. Wolf ordered the ending of Emanuel's special watch. That evening, a patient who shared the room with Emanuel noticed that the bathroom door in the room had been locked for more than 15 minutes. Worried, he knocked and banged on the door, heard nothing, and then ran to inform the nurses. The nurses and aides hurried into the bathroom and found Emanuel tied by his neck to a water-pipe. The psychiatric resident on night shift performed CPR, but to no avail. Emanuel was rushed to the general hospital where he was declared dead on arrival.

This is a tragic but a not all-too-rare occurrence in a closed ward. Everyone on the ward, patients, and staff alike, were shaken by what happened. During the morning report, Dr. Wolf spoke about Emanuel Cooper's suicide, emphasizing that "we as a team did everything by the book." Carmen echoed him, stressing the whole treatment of Emanuel had been conducted with total collaboration between sectors. Dr. Wolf added that Emanuel's family was coming to meet him eight days later, at the end of the seven day "Shiva" (the customary Jewish mourning period). Dr. Wolf then held a special community meeting with everyone on the ward, informing those who had not heard about the tragedy, and urging patients to approach staff members on feeling distressed. During the weekly staff meeting, Dr. Wolf stressed that "the show must go on," and everyone should continue as usual. Everyone agreed.

What is the ward clinical psychologist to do in such a situation? At first, Dr. Rachel entertained the idea of conducting a special staff meeting for the purpose of ventilation and working through the traumatic event. However, her familiarity with her colleagues convinced her that they were not natural candidates for such a group intervention. She recalled an insightful remark made by one of the psychiatric residents: "every morning, upon entering the ward, I put on a mental sheath so as to desensitize myself to the effects of the intense madness that goes on." Rachel knew better than to abruptly take off the ward staff's "mental sheath." The anxiety that might be caused by the clinical psychologist's wish to encourage "group ventilation" or "sharing" could backfire; nobody thanks the messenger of bad news, the one who pushes too hard toward emotional self-revelation. In the ward's collective unconscious, such a person might cause staff members to regress, to identify with patients' psychosis and/or suicidal tendencies. Dr. Rachel kept her fantasy of conducting such a special staff meeting to herself, understanding this as a rescue fantasy and as a wish, in the face of such catastrophe, to operate in a *doing* mode.

Several days went by, and things looked as if they were back to normal. Ten days after Emanuel's funeral, his parents and son came to meet Dr. Wolf together with Dr. Wolf's deputy, Carmen, and Dr. Rachel. Dr. Young, the psychology intern who had Emanuel for case management, had called in sick. The Coopers looked sad, with a hint of anger in their eyes. Dr. Wolf expressed his condolences. Emanuel's son gazed at the floor and kept rubbing his leather bag. Mrs. Cooper did most of the talking on the family's behalf: She began by stating politely that they wished to investigate what their son's last hours were like. She added that she expected to receive the full cooperation of the ward. Dr. Wolf assured her that he and his staff would do anything they could to help, and that in these very sad circumstances, he could at least report that to the very tragic end, their son and father was treated in the best possible way. Mr. Cooper began coughing loudly, and Mrs. Cooper said, "Yes, well, that remains to be seen." Carmen interrupted, saying that she and her staff had nothing to hide. Looking Carmen straight in the eye, Mrs. Cooper asked, "Who exactly gave the order to take Emanuel off special watch?" Carmen said that with all due respect if Mrs. Cooper had come all the way to throw around accusations, that was too bad. At this point, all hell broke loose. Mr. Cooper said: "You guys didn't even come to pay your respects, either at the funeral or at the 'Shiva.' What kind of professionals are you?" Dr. Wolf said, "Look, let's not get personal here." Mrs. Cooper raised her voice. "This is OUR SON we are talking about here; we don't have the privilege of not getting personal here." Everyone was talking at once. Dr. Rachel then said she wished to say something. She turned to Mrs. Cooper: "I am Dr. Rachel, the ward psychologist. Since I heard of Emanuel's suicide, I have found it difficult falling asleep at night. Certain questions keep me awake: how could this happen under our very noses? Was there anything we could have done differently?" "Dr. Rachel ...!" Carmen started to say, hinting that she should stop. The psychologist continued, "You see, I am sure you want to do everything you can to find out what happened prior to your son's death. I'm even taking into account that this conversation is being recorded." Emanuel's 15-year-old son immediately stopped rubbing his bag and lifted his gaze for the first time." Dr. Rachel continued. "But my point is – if I find it hard to deal with what had happened, I cannot imagine what you are going through." "That's true," replied Mrs. Cooper, "you cannot imagine." However, the general affective tone in the room had changed significantly. Mr. Cooper started sobbing. Emanuel's son said to Dr. Rachel, "It's a nightmare." "It is a nightmare," said

Dr. Rachel, "and it's impossible to wake up from it now." Mrs. Cooper wiped her eyes and handed her husband a tissue. "We will be in touch," she said to Dr. Wolf, who answered, "Indeed. I guess that your lawyers will speak to the hospital's lawyers. But please note that we, the staff, are here for you whenever you see fit."

When a suicide occurs on the ward, a high priority of senior staff is to make sure that staff cannot be accused of malpractice. But this concern actually screens the deep, hidden guilt that inevitably arises when a patient makes the worst fear of every helping-professional come true: the fear of their efforts resulting in the opposite of rescuing, of having a patient take his own life while on the team's watch. Dr. Rachel knew this. By disclosing her self-doubts and guilt feelings, she made legitimate the parents' own guilt feelings over losing their child to suicide. Dr. Rachel also voiced the underlying atmosphere of suspicion, by pointing to the possibility that they were being recorded. She noticed that Carmen was "protesting too much" about her part in the decision to cease the watch prior to Emanuel's suicide. What Dr. Rachel did not grasp at that time was that the atmosphere in the ward was turning darker by the minute.

Two days after meeting the Coopers, Dr. Wolf ordered Dr. Rachel to go into Dr. Young's office and look for any file that might contain information on Emanuel's case management. "Why don't you tell her to provide you with the material yourself?" asked Dr. Rachel. Dr. Wolf said he did not want Dr. Young to know that he was after this data. Dr. Rachel said that she found it difficult to follow this order. She was not prepared to spy on a co-worker. "Stop exaggerating," said Dr. Wolf, but he did not repeat his request. Dr. Young, for her part, had not yet returned from her sick leave. When Dr. Rachel called to ask her how she was doing, Dr. Young said she was seriously considering leaving the field of clinical psychology.[1] Meanwhile, one of the aides told Dr. Rachel that Carmen was making mean comments about Dr. Rachel to the other nurses. "She said that you are not available for patients' parents when they call and that your DO NOT DISTURB sign is inappropriate in a closed acute ward such as ours." Dr. Rachel was furious. It took a while before she realized what was going on. She asked to talk to the aide again, and told her, "I trust that every word you said was true. But if *you* have any criticism you want to articulate to me, or if *you* are angry with me for some reason, tell me openly. Don't use Carmen's efforts to tarnish my name as an excuse." Now it was the aide's turn to be offended. "I only

> wanted you to know. I was acting as your eyes and ears in the nurses' forum. I thought you would thank me for informing you." "Well," said Dr. Rachel, "Let's make a deal. From now on, please refrain from informing me about bad things people say behind my back, and I will refrain from telling you what people say about you. Please don't take offense from what I'm saying, just think about it."

We can see how paranoia pinball and the Iago effect were at play at this stage. But the story was not over yet:

> A week had passed since the Cooper's visit, and a new patient, M., was hospitalized. He did not cooperate with the police who picked him up for a minor offense. M. did not seem psychotic by any means. As the weekend approached, the word spread in the ward that M. was actually an informer planted by the private investigator hired by the Coopers to obtain evidence regarding malpractice on the ward. Dr. Rachel was shocked when she heard a nurse whom she always considered as cool and resolved, telling her seriously about M's secret mission. But Dr. Rachel could not help wondering, as she noticed his eyes following her as she walked to the canteen …

To the extent that the ward clinical psychologist can manage her own paranoia, she will be able to recognize and neutralize its poisonous effects by pointing out its various manifestations. In our example, Dr. Rachel refused to succumb to Dr. Wolf's request to spy on her teammate. She called "a spade a spade" when faced with hearsay about her poor functioning, as relayed by a messenger from the head nurse. It was actually aimed at fending off both the nurse's and the aide's own persecutory anxieties by depositing them inside herself.

Parenthetically, it is worth mentioning that another fruitful way of regulating the ward's climate may be by using humor. Following the rule that jest often hides the truth, subtexts or hidden meanings can find their way into spoken language by way of a quip, a joke, or a pun. Humor, however, is always context-dependent; it is difficult to come up with a joke that will ease the frightening atmosphere surrounding Emanuel Cooper's suicide.

Finally, let us turn to one more manifestation in the aftermath of Emanuel's suicide.

The Mysterious Somatic Symptom

> Dr. Spock, a highly motivated and energetic resident, developed some irritating pains in his left foot that soon made it impossible

for him to walk properly. Although he underwent various tests, no physical diagnosis was found, and everyone got used to seeing Dr. Spock limping about. Nobody, including Dr. Rachel, seemed to remember that Dr. Spock was on call the day of Emanuel's suicide. One day, over lunch, he mentioned in passing to Dr. Rachel that he thought he could trace the beginning of his pains to the morning after his CPR failed to save Emanuel. "It reminds me of when my dad had a heart attack 4 years ago, and I had to persuade the doctors in the ER to pay closer attention to him. He could have died while in hospital. Scary!" After lunch, Dr. Rachel called Dr. Wolf urgently, told him of her conversation with Dr. Spock, and asked to give Dr. Spock some days off work. Dr. Wolf was reluctant to agree, but Dr. Rachel argued that Dr. Spock's state might get worse. Dr. Wolf called Dr. Spock, told him that he thinks his pains might be connected to his role in trying to save Emanuel's life and that he wants him to take the week off, non-negotiable.

Paul Williams observed that staff members on a psychiatric ward tend to take many days of sick leave (Williams, 2010). In our example, Dr. Spock continued to work despite his pains. This could be understood as post-traumatic symptoms, dissociated from their source (see Rubin, Malkinson, & Witztum, 2010, pp. 55–70 for a fuller discussion). Dr. Rachel did not think of it until Dr. Spock mentioned in passing the timing of his ailment. Her intervention brought about considerable change: Dr. Spock came back from his leave with no pains in his foot. A couple of months later, he asked Dr. Rachel to recommend a therapist, "... because I'm starting to do psychotherapy, and it is high time I found out for myself what this thing is about."

Concluding Remarks

The word "madness" has a two-fold meaning. It refers to insanity, but it also refers to anger. This gives us a clue as to what might at times characterize the atmosphere of the closed psychiatric ward. Anger, exasperation, guilt, anxiety – these emotions are part and parcel of any professional working with acute psychiatric patients. Indeed, if it were not also for the hope and the satisfaction of helping these patients, no one in his right mind would last long in such a job.

The Biblical quote heading this chapter asks whether a shield or spear was seen. The focus of this chapter is on unseen spears and shields: spears, in the form of harmful rumors and gossip (explained here in terms of projective identification, etc.) that lead to paranoia, and shields that protect the ward from the anxiety this may produce. In this chapter, Dr. Rachel's character served to illustrate the clinical psychologist's roles on the ward as hidden protector. The clinical psychologist is more human than otherwise, and as such she is prone to fall into the traps of concrete-thinking, paranoia pinball, as well as playing unwittingly the part of Iago in the ward's dynamics. She has to be aware of these traps, and she has to invest special effort in avoiding them. She will then gain the satisfaction of serving as interpreter, silent organization consultant, and climate regulator.

A well-known proverb states "no good deed goes unpunished." One should not expect ward's staff members to express their heartfelt gratitude to the psychologist for her efforts to facilitate patients' subjectivity, handle family members' crises, contain the manager's anxieties, and monitor the ward's atmosphere. However, next time someone asks (and they are likely to do so), "who needs a psychologist in the acute closed ward?" she can smile to herself and keep up the good work.

Note

1 See Daza & Sharma (Chapter 21, this volume) on supervising psychology interns on inpatient suicide.

References

Adizes, I. (2016). *Mastering change: Introduction to organizational therapy*. Carpinteria, CA: The Adizes Institute.

Evans, M. (2016). *Making room for madness in mental health: The psychoanalytic understanding of psychotic communication*. London: Karnac.

Laing, R. D. (1960). *The divided self: An existential study in sanity and madness*. London: Karnac.

Mitchell, S. A., & Black, M. (1995). *Freud and beyond: A history of modern psychoanalytic thought*. New York, NY: Basic Books.

Rubin, S. S., Malkinson, R., & Witztum, E. (2010). *Working with the bereaved: Multiple lenses on loss and mourning*. New York, NY: Routledge.

Saint-Exubery, A. de. (1943). *The little prince*. New York, NY: Harcourt Inc.

Searles, H. F. (1961). Schizophrenia and the inevitability of death. *Psychiatric Quarterly*, *135*, 631–665.

Searles, H. F. (1965). *Collected papers on schizophrenia and related subjects*. New York, NY: International Universities Press.

Searles. H. F. (1979a). Countertransference and theoretical model. In: H. F. Searles, (Ed.) *Countertransference and related subjects* (pp. 373–379). Madison, WI: International Universities Press.

Searles, H. F. (1979b). Feelings of guilt in the psychoanalyst. In: H. F. Searles, (Ed.) *Countertransference and related subjects* (pp. 28–35). Madison WI: International Universities Press.

Searles, H. F. (1979c). Paranoid processes among members of the therapeutic team. In: H. F. Searles, (Ed.) *Countertransference and related subjects* (pp. 89–108). Madison, WI: International Universities Press.

Segal, H. (1979). *Introduction to the work of Melanie Klein*. London: Karnac.

Shakespeare, W. (1987a). *Henry IV*. D. Bevington (Ed.). New York, NY: Oxford University Press.
Shakespeare, W. (1987b). *Othello*. S. Wells, & G Talor (Eds.). Oxford: Clarendon Press.
Sharfstein, S. S. (Ed.). (2009). *Textbook of hospital psychiatry*. New York, NY: American Psychiatric Association.
Silver, A. L. (2014). Intra-staff openness; "What's a nice girl like you doing in a place like this?" *Psychosis: Psychological, Social and Integrative Approaches, 6 (4)*, 297–305.
Sterba, R. (1938). The fate of the ego in analytic therapy. *International Journal of Psychoanalysis, 15*, 117–126.
Sullivan, H. S. (1956). *Clinical studies in psychiatry*. New York, NY: Norton.
Williams, P. (2010). *Invasive objects: Minds under siege*. New York, NY: Routledge.

7 The Development of a Recovery-Oriented Tool for Work with Patients in the Closed Forensic Ward

Enav Or-Gordon

In this chapter, the author describes a therapeutic intervention technique developed on a closed men's forensic ward in a public psychiatric hospital in Prague, Czech Republic. The target group included patients diagnosed with schizophrenia, some with concomitant substance use disorder. The intervention technique was developed by the head psychiatrist and the psychologist, in an attempt to better adapt therapeutic efforts to patients' individualized and holistic needs and to promote recovery.

The Starting Point: The Situation on the Ward

Immediate goals of hospitalization in a forensic ward include diagnosing the individual, stabilizing his mental state, adjusting medication accordingly and distancing the potentially dangerous individual from society. The aims of *continued* hospitalization are to increase the patient's awareness of his illness and its associated risk factors, to establish treatment that will effectively lead to stable remission, and to assess and reduce potential future risks while striving for the patient's safe return to the community. For patients with concomitant substance addictions, an additional goal is to be drug-free. The court decides when a patient can be discharged based on the hospital's recommendation following the achievement of treatment goals.

The ward on which the treatment described in this chapter took place had two main groups of patients: patients with a primary diagnosis of schizophrenia (henceforth referred to as "psychiatric patients") and patients with a primary diagnosis of substance use disorders (henceforth referred to as "patients with addictions").

The latter group of patients participated in a forensic rehabilitation program following incarceration in prison (Švarc, 2008). This program was dynamically oriented. It dealt with behavioral, emotional and social aspects of addictions by presenting patients with a fixed series of assignments, completion of which advanced the patients toward a recommendation for discharge (Kalina, 2013).

In contrast, although psychiatric patients were obliged to attend some activities such as group psychotherapy, art therapy and chores, prior to the development and use of the therapeutic tool to be described in this chapter, they were not expected to actively engage and were not presented with a comprehensive therapeutic plan. Progress was determined according to the multi-disciplinary team (MDT) members' assessments of their mental state and basic functioning.

The Need for a Change

A psychologist working in a psychiatric ward has the privilege of seeing patients in multiple contexts: during doctors' rounds, in common activities, in case presentations and also in individual and group therapy. Through his or her therapeutic efforts the psychologist continuously strives to comprehend the patient's unique experience. These multiple perspectives of patients in my psychological work enabled me to gain a broader understanding of patients' functioning in different situations, and also to better understand their subjective experiences in the ward. While listening to patients, it became clear to me, that the psychiatric patients perceived their hospitalization distinctly different than patients with addictions. There were also notable between-group differences in the levels of functioning and the nature of dialog with the team.

Patients with addictions tended to have a more active approach; they set personal goals and knew where they stood and what they had to do to advance within their programs. They maintained continuous therapeutic relationships with team members and approached their therapists in times of need. Despite frustration with obligatory participation in the forensic program, they had a relative sense of orientation and control over the therapeutic process.

In contrast, the psychiatric patients tended to be frustrated, passive, invested less time in discussing their medical treatment and had difficulties describing their therapeutic plan and signs of improvement. They tended to grasp the therapeutic process as medical or punitive and passively waited for a change in their mental state that would allow them to be discharged.

These between-group differences might have stemmed from differences in pathologies and ego strengths; however, my colleagues and I believed that they were also a consequence of the different therapeutic programs, and patient and team expectations.

We sought to develop a therapeutic tool that would structure the work with psychiatric patients and help them develop a greater sense of ownership and investment in their therapeutic plans and goals. We wanted to establish patient-friendly criteria to motivate greater involvement and cooperation of patients with the MDT in order to promote the therapeutic process and optimize therapeutic gains.

Following is the case of S., which demonstrates the influence of the therapeutic paradigm on psychiatric patients' functioning on the ward:

S., a 32-year-old man with schizophrenia, was hospitalized numerous times in other hospital wards. He was first admitted to the forensic ward after severely attacking a night guard in a city parking lot. At that time, S. was under the influence of drugs and had severe paranoid symptoms. In the ward, he was assigned to the psychiatric program.

S. showed interest regarding his condition and had good insight that was expressed when he accurately described psychotic states, drug-induced experiences, and remission states. In the ward, S. generally slept or passively stared into space. He rarely watched television, or opened the books at his bedside, and did not initiate conversations with team members. He took very little care of his personal hygiene and explained the reason for his behavior to be that he was waiting for an improvement in his mental condition in order to be discharged. A few months later, S. was transferred to a different open ward, only to be re-admitted to our ward following recurrent substance abuse. It was then decided to assign him to the program for patients with addictions. His functioning in the drug rehabilitation program was markedly different. He addressed personal themes and actively participated in group sessions. Though his personal hygiene was still lacking, he discussed this problem in group and individual sessions and tried to improve himself in that domain. Upon discharge from the hospital, he was more organized, and was able to discuss his achievements and current goals. His relationship with his family improved, and his plans for the future seemed more cohesive than in the past.

In recovery-oriented rehabilitation models, the therapeutic process is aimed at enabling both external and internal changes. The internal changes revolve around hope, healing, empowerment, and connection:

Hope – is based on the belief that recovery is possible. It is characterized by acceptance of difficulties while searching for strengths and abilities, emphasizing success and maintaining an optimistic feeling regarding opportunities for improvement.

Healing – is achieving the ability for self-help and living a meaningful life. Two components of healing are the definition of the self apart from illness, and control. The first is reached when one's self-perception is not reduced to the role of being ill, but rather includes characteristics and roles that promote self-esteem and respect. Control is the ability to recognize symptoms, know the course of the illness, actively seek support, properly use medications and maintain a balanced lifestyle. Perception of the focus of control within rather than outside the individual is important.

Empowerment – patients with mental disorders often experience feelings of helplessness, dependency and a reduced ability for effective functioning and self-regulation; they struggle with inner changes and with changes in their social functioning, status and support systems. The rehabilitative process should aim to find new ways to achieve autonomy and assist in finding new strengths and ways to assume responsibility.

Connection – recovery is a social process in which it is important for the patient to reintegrate into former social frameworks such as family, friends and work as well as finding new roles and relationships appropriate to one's current abilities and needs(Jacobson & Greenley, 2001).

The therapeutic tool we envisaged would help patients find their way in the therapeutic process, offer them a greater sense of control and orientation and motivate them to become active agents of their rehabilitation.

The tool we thus created was a "workbook" that was flexible enough to fit the needs of a variety of patients and a wide range of functioning levels. With the aid of this workbook, patients were able to examine their progress, better conceptualize and communicate regarding their rehabilitative process, identify strengths, difficulties and needs and set goals. The workbook was designed to encompass various dimensions of the individual patient's life rather than focus specifically on pharmaceutical treatment or illness course.

The Workbook

Following admission to the ward, once the patient was no longer in an acute psychotic state, and was free of drugs and able to communicate with the staff, he was given the workbook. The workbook's layout corresponds with stages of hospitalization: At stage 0 the patient is confined to the ward and its adjacent courtyard. Family visits take place in the visiting room. At stage 1 the patient is allowed to go for walks on the hospital grounds, at first accompanied by a family member and later on his own. At stage 2, short leaves outside the hospital are allowed. At stage 3, in addition to short leaves, recommendation for discharge is submitted by the hospital, and the patient awaits court ruling for discharge.

The first section of the workbook includes a general list of subjects related to stages of patients' treatment during hospitalization. A separate page is dedicated to each stage, with stage-related subjects and space to write down specific tasks that will advance the work on each subject. For example at stage 1, for the subject "diagnosis," the first assignment might be to discuss one's diagnosis with the psychologist. The second task might be to read a booklet about mental disorders. The third task could be to prepare a short lecture about the diagnosis for presentation in group therapy.

At the early stages, a staff member must sign to verify that the patient has completed his assignments. As the patient progresses through the various stages, he can monitor himself, for example, by signing the workbook each time he attends an Alcoholics Anonymous meeting outside the ward. The duration of the different stages varies, with a minimal duration of one month. Some patients may remain at the same stage for a number of months or even years.

Dialog between patients and team members is aimed at discussing the patient's current state, and to formulate new goals and assignments for further advancement by identifying current important themes and considering the patient's level of motivation and functioning.

The subjects that were chosen as guidelines for the patients to attend to represented the team's general expectations for patients at each stage of hospitalization. Thus, during the first weeks on the ward, the patient was expected to work on orientation, hygiene and the ability to deal with the reasons for his hospitalization. He was then expected to gradually cope with subjects that are more complex. Prior to going on leave to visit family, the patient might need to deal with family relationships, and how to spend his leisure time. Before discharge, the patient needs to have sufficient insight and knowledge about his disorder and medical treatment. In case of concomitant mental illness and drug dependency, the patient needs a plan for supporting abstinence.

Effort was made to adapt themes and work methods according to individual patient needs and interests. However, as a forensic ward, there are also specific security-related issues that must be addressed. Thus, for a patient with a high-risk potential, compliance with pharmaceutical treatment during and after hospitalization is essential. The patient's attitude regarding the use of addictive substances must be responsible and safe.

The workbook's flexibility is reflected in the various ways a theme can be adapted to specific patient's needs. For example, a subject such as "leisure time" can be dealt with on different levels – how to spend time in the ward or in daily life, the relationship between hobbies and mental health, the relationship between boredom and the use of addictive substances. The patient might choose to present a lecture on leisure time during group therapy or prepare a concrete list of suggestions for leisure time activities. During leave from the ward, patients might explore different possibilities for spending leisure time. Assignments are individualized according to the patient's goals, personal preferences, and abilities.

A similar theme might have different implications for different patients. The theme "life story" might be significant for some patients to communicate with others in group therapy as they might describe important life events, receive feedback and form relationships. For other patients "life story" may offer an opportunity to organize one's personal narrative and work toward integration of the self.

Presentation of the Workbook

Cover page – Hospital logo, ward, patient's personal details, date receipt of notebook, and signature.

Page one – Explanatory list of subjects.
The personal program refers to:

Psychiatric treatment: Diagnosis, reasons for medications, dosage and side effects.
Functioning: Personal hygiene, adherence to ward regulations, leisure time, relaxation techniques, housekeeping chores, work.
Insight: Mental disorder, me and my surroundings, illness process, symptoms, relapse, remission.
Social abilities: Communication with the psychiatrist, the team, other patients, relationships within the family, social life.
Addictive substances: Drugs, alcohol, and mental disorders.

As the various subjects in the workbook are loosely defined in order to allow for flexibility, this list aims to provide the patient with an idea of the areas expected to be addressed.

Page two – stage 0, date:
Personal weekly assignments:

The patient is asked to list which weekly assignments he will perform on a regular basis. There is space for staff signatures to verify the performance of the assignments such as writing a diary, exercising in the gym, playing ping pong or chess, individual psychotherapy.

Suggested topics to work on in this stage:

How can I improve my orientation in the ward?

How can I achieve a good level of personal hygiene and basic functioning?

How do I train my cognitive skills?

With whom can I discuss why I am hospitalized in this ward?

Which additional topics should I work on?

Under each topic heading, either the team members or the patient record concrete tasks to be performed.

Completed tasks are dated and signed.

Page three – stage 1, date:
Personal weekly assignments:
Suggested topics to work on:

Where and how can I work on the topic of my diagnosis?

Where and how can I work on the topic of addictive substances and dependency?

How can I address the topic of relationships with my family?

What can I do to improve the way I spend my leisure time?

Which additional topics should I work on?

Page four – stage 2, date:
Personal weekly assignments:
Suggested topics to work on:

Where and how can I work on my life story?

Where and how can I deal with the reasons for my hospitalization?

Where and how can I address the subject of planning for after my discharge?

How can I make sure that I will have housing after my discharge?

How should I look for a psychiatrist in the community and how should I discuss cooperation with him?

Which additional topics should I work on?

Page five – stage 3, date:
Personal weekly assignments:
Suggested topics to work on:

How can I improve my knowledge about my illness?

Did I deal with economic issues and what should I do about my financial situation?

How can I work on constructing a plan for after my discharge?

How can I work on constructing an emergency plan?

Which additional topics should I work on?

The transition from one stage to the next is accompanied by a doctor's signature confirming that the "patient is in a mental state that enables him to move up to the next stage." This confirmation was added in order to ensure that patients advance only when their mental stability is adequate for progression to the next level. This additional criterion was found relevant especially for motivated patients whose insight was lacking. Prior to the requisite confirmation, difficult situations arose in which patients completed numerous assignments but failed to gain insight about their illness. Patients sometimes avoided the subject of their mental state and diagnosis altogether. For these patients, progression in hospitalization stages with the associated increased levels of freedom in preparation for discharge was considered dangerous.

Last page – checklist:
Official documents (identification papers, health insurance card), housing, sources of income, debts, a psychiatrist in the community. The purpose of the checklist is to help the team, and the patient ensure that the patient has solved crucial technical issues prior to discharge.

Strategies in the Development of the Tool – The First Year

The ward team includes division chairperson, department head and one resident (psychiatrist), four psychologists, one art therapist, one social worker, chief nurses and nursing staff. We identified many communication opportunities between patients and staff in different activities and settings. We had the impression, that although the ward activity program was binding, psychiatric patients' requests regarding their activity plans were positively considered. Changes in pharmacological treatment were initiated with patients being informed, explained and preferably with their consent. Patients described relationships with psychiatrists and psychologists as basically respectful and many times helpful. In psychotherapy, patients felt they were encouraged to raise topics for discussion. Most requests for individual sessions were answered positively. We thus aimed to encourage patients to be active and to take advantage of the therapeutic opportunities on the ward. Together with the head psychiatrist, we continuously developed and adjusted the tool in response to feedback from the team and patients.

After deciding on the workbook's format, content was considered. We clearly defined several important dimensions for work with patients in their various stages of hospitalization. Initial versions of the workbook were drafted and offered to a limited number of patients who provided feedback. Based on that feedback, the workbook was modified. We sought to formulate a flexible plan that could easily become individualized in order to enable, empower and promote active patient participation. To that end, we presented a list of general subjects on the first page of the workbook and added the question "Which additional topics should I work on?" to encourage delineation of patient-specific needs. We formulated questions and topics together with the patients using simple language. The workbook as a means to promote effective dialog and track patients' progress was readily accepted.

> P., a 27-year-old patient in long-term hospitalization, was diagnosed with schizophrenia and drug addiction. He was re-admitted to the forensic ward after running away from an open ward. A week after his return to the ward P. asked for a workbook like the other patients had. He noted that in the past he did not have one. He immediately wrote assignments to be completed each week. He also asked for weekly sessions with the psychologist, something he had not done before. He explained that with the workbook he understood what he could do to promote his therapeutic process and advance discharge.

Contrary to preliminary doubts, we happily discovered that most patients managed to responsibly take care of their workbooks. There were very few cases of lost workbooks or refusals to use them. Patients with a higher level of functioning, such as P., used it to plan and systematically advance their therapy and relate to issues outside of the ward. For less well functioning patients, such as N., whose description will follow, the signatures in the workbook confirmed their achievements or efforts. N. stopped saying he did "nothing" during the previous week, and began referring to small activities he had performed – such as a short conversation with the psychiatrist. Cooperation with the patients positively contributed to the ward atmosphere and to therapeutic relationships.

> O., aged 23 with schizoaffective disorder, substance use disorder and a history of long periods in youth detention institutions, began to show interest in the workbook. During individual therapy sessions, he was glad to assist me in formulating questions and clarifying terms that I thought should be added. He was one of the first to receive the workbook and was very conscientious in using it. During group therapy sessions he volunteered to explain how to work with it. It became apparent that he had a talent for suggesting original suitable assignments for other patients as well as for himself. A year later, when the workbook was integrated into the ward routine, he volunteered to help prepare copies of it while referring to his contribution in creating it. In future therapy sessions, we both felt a sense of positive cooperation, even when addressing other issues.

The introduction of the workbook helped the team identify adjustments that needed to be made to better adapt the ward to patients' needs. We increased the number of hours dedicated to individual therapy. A new group therapy for patients with dual diagnosis of schizophrenia and substance use disorder was developed; an elective art workshop was added, and an array of booklets with crossword puzzles, etc. was presented to patients, to enrich cognitive training and leisure time activities. A list of appropriate themes was created by patients during group therapy and added to optional activities. During routine meetings with patients, in addition to the question "how are you," we added, "what are you currently working on as part of your personal work plan?"

> Y., a 46-year-old patient with schizoaffective disorder and alcohol dependency, was re-admitted to the forensic ward because of violent behavior. He had a history of hospitalizations beginning at age 18. Y. had good insight and he dealt with complex and symbiotic family relationships and traumatic life experiences. Y. used the workbook to make a precise plan of activities. Every week he added to the list new concrete assignments and strove to fulfill them. He came to meetings with the psychologist and the psychiatrist, and to the doctors' rounds with his workbook, and with an exact record of what he had accomplished as well as a list of his future goals, tasks and plans. The assignments he chose included finding a new psychiatrist in the community and beginning to attend AA meetings. He added to his workbook a short article defining schizoaffective disorder and a card with sentences of encouragement to avoid the use of alcohol. He prepared for moving in with his father by preparing a list of his expectations and the duties he was willing to undertake, and presented it to the psychiatrist. Y. commented that using the workbook calmed him and enabled him to gradually prepare for discharge.

A year after implementation of the workbook, we observed that the psychiatrists, psychologists and patients considered it an integral component of treatment. In contrast, perhaps owing to their different interactions with the patients, nurses were at first less involved with the workbook. The department's head nurses recognized the benefits of the tool and were willing to incorporate some nursing tasks in the workbook. We identified a motivated patient who tended to neglect his personal hygiene and suggested that he would get the concrete task of brushing his teeth. The nurses were to sign the workbook every evening, when the task was completed. The head nurse and I presented this in a team meeting and discussed how the workbook could be used in rehabilitative and behavioral work. Nurses responded positively, describing various progressions in functioning they noticed throughout the past year among patients who were using the workbook, and we decided to involve the patients in formulating assignments related to tasks associated with nursing care.

Thoughts Regarding Work with the Workbook – the Second Year

The workbook became a meaningful tool for organizing various levels of work with the patients. During the first stages of hospitalization, the workbook offers a well-defined method for the psychiatrist to explain the course of treatment and to delineate the team's expectations in terms of specific steps and goals presented in the therapeutic program. During these first stages, the nursing and MDT concentrate on basic functioning, hygiene and orientation. Working on clear assignments calms the patient and allows for a more positive attitude toward involuntary hospitalization.

Throughout the hospitalization, the workbook enables a continuous dialog with reference to defined themes and areas of functioning, while reflecting on the patient's progress. Terms such as insight, understanding the reason for hospitalization, cognitive functioning, hygiene and general functioning are presented in the workbook as tasks that need to be completed. The open format encourages the formulation of individualized assignments, thus enabling the patient and the team to work together to develop patient-specific tasks according to each patient's strengths and need for assistance.

The patient and team develop constructive cooperation, with a growing sense of optimism. In cases of resistance, difficult issues can be postponed, and more compliant areas worked on, thus strengthening a positive relationship.

> B., a 22-year-old patient with schizophrenia, was in an acute psychotic state and had difficulties coming to terms with hospitalization. During his first few weeks in the ward, he actively resisted talking about his mental state. B. kept himself busy with intensive sports activities. He doodled in his workbook and was especially keen on painting over the title page, changing the words to words with different meanings. After a few weeks of hospitalization and pharmacological treatment, his condition somewhat improved. He agreed to record in his workbook the tasks he was fulfilling, such as going to the gym, and he confirmed completion with the appropriate signatures. Fulfilling the tasks gained positive reinforcement. Gradually, he became more

> cooperative, started to go to therapy and agreed to read a booklet about schizophrenia.

With the use of this simple tool, patients become partners in their treatment and actively participate in assessing the various dimensions of their well-being. Flexibility and the option of adding more subjects allow the patient to choose what is most suitable for him. Working with the workbook helps improve patients' awareness and insight regarding their mental states and the mental disorders with which they are coping. The workbook promotes a better understanding of the therapeutic process and helps patients gradually realize the different aspects of their functioning, life, and social situations. By using the workbook patients are able to describe what they are working on, and this contributes to their awareness and self-confidence and promotes self-advocacy.

> K. was a 23-year-old patient with schizophrenia and drug addiction. When he was admitted to the ward, he exhibited mainly negative symptoms such as blunted affect and poor motivation. The dialog with him was on a simple and concrete level. Treatment focused on his relationship with his family and later on his returning to the community. Short visits to his family led to talks about his functioning at home. He worked on becoming more independent by going home on leaves by himself using public transportation rather than having his brother pick him up. Later on, K. began to think about sheltered housing. He discussed this option with his parents and started attending a preparatory group. He used the workbook as an anchor, read his assignments a few times during the week and expressed satisfaction when he made progress. He was able to describe the stages of his rehabilitation and regarded the appointed time for his discharge as his entrance to the sheltered housing. The workbook provided a number of important themes to work on and enabled the team to adjust different activities, such as individual and group psychotherapy to K.'s current needs.

Many patients preferred to work on their themes in individual therapy. As a result, more patients entered a routine of weekly psychotherapy. Using the workbook, patients gradually learned to complete their assignments and thus advance themselves. Group therapy provided an opportunity for patients to become more active and self-advocating. It was often chosen as the best setting for working on social issues and issues of insight into illness and substance dependency. However, the therapeutic team avoided determining when or in which group patients should discuss these personal issues. In practice, most patients directly communicated with the group therapist and explained what topic they should work on and when. Some more competent patients arrived at their group session with a well prepared written theme, while less active patients remembered their allotted time and theme, and then spoke freely.

Thus, the workbook also influenced the nature of group therapy on the ward. More sessions than before revolved around specific subjects or specific patients and were led by the patients themselves with participants showing more motivation and interest. It was also our impression that when a group discussed a theme brought up and prepared by a patient, group members became more actively involved.

Patients' work on the ward was also enriched by the addition of writing a diary, processing certain subjects in writing, preparing short lectures about different subjects, especially concerning diagnosis, pharmacological treatment and addictions. We noticed, that gathering signatures for various completed activities created motivation and contributed to the patient's feeling of making progress and self-agency. Many patients talked about a better feeling stemming from being more active and having both general goals and concrete assignments.

> N. was a 32-year-old patient hospitalized in the ward for many years. He had a diagnosis of schizophrenia, exhibited borderline intelligence and had a complex symbiotic relationship with his father. For many months he refused to acknowledge the existence of the workbook, which represented a change and need to deal with new demands. After almost a year-long negotiation, N. agreed to accept the workbook and sign his name in it. When he entered stage 1, the psychiatrist added one assignment – weekly conversations with her. These sessions had already been taking place, but were now introduced into an organized work schedule and required the psychiatrist's signature in the workbook. N. remembered to ask for a signature after every weekly session, and later used them to demonstrate his cooperation when he asked for short leaves with his father. The psychiatrist added small concrete assignments such as writing a list of his weekly activities in the ward. After a while, they started planning the topic for the next conversation – at first the psychiatrist suggested topics, and later N. recommended topics for forthcoming sessions. After a year of working in this format he wrote a short poem about winter, and later wrote a few lines about his experiences during hospitalization. These activities helped N. gain a sense of personal strength and improved the therapeutic process.

Working in various domains with a tool that organizes the patient's work motivates the team to cooperate in supporting the patient's progress. A psychiatrist who sees the need to work on the patient's insight can encourage him to lecture about his diagnosis in the group session with the psychologist. A psychologist who discusses cognitive training with the patient can direct him to solve labyrinths or Sudoku in his spare time, together with a nurse. A nurse working with the patient to improve orientation on the ward can encourage him to practice writing his daily activities in a diary which the psychologist will later read. All of the patients' assignments are written in their workbooks, which the patients work on continuously in various settings and with different team members, promoting continuity of care.

The work with H. demonstrated this growing potential for working through a wide variety of topics with different team members.

> H. was a 30-year-old patient with a diagnosis of schizophrenia and substance abuse. His insight was poor. For years he attempted to live an orderly life in the community but failed to hold a job, abstain from drugs and cooperate with medical treatment. This was his third hospitalization in the forensic ward. The psychiatrist offered to work with him on improving his everyday functioning and sense of reality. Together they chose the assignment of recording his daily expenses thus creating a weekly list of expenditures. During doctors' rounds, the list was discussed, and the patient talked about difficulties in following and planning his expenses. The psychiatrist encouraged the patient to set a meeting with one of the staff members in order to discuss concrete details of weekly financial planning. It was decided that a group therapy session with the psychologist should focus on the gaps between planning and reality.

Cooperation and the ability to follow up themes with different team members enables more holistic and effective work. It also increases integration, thus counteracting forces of disintegration typical to mental illness and psychosis. An integrative and structured ward has a calming effect and advances processes of reconstruction and reorganization. Very often these processes of integration not only counterbalance processes of inner disintegration, but they may also provide a therapeutic experience on the ward different from the patients' experiences with their families and in their natural surroundings.

> M. was a 41-year-old patient diagnosed with schizoaffective disorder. He was repeatedly hospitalized for long periods of time, regaining inner integration very slowly with the help of intensive medication and psychotherapy. During one of his hospitalizations, after gaining

some integration and insight, a meeting was held with his parents and sister regarding future plans for returning home. The issue was processed and prepared by M. using the workbook. He worked with the psychiatrist on establishing goals and expectations and making a list of topics to discuss. The same issue was discussed in individual therapy with the psychologist and also raised in group therapy. Owing to the intensive and diverse dealing with the subject, M. felt prepared to meet his parents. He also asked the psychiatrist and psychologist to be present at the meeting.

The meeting with M.'s parents and sister demonstrated the levels of disintegration that characterized his family. Each family member gave a different, contradicting message, and mother and father "took turns" representing contradictory attitudes regarding how to support M., in a very confusing way. For example, the father invited him to come home, and at the same time the mother sent a strong message that he was unwanted. A minute later it was the other way around. When the psychiatrist reflected the confusion she witnessed, both parents denied the messages they conveyed and had difficulties seeing the dynamics she was describing, or recognizing their son's distress.

At the end of the meeting, the patient preferred to postpone having contact with his family for a while and to stay in the ward, where the system was better coordinated and more comprehensible to him.

In his article "Self-determination theory: A framework for the recovery paradigm," Mancini (2008) portrayed the main aspects of controlling vs. recovery-oriented practices along a continuum. Recovery-oriented practices promote individualism; set goals outside the treatment process such as improving family relationships or finding housing; are client-driven, creating a unique plan for each patient according to his needs; are based on patients' feedback; promote self-motivation and autonomous functioning and allow a variety of choices including medication.

I would like to stress elements of the workbook approach described above, that are in line with the principles of recovery. The workbook presents the patient with openly defined dimensions and no fixed assignments, along with an invitation to seek and define topics that are important for him. This leads to the construction of a unique individual plan for each patient. The process of gradually identifying relevant issues and tasks in cooperation with the team enables the patient to initiate and become active in the process.

Individual and group therapies present opportunities for working on subjectivity, thus promoting individualism. The subject of "life story" that is emphasized in the workbook aims at developing self-cohesion while working on the individual narrative. The simplicity and practicality of the tool, together with the team's orientation, encourage patients to reach higher levels of responsibility and independence regarding their therapeutic processes. This enables patients to acquire and practice skills that will benefit them after discharge. Finally, the presentation of a broad spectrum of issues that the patient and team members address together broadens the scope of therapy and encourages exploration of themes other than medication and illness.

Challenges

Two areas of difficulty to be tackled with when implementing this type of intervention in a hospital ward:

1. Correct use of the workbook to maintain its positive spirit.
2. The scarcity of community facilities that ensure its continuity beyond the period of hospitalization.

Jacobson and Greenley (2001) refer to the recovery process as being complex and requiring motivation, along with a combination of both internal and external needed conditions. As discussed above, the main internal factors are hope, healing, empowerment and connection. External factors important for recovery are a positive culture of healing, the implementation of the principle of human rights and recovery-oriented services.

A positive culture of healing in the health care environment is characterized by empathy, listening, respect, safety and informed consent. Patients and professionals alike are engaged and empowered. They cooperate and acknowledge not only the illness but also strengths, hope and the person as a whole.

Recovery-oriented services deal with the individual, his family and his social context, and are aimed at empowerment and personal meaning. This is achieved in cooperation with the patient through discussions and in the framework of the patient's complex relationships (Jacobson & Greenley, 2001).

In practice, a tool such as the workbook, designed with cooperation and empowerment in mind, can easily become a means of authoritative assignment and supervision. Professionals might be used to being paternalistic. Patients tend to take a passive role because of system expectations and education. Team members might also be inclined to be more authoritative in times of greater workload or burnout.

In working with psychiatric patients diagnosed with severe mental disorders, the tendency to lead the patient correlates with the fact that these patients generally have a weaker ego structure and more negative symptoms. Forensic hospitalization because of a patient's failure to function in a socially acceptable manner might strengthen the tendency to rationalize such approaches.

In attempting to minimize these tendencies, it is important to actively encourage a dialog that promotes healing, respects human rights and is recovery-oriented. As psychologists on the ward, it is our continuous role to promote and develop the use of the workbook and support positive ways of using it. This can be accomplished during weekly rounds and on other occasions, and can thus influence the team's approach and the patterns of communication between team and patients.

We encourage patients to take more responsibility for their rehabilitation process. We teach them to use the workbook, identify and advance goals important to them. In group sessions, we raise subjects of free choice, rehabilitation, stigma, relationship with the psychiatrist and subjective experiences as medication consumers. From time to time, the ward psychologists hold therapeutic group sessions that are dedicated to patients' work with the workbook. In these sessions, the group discusses each patient's therapeutic plan. Patients discuss each other's themes and suggest additional important areas for work or assignments that can suit each patient's needs. Such sessions with the psychologists encourage patients' self-advocacy and awareness of ownership of their therapeutic plans. Internalization of this method of work is crucial to the added therapeutic value of the workbook.

A second area of difficulty is the lack of continuity following discharge from the ward. Sufficient services beyond the boundaries of the ward are lacking, both during hospitalization (for example, a range of training programs or sheltered employment) and following discharge. Community mental health services are scarce, and psychiatrists have considerable workloads. Sheltered employment services, sheltered housing and support systems of case management and psychotherapy are neither varied nor sufficiently accessible (Hoschl et al., 2012).

Summary

As a clinical psychologist in a psychiatric hospital ward, I see great importance in working with patients individually, and according to their unique personalities, strengths, needs and problems. It is my belief that a therapeutic process can only take place within a framework of meaningful dialog. I consider it important to allow room for working through internal processes, providing information, developing insight, strengthening the ego, working on skills of self-advocacy and the ability to find support and help in the community.

On a psychiatric ward, where hospitalized people tend to comply with the role of an ill and disempowered patient, it is important to preserve the patient's subjectivity and to revive, time and again, questions of meaning and choice. I strive to act against stagnation, to encourage the search for strengths and to advance the processes of integration and recovery.

The ward and its team are subject to constraints in ways parallel to those that affect patients: The hospital structure, the well-defined hierarchy, the uniformity of regulations, the need to maintain a fixed routine and clear boundaries between the ward and the external world, and between therapists and patients, all promote a view that the patient is one of many. The psychologist's contribution is in his ability to see each patient as an individual with subjective experiences and needs. Working together with staff through the process of developing and implementing the workbook allowed us to advance this view of the patient as a subjective individual on the ward. My impression is that for most patients, working with this tool encouraged a more positive and active approach, and enhanced creativity and flexibility. Most important, the introduction of the tool strengthened patients' feelings of control and of hope throughout hospitalization.

References

Hoschl, C., Winkler, P. & Pěč, O. (2012). The state of psychiatry in the Czech Republic. *International Review of Psychiatry*, *24*(4), 278–285.

Jacobson, N. & Greenley, D. (2001). What is recovery? A conceptual model and explication. *Psychiatric Services*, *52*, 482–485.

Kalina, K. (2013). Terapeutické komunity v adiktologii. *Psychoterapeutické Systémy a Jejich Uplatnění v Adiktologii* (pp. 461–468). Prague, Czech Republic: Grada Publishing.

Mancini, A.D. (2008). Self-determination theory: A framework for the recovery paradigm. *Advances in Psychiatric Treatment*, *14*, 358–365.

Švarc, J. (2008). Omezující prostředky v psychiatrii. *Psychiatrie pro Praxi*, *9*(5), 243–245.

8 On Trying to Stay Sane in Insane Places

A Personal Account of a Clinical Psychologist's Challenges on the Psychiatric Inpatient Ward

Jim Geekie

Curiosity about the human condition was the driving force behind my becoming a clinical psychologist. From as far back as I remember, I have found myself wondering about what goes on in other people's minds, about the nature of consciousness – other people's as well as my own – and, among countless other things, about how we go about the business of navigating our way through the murky, uncertain social worlds that we find ourselves in. As a child, my personal circumstances were such that I had very good reason to want to understand, and, if possible, predict the behaviour of others in my immediate environment. I also needed to find a place to retreat to following those occasions when, despite my best efforts, I was unable to anticipate events sufficiently to allow me to avoid the violence that I was subjected to on a fairly regular basis. The natural – or perhaps the only available – place to retreat to at these times was my own internal space, where I cultivated a rich inner world that both afforded me some protection and provided me with further material to feed my curiosity about the human condition.

Looking back, I can see that this state of affairs was conducive to nurturing my interest in understanding human experience. Though my route to university was somewhat unconventional, having left school at 15 years old, when I did reach the point of applying to obtain a degree, I had no doubt at all about what I wanted to study: philosophy and psychology, both of which at the time I saw as being congruent with my drive to further explore the nature of being. Despite a few disappointments along the way, I am happy to say that I am now some 25 years plus into my career as a clinical psychologist (having made a pragmatic decision to prioritise psychology over philosophy in the latter years of my undergraduate studies). I feel fortunate indeed that I have been able to find a profession that not only provides me with sufficient income for a comfortable enough life but more importantly does so while allowing me to continue to explore the questions about being human that have been my preoccupations since childhood.

Working as a psychologist afforded me opportunities to explore human experience in ways that may otherwise have been impossible for me. Fairly early on in my working life, I realised that I was particularly drawn to working with those who have out of the ordinary experiences. Where the very nature of what constitutes 'reality' seems to be called into question: seeing or hearing things that others can't or don't see or hear; believing things that others view not only as false but as patently impossible and so absurd. In short, I found that working with those who experience psychosis felt, quite simply, like a natural fit for me. My curiosity was piqued, and I found I had unbidden, but entirely welcome, feelings of empathy and compassion for those who found themselves troubled by experiences of this nature. I have written elsewhere about my work with those who have such experiences (Geekie & Read, 2009; Geekie, Randal, Lampshire & Read, 2012).

It took me a good 10 years of working in this area before, as a result of a particularly helpful discussion in clinical supervision, it suddenly dawned on me that my comfort with, curiosity about – and indeed attraction to – psychotic states of being, may be at least partly attributable to my having spent a significant portion of my critical childhood years being cared for by my mother who, at that time, was clearly psychotic, a position she retreated to as her way of surviving a physically abusive relationship.

After just short of 20 years of working almost exclusively with those who experience psychosis, primarily in community settings, within early interventions for psychosis services in both New Zealand and in UK, I decided to move out of what had become a clinical comfort zone for me and to work in an area with which I was less familiar and which I expected to be far more challenging. I took a job in an acute inpatient unit in the southeast of England. That was 18 months prior to writing this chapter, which is my attempt to summarise my subjective experience of working in this setting over this time. By way of context setting, I should mention that this is a National Health Service (NHS) mental health unit, with four wards and around 70 beds in total. Geographically, the region covered by the unit consists of a predominantly working-class area, including some pockets of significant socio-economic deprivation. It was with considerable trepidation that I accepted the post as I anticipated, rightly as it turned out, that there would be much that I would struggle with in terms of the nature of the working environment, including what I can only refer to as the extreme medicalisation of human distress and the commonplace deprivation of liberty through the almost casual (as it seemed to me) use of mental health legislation to compel service users to accept the overwhelmingly medical treatment. I should point out that this was not my first experience of working on an inpatient unit. I have had reason to visit many inpatient units as part of my previous jobs and had worked part-time for six months in a similar setting in Auckland, New Zealand. However, this time felt different, as this was to be my full-time, permanent occupation, so I expected to feel more immersed in the unit.

The Inpatient Job

My motivation for taking this post was more than just to test myself in a new working environment. It is reasonable to postulate that if we want to understand anything about the human condition, then attending to the stories of those who experience extreme states of distress or confusion must be fairly high up our agenda. Similarly, looking at how we as a society have chosen to care for those in such states must, it seems to me, involve grappling with some difficult and delicate ethical and social questions relating to the nature of this care and, in particular, to consider what role, if any, legislation should have in the provision of such care. Here, I concur with Jaspers' (1963, p. 309) argument that 'In psychotic reality we find an abundance of content representing the fundamental problems of philosophy', though to this I would add that profound ethical, moral and social considerations are unavoidable the moment we consider if and how, as individuals, as families and as a society, we ought to relate to those who may experience these extreme states. As cogently argued by Bentall (1992), classifying certain human experiences as 'mental illness' inevitably involves value judgements which, ultimately, are impossible to justify on scientific grounds alone.

However naively, I was drawn to working in an inpatient setting because I thought of this setting as the frontline where these fundamental problems would be manifest. Not for a second do I wish to suggest that in this chapter I will do much more than merely acknowledge these challenges. They are, I believe, inherent in all areas of mental health care, though nowhere are they more blatantly obvious than in acute inpatient settings. My ambitions in this chapter are more modest. I hope to give something of the flavour of what it feels like (or at least, what it felt like for me) to be a clinical psychologist working in the kind of setting described by Isabel Clarke (2009, p. 2) as 'the last bastion of the medical model in its pure form'. Rather than try to give a comprehensive overview of my experience, in this chapter I will instead focus primarily on two specific aspects of my experience that made a significant impact on me: the ward atmosphere and the clinical work, particularly how being part of a multidisciplinary team impacted on this. I happened to keep a journal over my time working in the wards and will, from time to time, quote directly from this as it best conveys my experience at the time.

The Ward Atmosphere

Reflecting on my initial impression of the wards, gathered as I was being shown around by a colleague, I am struck by memories that are predominantly non-verbal in nature, relating, as they do, to my sense of the atmosphere of the ward. Of course, I noticed, and could easily describe to you some of the objectively observable 'facts' of the ward – the physical layout, the number of staff, the interior design – all of which did make an impression on me. But, my overarching recollection of my initial experiences on the ward is something more ethereal, less tangible. 'Atmosphere' may be difficult to operationalise or quantify, though that makes it no less real and certainly no less central to what it was about the ward that made the greatest impression on me. It was an atmosphere of hopelessness. At times an angry hopelessness. Anger fuelled by the person's conviction that he or she should not be there. A deeply felt and sharply expressed sense of injustice. Hopelessness fuelled by the recognition, based no doubt on experience that expressing opposition to the legitimacy of being detained is futile.

My first few visits to the wards often involved service users rushing up to me, recognising me as a new face and possibly assuming from my age, dress and gender that I might be someone with influence on the ward. Many seem hungry for something and immediately try to impress upon me the legitimacy of their story and the illegitimacy of their detention in hospital; others, perhaps a little more experienced in the ways of the ward, first endeavour to establish who I am and whether or not I can help them to achieve their goal. Most commonly, this entails asking me 'Are you a doctor?' My answer to this question determines what will happen next. Most commonly, the person then lets me know, one way or another, that as I'm not a medical doctor I'm not much use to them. From this, I learn very early on that the service users – 'patients' here – see power as residing within the medical staff. In fact, most service users do not approach me in this way; though the few who do, have the most immediate impact on me. I also see other patients – am I already using that term? – who watch me and are clearly weighing me up, getting a sense of who I am and what I do, but are not about to approach me. Not yet anyway. Others still are, or at least seem, oblivious to my presence. Indeed, oblivious to their own surroundings. I wonder why. It is early morning: are they already sedated? Those seemingly passive and docile service users trouble me the most. I wonder what I might be able to offer people who are struggling to stay awake.

Images from *One Flew over the Cuckoo's Nest* flash before me. At the time, that felt clichéd. It still does. But, as I looked around, I found it difficult to see any significant differences between the depiction in the movie and what I was seeing around me on this ward. In truth, I felt despondent. Not too surprised, but nonetheless dejected. I also worried that I might be projecting my own prejudices on to this place. I came expecting to find somewhere I would be critical of: what is the surprise in my finding that? I considered the possibility that my expectations were colouring what I was seeing. With all of those doubts in mind,

I still could not shake off that initial impression that the environment, the atmosphere, in this place was permeated with a sense of hopelessness. I wanted to immunise myself against that, as I feared it would be easy to absorb and reflect the very same attitude. I doubted that I could fully prevent that from happening.

These initial impressions of the ward never completely left me, though over time I became more accustomed to them: this worried me, lest I became blasé about something I actually found intolerable. I also became more sensitive to subtle but important variations in the ward atmosphere, which could fluctuate from tense and volatile to lethargic and lifeless. What remained constant though was my sense that focussing only on the 'patients', while ignoring the environment, was problematic. In fact, as I look over my journal, I see that there were times when I was deeply troubled by the environment. After four months into the job, I wrote:

> Truth be told there are times when I find the ward absolutely abhorrent. That's not an overstatement. I find it a horrendous place, filled with a toxicity that reaches my very soul. How can I stay working in a place that I feel that way about? My not working here will, of course, have no impact on the place continuing to exist, only it will not exist as part of my world. Is that OK?

A few months later, clearly concerned that I would become so acclimated to the ward that I would fail to notice what it was actually like:

> How do you protect yourself from such a toxic environment? Would you even recognise when you've been infected? What are the early signs?

I was not alone in struggling with the ward environment. Service users consistently told me they found the wards very difficult places to be: unpredictable yet boring, restricted in the range of activities available and – most damning of all – lacking in compassion. I struggled to establish how I could work therapeutically in such a counter-therapeutic environment. I tried to change it, but I also recognised that my strengths, such that they are, involve working with individuals rather than systemically. I felt ill-equipped to address what I came to see as the underlying problems:

> It feels more and more that we are treating the patients (as they're called here) when the real problem is with the environment. Is my job simply to help people endure an intolerable environment?

Perhaps one could argue that some of the contradictions within psychology are simply laid bare in inpatient settings: if psychological struggles are largely attributable to being subjected to harsh environments, what is the value of an intervention that aims to modify a few intra-psychic processes (be they cognitive, emotional or dynamic)? Profoundly troubling though this proposition is, for better or worse, I found myself working in an inpatient setting, with the expectation that I offer input to the care provided to service users on the ward and this was a major component of my work on the wards. So, what can I say about my actual clinical work on the ward?

The Clinical Work

When I reflect on this, I find it necessary to distinguish between the direct clinical work – by which I mean immediate involvement with service users (and occasionally family/carers) – and my work as part of the multi-disciplinary team (MDT) responsible for providing care on the ward. I have, over the course of my career, worked in many multi-disciplinary teams and, overall, I think I can say that while there are always tensions between different perspectives on and approaches to working with distress, generally speaking I think these tensions can be acknowledged and addressed, sometimes leading to very effective interventions for the service user. My experience is that in inpatient settings, and certainly in the one discussed here, achieving this effective MDT working is much more difficult. Before considering why this might be so, let me first describe my experience of working in these different domains.

I can say without hesitation that I love – really love – the direct clinical work. The conversations I have with service users are incredibly varied, poignant, intense, sometimes difficult, often distressing but always engaging, always human. I have no doubt that this is the part of the work that has sustained me over my time working on the wards. I feel truly privileged to be trusted, as I often am, with stories of great struggles; to be witness to such a vast array of intense human experience; to be privy to at times overwhelming and almost tangible existential angst; to hear tragic, sometimes as yet untold, stories of abuse of trust, abuse of power; and alongside all of this to see – even if sometimes the service user cannot – the great courage that has been shown in the face of such adversity. The human, all too human, endeavour to find a way of being and of relating to others and the world around us that provides meaning, purpose and – if we're fortunate – something resembling pleasure. For me (and I hope that this doesn't sound too corny or pious, though I fear it might be a bit of both), working with people detained in an inpatient unit is to have the honour, and the responsibility, of operating on the coalface, the front line of the essence of what it is to be human. What I mean by this rather glib statement is that

I believe that if we are truly interested in the nature of what we mean by and how we construe reality, if we want to understand what it means to be a 'self', if we want to appreciate the impact that trauma can have on our well-being; in short if we want to better understand some of the fundamental problems of philosophy referred to by Jaspers (1963) then we have to be prepared to listen to and learn from those who experience the kind of extreme states that are commonly associated with being admitted to an inpatient unit. And for me, to fail to acknowledge this is a great tragedy. To reduce these experiences to little more than symptoms of a putative 'mental illness' is to completely overlook the potential for enriching our understanding in the broadest sense of what it means to be human. Worse, it is, I believe, to compound the struggles of those who have such experiences by locating the cause of these troubles firmly within the individual, decontextualised, ahistorical and meaningless.

With the above position as my starting point, it will come as no surprise to hear that I have found it difficult to fit within the MDT. The unit where I work, which I take to be fairly typical of inpatient units in UK and, I assume, much of the rest of the world, operates within a strongly medical framework, both in terms of the conceptualisation of distress, but also, importantly, in terms of the power dynamics within the unit, where the dominant, decision-making narrative is that of psychiatry. Here, from my journal, one of the many entries I made on the struggle I had in reconciling my view with the model of care in the unit:

> Everything seems to revolve around diagnoses and medication. As if we are treating brains, not people; neurotransmitters not whole living beings. The impression is that people are little more than vehicles for neurotransmitters, neuro-receptors and putative brain states that are best understood as diagnoses. It's bad enough when it feels that the person is reduced to a diagnosis, but worse when the person is reduced to a brain state which itself is reduced to or explained in terms of a diagnosis and nothing but a diagnosis.

I endeavoured to shift this narrative through my contributions to the MDT discussions, sometimes by doing little more than drawing attention to some of the life events – and often these included extensive trauma histories – that the service user had been subjected to. It felt to me that I was doing little more than pointing out that we were discussing an individual with a history and a context, both of which would need to be taken into account if we hoped to make any useful sense of what it was that was troubling the individual. Over time, I believe there was some recognition that being aware of and sensitive to the individual's personal history and circumstances were necessary considerations in engaging the service user in treatment. Indeed, there was often a request for psychology input from the MDT when it was clear that there were things that had gone on in the service user's life that contributed to how the individual was presenting and in particular to how he or she was relating to other members of the MDT. Not infrequently, this would lead to my meeting up with the service user who would commonly express great relief that at last there was someone interested in listening to his or her story. And, this in turn did, I believe, at times lead to a psychological intervention that was valued by the service user – as well as by the MDT. What I struggle with though is the question of if and how this psychological approach, effective and appreciated by the service user though it may be, sits within the overarching model of the medicalisation of distress.

Newnes (2011), drawing from the work of Goldie (1977), has written about the positioning of clinical psychologists within psychiatric settings, characterising this as 'compliant, eclectic or in radical opposition', going on to suggest that the latter 'might take up a public opposition to the dominant medical discourse or leave the conflict zone' (p. 217). Reading this led to me reflecting on the position I adopted within this particular psychiatric setting. While confident that I do not endorse the biomedical conceptualisation or treatment, I fear that my ability to articulate an alternative to this has been limited, particularly on a systemic level. Working 1:1 with service users, I have had little trouble in considering, even encouraging, ways of understanding and relating to distress that is not limited to the dominant biomedical discourse. I know too that this approach was often valued by service users who found it helpful to have the opportunity to explore the meaning of their experience. But, if I am honest with myself, I feel obliged to admit that the position I have adopted is one where I operate 'under the radar', away from the direct gaze of the medical model and so avoiding direct confrontation. No doubt, there is an element of self-preservation in this: I suspect that were I to be more confrontational, I would find myself even more isolated, potentially even jeopardising my position. This is not to say that I have not made efforts to contribute to systemic change: I repeatedly draw attention to the role of trauma in contributing to distress; I argue for increased service user involvement in the unit; I try to encourage more compassionate approaches based on understanding service users' troubles in the context of the lives they have led. But, ultimately, I feel such efforts have been largely fruitless. Hence, I have retreated to what I think of as working more in parallel to rather than within the MDT. This may not be an entirely satisfactory state of affairs; certainly, I don't feel comfortable with this myself, but, for better or worse, I think this is a fairly accurate description of how I have come to position myself with the team and in relation to service users.

Conclusion

As I approach the end of this chapter, I find myself reaching for a satisfactory way of summarising my experience of working as a clinical psychologist in an inpatient setting. That may prove impossible, but I do hope I have drawn attention to some of the challenges I have had working in this kind of environment and I hope that some of my personal struggles will resonate with others and may shed some light on what it feels like to be an inpatient psychologist, even if I am short of solutions to the dilemmas raised. I am somewhat reassured that when I look at the literature which investigates the subjective experience of working in this area, psychologists and other professionals make observations not too dissimilar to my own. In an unpublished thesis exploring clinical psychologists' experiences of inpatient work, Bentley (2014) reported dominant themes that emerged from her qualitative analysis including feeling unable to 'fight the system' and finding no easy resolution to the mismatch between their professional and personal values and the model of care in the units they work in.

My own personal view is that the question of how clinical psychology positions itself vis-à-vis a dominant psychiatric discourse is a critical one; my experience suggests to me that this is nowhere more pronounced than in inpatient settings where the medicalisation of distress continues to have a relative hegemony. As a profession, I believe clinical psychology has to give serious consideration to the question of how to position itself: as an adjunct to medicalisation or as an alternative approach to thinking about and relating to the experience of distress. On a personal level, based on the experiences described in this chapter, I have reached the position that, ultimately, working within the system, I have been ineffective at making the kinds of changes that would make it possible for me to remain in post. My resolution to the many ethical, clinical and personal dilemmas that working within this particular inpatient setting entails for me has been, to quote Newnes (2011), 'to leave the battlefield'. At least to leave the immediate battlefield of working in an inpatient setting, having decided over the course of writing this chapter that the personal and professional compromises required to survive in this environment are intolerable to me. Ultimately, I found it impossible to persuade myself that working within a system that clashes in such a fundamental way with so many of my personal values was a tenable possibility. Believing, as I do, that human distress is better understood and related to as a response to painful and confusing life events, I was unable to reconcile this with working in an environment that seemed to replicate many of the experiences that had led to the individual being so troubled in the first place.

I hope to find another way of fighting for mental health services – including residential or inpatient services – that are informed by curiosity and compassion and that recognise that people, service users and clinicians alike, are shaped by their personal histories and social contexts. I have now moved on from this inpatient post, having resigned myself to the impossibility of reaching any reconciliation between my values and those that dominate on the unit. In hindsight, this outcome was perhaps inevitable, as indicated in the entry below, taken from my journal and written after only three months in the job:

> I picture myself as witnessing the sledgehammer of psychiatry struggling but failing miserably to come to terms with the unpredictable vicissitudes of our precarious human existence. Does shoehorning people's existential dilemmas into psychiatric nosology shed any light on our suffering? I think not.

References

Bentall, R.P. (1992). A proposal to classify happiness as a psychiatric disorder. *Journal of Medical Ethics 18*(2), 94–98.

Bentley, M.C. (2014). *How clinical psychologists experience working in an acute mental health inpatient setting*. Unpublished thesis, University of Hertfordshire. Retrieved from: http://uhra.herts.ac.uk/handle/2299/14328.

Clarke, I. (2009). Introduction. In I. Clarke & H. Wilson (Eds.), *Cognitive behaviour therapy for acute inpatient mental health units. Working with clients, staff and the milieu* (pp. 1–9). London: Routledge.

Geekie, J., Randal, P., Lampshire, D. & Read, J. (Eds.) (2012). *Experiencing psychosis: Personal and professional perspectives*. Hove, UK: Routledge.

Geekie, J. & Read J. (2009). *Making sense of madness: Contesting the meaning of schizophrenia*. Hove, UK: Routledge.

Goldie, N. (1977). The division of labour among the mental health professions. In M. Stacey, M. Reid, C. Heath & R. Dingwall (Eds.), *Health and the division of labour* (pp. 141–161). London: Croom Helm.

Jaspers, K. (1963). *General psychopathology*. Manchester, UK: Manchester University Press.

Newnes, C. (2011). Toxic psychology. In M. Rapley, J. Moncrieff & J. Dillon (Eds.), *Demedicalizing misery: Psychiatry, psychology and the human condition* (pp. 211–225). Basingstoke, UK: Palgrave MacMillan.

9 A Path Taken

A Psychologist's Professional Journey Within the Psychiatric Inpatient System

Michael Siglag

Historical Perspective

During the mid to late 1800s, Dorothea Dix, a former superintendent of nurses during the American Civil War, and like-minded political and social leaders sought to provide humane settings for people who were seen as presenting with emotional and behavioral disturbances. These individuals were often isolated, and sometimes treated in brutal ways. Improvements in treatment promoted by Dix and others during this time were influenced by the 'moral treatment' model. 'Moral treatment' was characterized primarily by care and treatment guided by attitudes of kindness and compassion. In addition, under the 'moral treatment' model, individuals presenting what we now call severe behavioral or psychiatric disturbance or psychological distress were considered capable of recovering and returning to productive lives in society. Aspects of the moral treatment model have continued to influence treatment to the present time, but the predominance of the moral treatment movement in shaping psychiatric hospital treatment has declined over time.

Multiple factors led to shifts in treatment emphasis from the 'moral treatment' model. Among the most significant circumstances driving changes between the nineteenth century and mid-twentieth century was the tremendous expansion of the number of people housed in the large facilities that were built during that time period. Among other factors, increasing numbers of people needing to be cared for in these facilities eventually stimulated an increasing emphasis and reliance on biologically based treatments. This expanded use of biologically based treatments was generated by the perception that such treatments could help provide relief to the increasing number of patients crowding the facilities. Biologically-based treatments included approaches that currently seem extreme, but that for a time were seen by many as 'state of the art' medicine. For example, biological interventions that were widely practiced included bloodletting, purging, prefrontal lobotomy, intentional initiation of seizures, and a focal infection model which posited that physical organs contained toxins that were the source of mental disturbance and that to cure the patient the affected organs needed to be removed. Many individuals died or were maimed as a result of such procedures, and such treatments became generally discredited over time. Current 'state of the art' biologically-based treatments primarily consist of psychotropic medication and electroconvulsive therapy (ECT). Many vouch for the benefits of these biological treatments, including both practitioners and patients. However, ongoing debates exist among professionals and consumers regarding the validity, effectiveness, and both positive and negative impacts of the current biologically based approaches to treatment (Whitaker, 2010).

Echoing ideas articulated in nineteenth-century moral treatment, recognition has grown that many people suffering from psychosis and other severe emotional and behavioral disturbances can recover when engaged in adequate treatment and provided with needed support. In many instances, people suffering such disturbances are able to return to successful lives in the community. It is now also recognized that severe disturbance and life-disrupting symptoms could be related to traumatic life experiences. Many therapeutic approaches focusing on interpersonal and emotional dimensions of experience have been recognized as effective, at times in conjunction with and at times without biological interventions. Interpersonal and other psychological and rehabilitative treatments have reasserted an important role in psychiatric hospital or inpatient mental health treatment and follow-up treatment. Most recently, factors such as an increasingly vocal and sophisticated consumer movement, the 'recovery' movement, gradual influence and incorporation of biopsychosocial models, recognition of trauma as a significant factor in emotional disturbance, and an effort to establish and utilize a broad array of evidence-based psychological treatments have all played roles. These and other factors, including a trend toward the reduction in the number of public institutions, and a greater concentration in these institutions of individuals presenting with more severe disturbance and co-occurring legal issues, have led to shifts in treatment approaches.

For psychologists working in psychiatric hospital environments, it can be helpful to know about the history of treatment in such settings, and the shifts and cycles that have taken place in the types and expectations of treatment. Knowledge of the historical shifts in purpose, function, and hoped for results that have changed over time in such facilities can influence how we perceive the facilities, the individuals who reside and are treated there, current treatment emphases and trends, and current political and administrative pressures. Such awareness can contribute, and one could argue should contribute, to the ways we perceive and carry out our roles.

A Spectrum of Experience

An interest in working with people presenting serious, life-disrupting emotional and behavioral problems motivated me to become a psychologist and led me to take the professional path I have pursued for over 30 years. From early on in my career, my interests led me to seek training and then to work with adults in inpatient psychiatric settings, particularly public institutions. For more than 30 years, after my initial training practicums and internships, I served as a psychologist in public psychiatric institutions. While doing my best to benefit the individuals I worked with in treatment, I also recognized and experienced many of the obstacles inherent to treating people in these settings.

My pre-doctoral internship in the early 1980s was at Essex County Hospital Center (ECHC). ECHC was the largest functioning county psychiatric hospital in the country at the time and served a population similar to those in state hospital settings. Following my internship, I accepted a position as a staff psychologist at Trenton Psychiatric Hospital (TPH), founded in 1848, one of the many hospitals founded by Dorothea Dix. The building housing Dorothea Dix's office there had been dismantled, but some of her memorabilia remained. Trees Dorothea Dix had planted during the 1800s grew throughout the expansive grounds more than a century later.

Over time, my roles varied. I worked as a unit psychologist and later as 'Chief of Psychology Services' in a community transition unit, unit psychologist in an admissions unit, 'Director' of an American Psychological Association (APA) accredited pre-doctoral internship program, and 'Acting Director' of the psychology department. After almost 30 years working at Trenton Psychiatric Hospital, I took a position at New Jersey's Ann Klein Forensic Center (AKFC) to pursue more specialized work with the forensic psychiatric population there. As a psychologist at Ann Klein, I worked on a forensic admission/ITU/crisis unit and carried out evaluations inside the hospital and in correctional settings in New Jersey. Each of these positions provided different challenges and rewards.

Applying Training to Experience

When I began working as a staff psychologist at TPH during the 1980s, I was lucky enough to provide services on a unit that was unusual, in both its' function and physical setting. The unit functioned as a 'biopsychosocial rehabilitation' program. While this unit was on the grounds of the hospital, and was considered a hospital unit, the unit was structured physically as a kind of neighborhood. Twelve houses that formerly had served as homes for hospital physicians were arranged in a circle. The houses were not locked, but patients who lived in them were supervised by staff 24 hours a day, similar to the way many group homes were managed in the community. Patients shared chores, largely based on willingness and ability, including cooking meals. Each resident had a schedule of therapeutic activities and groups that were mostly provided outside the homes, including psychological therapies. Some attended occupational therapies or vocational training activities in the hospital's greenhouses. Many took part in a vocational rehabilitation program which involved working in a variety of positions under staff supervision on the hospital grounds. Patients were encouraged to participate in selecting the activities and groups on their schedule. There was a 'level system' allowing many patients to leave the hospital either accompanied or unaccompanied. Many patients or residents went on visits off-grounds accompanied by family or approved friends. Visits could be as brief as several hours to as long as several nights. Overnight visits were expected to prepare residents for discharge. A small but significant number of patients were allowed to leave the hospital on their own for preauthorized periods of time, usually during the weekend. They would typically take buses into the local community in order to attend movies, eat at inexpensive restaurants, and buy personal items at shopping malls. These visits helped reorient residents to the community. An explicit goal of the program at that time was to help people hospitalized in our setting to make successful transitions back into the community.

Staff who supervised the homes were mostly from the nearby Trenton community where many patients on the unit also had lived. The ages and personalities of staff varied, and the patients came from diverse backgrounds and different localities in New Jersey. Many staff members were middle-aged and behaved in a parental manner toward the residents. There was a familial feeling in many of the cottages.

The process of filling beds when vacancies occurred generally involved screening and selecting patients from locked units in other parts of the hospital. The screening process included reviewing clinical records, speaking to treatment team members, and interviewing the patients themselves. In carrying out these screenings, efforts were made to find potential residents who would fit best into the cottages where there were vacancies. We developed expertise at determining what made it likely that someone would do well in the more open setting and whether they would fit best into a particular cottage.

Psychologists in the early to mid-1980s served as treatment team members, assisting with treatment planning and other team functions such as addressing emergent crises, and creating documents in preparation for court hearings. We also provided individual therapy, ran therapy groups, and carried out a variety of assessments. Assessments typically were by referral and included evaluations of personality and intellectual functioning. For some patients, especially those who had previously harmed themselves or others, we also evaluated their risk of engaging in future aggressive or suicidal behaviors. In addition, some of our psychologists, including myself, testified at regular court reviews, primarily in connection with patients hospitalized after having been found 'Not Guilty by Reason of Insanity' in the New Jersey criminal court system. Psychologists' roles could vary depending on the unit one was assigned, and we had a broad array of duties.

I worked on the above-mentioned unit for more than 20 years. During that time, the program helped transition hundreds and possibly thousands of hospitalized individuals back into the community. Many patients who had functioned with difficulty on locked units got back on their feet while residing in this more open unit. This unit was given different names over time, including the Transitional Living Unit, and the Travers Complex. The latter name honored a woman I had been lucky enough to work with, Agnes Travers. Agnes was an impressive woman who had worked her way up from a nursing role to become the administrator of the unit before she retired. She embodied the warm, caring, and 'tough when necessary' qualities that were evident in many of the staff working at that time.

As a psychologist, I attempted to apply much of what I had learned in my training. When I began working on this unit, I was still working on a doctoral dissertation in which I looked at commonalities and differences between 'schizophrenic' and 'mystical' experiences. In my clinical work, I kept in mind my working hypothesis that people who were experiencing psychosis or were diagnosed as schizophrenic were struggling with profound emotional and spiritual crises. I considered the possible outcomes of such crises to include varying degrees of growth or decline and debilitation. The outcome for each individual depended on their resolution of the personal crisis with which they struggled. As a psychologist, I saw my role as listening to them, helping them understand what they were going through, and attempting to help them through their struggle.

I had been introduced to the idea that psychological therapies could be effective means of treatment for disturbance as severe as psychosis by working with supervisors who provided such services, and by reading about others who did such work. Perhaps the most influential work of professional literature for me was Bertram Karon and Gary Vandenbos' book, *Psychotherapy of Schizophrenia Treatment of Choice* (1981), a book introduced to me by an influential supervisor. I read this work when I was in graduate school, not long after it had been published.

I found the central idea asserted in this book to be powerful, and the rationale described in the book plausible. Karon and Vandenbos asserted that people who were psychotic could be helped by a verbal therapy that was based in psychoanalytic thinking. Over time, I applied the ideas and approaches described in this book, also incorporating other ideas and lessons. What I found particularly compelling about Karon and Vandenbos' assertions was that psychotic symptoms were to a large extent, for many individuals, a reaction to traumatic life experiences. Over time, other professional literature that

I read, and supervision and professional training opportunities all provided additional support for this idea. The more I worked as a psychologist and listened to individuals presenting with psychosis describe their experiences, the more links I heard between individuals' traumatic life experiences and their development of psychosis, as well as manifestations of other forms of emotional distress.

As my interest in the impact of traumatic experiences and issues such as protective factors and resilience grew, the more I heard many of the patients I worked with describe having experienced emotional, physical, and sexual abuse. I became interested in understanding and treating the consequences of a traumatic experience such as posttraumatic stress disorder (PTSD). When I had a hospitalized patient come into my office one day and ask if it would be okay if another person inside of him spoke with me that day, I knew that I better learn more about dissociative disorders such as Multiple Personality Disorder, which later became known as Dissociative Identity Disorder.

During this time, I became the unit's psychology staff manager, or 'Chief of Psychology Service.' It was important to me that unit psychologists utilize their expertise to provide individual therapy to the extent that was reasonable and possible. I also prioritized expanding group therapy offerings to reach more people in meaningful ways by establishing groups which addressed specific needs. I increased my education in group therapy through readings, obtaining supervision, and attending conferences. I worked to achieve the American Group Psychotherapy Association criteria for Certified Group Therapist status and met this goal. I found two works, quite different, but with similar titles, to be particularly helpful: *Inpatient Group Psychotherapy* by Irvin Yalom (1983), and *Inpatient Group Psychotherapy: A Psychodynamic Perspective* by Cecil Rice and Scott Rutan (1987). Yalom's book provided much useful information and practical guidance related to running groups utilizing a short-term focused model. And Rice and Rutan's book provided historical background and a psychodynamic and systems perspective that resonated strongly with my experience. Expanding beyond the general process group therapy model, I worked with my staff to provide therapy groups that addressed a range of issues including women's issues, men's issues, assertiveness, anger management, stress management, and psychological trauma. I also began to think about our hospital in a more systemic way, as a setting that was potentially healing on one hand but could also be traumatizing or re-traumatizing for many patients. For example, feeling ignored or neglected, or becoming the target of emotional, physical, and/or sexual violence in the hospital were repetitions of similar experiences that many patients had encountered in their families and/or in the community. For other patients, such traumatic experiences could be new experiences that they had never encountered before.

I studied literature, participated in the research, and published on the impact of traumatic experiences (Siglag, 1999; Lu et al., 2011). I became involved in a number of organizations to further educate myself, both for professional support and to find forums to share my ideas on a range of topics relevant to my work. For example, I presented papers and research at conferences held by the World Association for Psychosocial Rehabilitation, the American Psychological Association, the New Jersey Group Psychotherapy Society, and other professional organizations. I joined a professional study group on dissociative disorders. In some instances, I joined professional organizations whose members shared my interests, and I became involved in the leadership hierarchy of those organizations.

During that time, I also became the Director of our APA accredited pre-doctoral psychology internship training program. I served in that role for approximately 20 years. Directing the internship program provided me with an opportunity to initiate developing professionals into psychiatric hospital work. This role also presented me with a chance to expose interns to research and work that I considered to be especially important, and that I saw as potentially influential on the work they might do subsequent to their internship experiences. I expanded an existing didactic training program, as well as initiating a group therapy seminar and a trauma issues seminar in order to provide more in-depth training for staff and interns. In these training seminars, I invited interns to also share their own interests and perspectives which were often well thought out and were consistently challenging and thought-provoking.

In order to succeed as director of the internship program, it was necessary for me to utilize and further develop my leadership skills. While my psychology department director was very supportive of me in the 'internship director' role, much work needed to be done with fellow psychology staff members and hospital administrators to make the program work. I needed to obtain institutional support for the time, work, and financial resources required for the program to flourish. Most psychologists enjoyed the rewards inherent in providing supervision and mentoring. It was generally easy to engage staff in aspects of supervision that they enjoyed. But I also had to find ways to engage the staff in some of the more tedious and time-consuming aspects of supervision. These included tasks such as completion of evaluation forms, screening application materials, and interviewing applicants. It was important to make the internship an investment shared by the whole department. While difficult and demanding in many ways, running an APA accredited internship program provided many rewards. The program was beneficial for the department and hospital in numerous ways. Our repeated successes with accreditation reviews were reinforcing and sustained the support we enjoyed from the hospital administration, and also from the state itself. Our program was an asset for patients and staff. Our accreditation review successes were feathers in the cap of the TPH psychology department, the hospital itself, and even for the New Jersey state officials who budgeted money annually in order to support our program.

Tectonic Plates Shifting

While I was focused on directing the internship program, and the work I was doing with the team and the patients residing in my unit, new legal and policy developments had been emerging on bigger stages that would profoundly affect the work my colleagues and I were doing, and thereby change my own trajectory. The agenda fueling these measures was to improve mental health services throughout the state. 'Wellness and Recovery' was the term given to the state's new approach to mental health services. Legislative and policy changes were enacted to improve mental health services for the state's most seriously disturbed citizens. Hospital administrations changed periodically, but the new administration seemed particularly aggressive about initiating changes in the way things were done. It was apparent that this was partly in response to pressures to conform to the state's new legislative agenda.

Simultaneously, there were new rulings on a federal level that had a direct impact on state psychiatric hospitals across the country, including in New Jersey. Legal challenges relating to patient length of stay in psychiatric hospitals were taking place nationwide—the 1999 federal Olmstead ruling related directly to this issue. The ruling led to new protocols and arrangements within each state, including New Jersey, and established new and more stringent requirements for discharging people from psychiatric hospital settings. Increasingly tighter timelines were put into place, with expensive fines and penalties on the facility and the state if the established goals and timelines were not met. Pressure to discharge people increased. Within the hospital, there was increasing pressure to improve and accelerate treatment results. More emphasis was placed on the implementation of evidence-based and evidence-supported treatments. This process helped fuel the expansion of community-based housing and services aimed at facilitating discharge of those ready for discharge. New community-based housing and support programs, and additional funding for previously established programs helped to increase the rate of discharge for those considered capable of succeeding in the community.

However, with increased success came added challenges. The patients who remained hospitalized tended to be more disturbed and more difficult to prepare for discharge. Many of these patients were more difficult to engage in treatment activities and were less responsive to the hospital treatments in which they did engage. The concentration of hospitalized patients presenting with concomitant serious legal issues and psychiatric issues increased. For these and other reasons, as the pressures to discharge hospitalized individuals intensified, many of those remaining in hospitals were more difficult to return to the community. As in other states, New Jersey's efforts to appropriately discharge people in reasonable amounts of time was complicated by the closing of some state psychiatric hospitals as well as some facilities which provided treatment for people with developmental disturbance or intellectual disability. Increasing numbers of individuals with developmental, intellectual, or cognitive delays, who were discharged from specialized facilities to group homes and other less restrictive settings, were struggling in the community. Many were then admitted to the lessening number of beds in the remaining psychiatric hospitals. As these and other pressures mounted, one of the psychologists in my department commented shortly after announcing her retirement, that 'storm clouds are gathering.'

It was in this changing and pressured environment that TPH's 'Director of Psychology,' who had led the psychology department for close to 30 years, retired. For many of the years that I had worked in the psychology department, he had supported my leadership of our internship program and the transitional cottage services. He was an important mentor for me and other psychologists. Under his leadership, the competencies and roles of psychologists were valued and supported.

After the psychology department 'Director's' departure, I was selected to serve as 'Acting Director' of the psychology department. I took on the leadership of the department at this turbulent stage, and my time in this role became increasingly tumultuous. Psychologists' and other departments' ways of contributing to patient care and hospital functioning were being re-evaluated. In a short time, it became clear that my ideas concerning how the psychology department could best continue to contribute to the hospital contrasted greatly with new ideas promoted by the existing hospital administration on the best ways to utilize psychologists.

As differences in our thinking became evident, I struggled to ascertain the source of our diverging priorities. Were they based on my sense of the importance of traditional psychologists' roles? It seemed apparent that the hospital administrators' desire for psychologists to take on different roles stemmed at least in part from a wish for psychologists to adapt to new hospital needs and priorities. Were psychologists' traditional therapeutic and assessment roles, and other treatment contributions, valued less by an administration that was more comfortable with a medical model tradition which emphasized biological etiology, rather than a model that emphasized psychological and psychosocial factors? A combination of these and perhaps other factors, appeared to play a role (Shur, 1994). The traditional roles that were historically valued by psychologists were minimized. Pressure increased for psychologists to take on additional roles and functions. Changes in psychologists' functions appeared to be seen by the hospital's administrative leadership as beneficial for the hospital. However, I did not always agree that the proposed changes represented the most beneficial or prudent ways psychologists could contribute to patient treatment and hospital functioning.

About a month after I was appointed as the Acting Director of Psychology, I was asked by the hospital management to explain my 'vision' for the psychology department. I saw our department for the most part as a group of well-trained psychologists who performed professionally, did excellent work that benefited the patients, teams, and hospital, and who were well-respected by their colleagues. When psychologists were supported in carrying out their core functions, patients benefited, and the team was most effective. Psychologists' core functions traditionally involved providing individual and group therapies and carrying out psychological assessments, although psychologists did much more. Additional functions carried out by psychologists included: providing consultation and support for other team members; developing and leading new treatment programs; and performing informal and unscheduled therapeutic interactions. While my vision for the department was still evolving, it included supporting psychologists to carry out the roles they were trained best to do, roles that were traditionally valued. Psychologists should also continue to build upon current services to provide an expanded repertoire of effective treatments and interventions to meet the needs of an increasingly diverse hospital population. I had led psychologists to expand services on a smaller scale when I was Chief of Psychology Services in the Travers Complex. In addition, I saw it as particularly important for psychologists to more effectively address the impact of emotional trauma on patients' experiences, presentations, and behaviors, issues to which I had been sensitized early in my career. Traumatic experiences were increasingly recognized and acknowledged as part of the etiological matrix that influenced and generated many individuals' disturbances. This broader recognition was evidenced by the federal government's Substance Abuse and Mental Health Services Administration's (SAMHSA) increasing emphasis on 'trauma-informed care.' In addition, I saw that trauma related to hospitalization itself could at times undermine a patient's treatment and healing. This was an aspect of hospital experience that needed to be more widely acknowledged by both clinical staff and administration in order to prevent or at least minimize its impact.

My efforts to follow through on these issues led to some collaboration and also some conflicts with senior hospital administrators. For example, I proposed and led a multidisciplinary trauma-informed care workgroup with an administrative colleague. This workgroup successfully carried out several important initiatives, including introducing a personal safety plan tool for patients, and increasing the number and types of groups addressing trauma throughout the hospital. And yet, at the same time, the provision of individual therapy sessions by psychologists, an intervention that I saw as crucial, was being discouraged by senior administrators in favor of group therapy interventions. Up to that point, psychologists had carried out a minimum number of group therapy and individual sessions, which particularly addressed the specific treatment needs they had identified on their units. The de-emphasis of individual therapy sessions, treatment that often reached different individuals than those who participated in groups, was one area of disagreement between myself and the hospital leadership.

Another hospital leadership agenda with which I disagreed was a change in the role of psychologists on treatment teams. I had noticed over the years that psychologists were frequently being pulled into the 'team leader' role. Psychologists could often be effective in such roles, although other professional staff could also be effective.

There was no 'team leader' title in the hospital, so staff from many departments could take on this role, although the duties were most consistent with our psychiatrists' job description. For many years, 'team leader' responsibilities were undertaken by people hired into civil service 'program coordinator' positions. These middle management positions required some degree of clinical training and background. In fact, some 'program coordinators' had graduate degrees in Psychology. At TPH, 'program coordinators' responsibilities included coordinating multidisciplinary teams. Many psychologists also had the skills and training to perform the 'team leader' task and excelled at integrating patients' and professional and paraprofessional staffs' perspectives into a coherent treatment plan. However, several problems arose with psychologists being drawn into team leader roles. The main problem was that the 'team leader' responsibilities took up much of the psychologists' time and decreased their ability to carry out the assessment and treatment services that were very much needed and in demand. Psychologists' training in group therapy and dynamics, and their generally good writing skills were seen as valuable assets that could be put to greater use in treatment team functions. Part of the vision of senior hospital administrators was to place psychologists in a central leadership role with regard to treatment team functioning; i.e., to make psychologists responsible for coordinating team interactions, and ensuring that documentation was satisfactory.

A third area of psychologists' functioning that was problematic in some ways, and led to some areas of disagreement with the hospital leadership, was the valued role of assessment. The assessment role, always significant, had become particularly important because an increasing percentage of our population had concurrent legal issues. The need for psychologists to provide risk assessments addressing violence risk, sexual violence risk, and other psycho-legal issues was increasing. Senior administrators saw the importance of psychological assessment, and wanted psychologists to expand their assessment roles in some ways; e.g., carrying out competency to stand trial assessments that had been the purview of our psychiatrists. However, there appeared to be little recognition of the amount of time required to carry out the assessments, nor willingness to allow for the flexibility or time accommodations that would ensure good work.

Pressure was being put on psychologists to carry out more functions. However, as I perceived it, this was being done without an adequate understanding of the time and other resources needed to perform additional roles being asked of psychologists. This appeared to stem from a failure to recognize the potential treatment impact that could result from limiting important aspects of the core work that psychologists had been originally trained to carry out.

Challenges and Achievements

Within this context of increasing pressures bearing down on the hospital, which included the pressures impacting the roles of psychologists, it was obvious that taking on the leadership of the psychology department provided numerous challenges. But also, opportunities to influence the department and hospital in positive ways were possible for me.

While serving as 'Acting Director,' I sought to support the psychologists' abilities to carry out their professional roles on a number of fronts that I had always deemed essential. I supported psychologists' working within teams as providers of group and individual therapy, and as leaders in initiating new programming that met patient needs. I considered treatment addressing sequelae of trauma as a highly important issue to address within the hospital population. I intended to expand psychologists' efforts to provide such treatment. I also wanted to maintain the support and integrity of the internship program at a time when it was likely to become vulnerable. Our program was due for an American Psychological Association review 2 years down the road, which meant that much work had to be done, including a lengthy self-study report that needed to be prepared.

In addition to everything just described were the many specific responsibilities that went along with the director role, which included participation in hospital committees and efforts to improve hospital functioning and systems. As 'Acting Director,' I was a member and participant on a committee that met weekly to review treatment team recommendations for changes in the status of patients who were hospitalized after committing violent or sexually aggressive acts.

I also participated in a weekly review of individuals identified by treatment teams for clinical review and recommendations. In addition, I had quality assurance and quality improvement data for my department to collect and report on. I also led the Research Review Committee, which evaluated research proposals submitted by hospital personnel and occasionally by researchers connected with local universities. I had multiple administrative meetings to attend on a daily basis. I had department meetings to run, supervision of staff to provide, positions to interview for and fill, and data to collect on department members' performance, which I reviewed and reported on monthly. Those were roles I knew about in advance. More responsibilities and challenges were to emerge.

In my role as acting director, I attempted to inspire and support staff in efforts to contribute to patient care in effective and creative ways, and in ways consistent with the hospital's mission. During my time as director, among the goals I set and actions I supported or initiated were:

(1) Many psychologists needed to develop additional skills in order to competently assess an increasingly forensic population. Particular competencies were needed in order to carry out risk assessments that were required as part of hospital review processes, and that were ultimately scrutinized by reviewers outside of the hospital. To assist psychologists with this, I arranged training programs on various types of risk assessment and initiated a monthly supervision session with one of the hospital's psychologists who had extensive forensic experience.

(2) In line with state-wide models for 'Wellness and Recovery' and 'trauma informed care' models, I supported and initiated efforts and training to help our psychologists to provide therapeutic interventions that explicitly were designed to address trauma issues. These included Dialectic Behavior Therapy (DBT), and other treatment approaches that were recognized as empirically supported, such as Cognitive Behavior Therapy (CBT). In particular, several psychologists were trained to use a version of CBT developed by psychiatrist Aaron Beck and his associates, which was specifically designed to treat psychotic patients (Beck, Rector, Stolar, & Grant, 2009; Chang, Grant, Luther, & Beck, 2014). Because people in treatment respond to a variety of approaches, and psychologists were trained in a range of treatment methods, I also advocated that we continue to provide treatment utilizing varied approaches including psychodynamic, psychosocial, and other treatment models. This was consistent with what I had learned and applied throughout my entire career. These were all treatment models that were supported by literature and research (Rosenbaum et al., 2012; Chien, Leung, Yeung, & Wong, 2013). Psychologists were well prepared to

provide both individual and group therapy services, and other therapy services consistent with these models of care.

(3) In addition to psychologists, the psychology department included what were called 'behavioral support technicians' (BSTs). These staff members generally had masters' degrees. They applied behavioral principles with patients to address specific problems identified by treatment teams. Common problems identified included aggressive and self-harming behaviors. Often the BSTs worked very closely with patients on an individual basis. Overseen and supervised by psychologists, BSTs worked with some of the most difficult patients to engage and treat who resided in the hospital. Nevertheless, the data that the BSTs collected demonstrated that despite many obstacles, they made measurable progress with most of those they treated. The BSTs were a tremendous resource that I considered essential for patients, treatment teams, and for the hospital. I made sure the data that revealed the BSTs value was presented clearly to hospital administrators. I advocated for resources needed in order for the BSTs to do their jobs well. I also ensured that the BSTs received appropriate supervision by psychologists.

(4) I led and supported psychologists in program development. Our psychologists took leadership roles in establishing 'best practice' interventions and innovative programming in a variety of modalities addressing patient needs. These included:

- DBT skills groups: a long time priority of the hospital, DBT skills groups were initiated and run by psychologists.
- A cognitive remediation program was developed with administrative support from a proposal submitted by psychology interns. This program incorporated the use of computerized video games in addition to a number of other innovations and won state-wide recognition, including an award from the governor's office.
- Groups that specifically addressed trauma treatment were initiated in several units in the hospital where they had not previously been provided. Some groups utilized original treatment models. Other groups utilized recognized 'best practice' such as DBT and the Trauma Recovery and Empowerment Model (TREM) (Fallot & Harris, 2002).
- Sex Offender treatment was initiated. In developing this program, expertise was provided by staff members with prior experience working in facilities in which they treated individuals who had engaged in predatory sex offenses.
- A 'Competency Restoration Group' to help restore legal competence when needed, for patients involved in judicial processes,

was developed and run by psychologists and one Psychology Intern.

- I supervised a psychologist functioning as the clinical leader of a program that incorporated social learning and behavioral reinforcement to help transition several patients with long hospital stays into community services and treatment.
- I initiated steps to begin using valid and reliable measures of therapists' working alliances with patients, patient satisfaction, and outcome measurement. Psychology and rehabilitation department staff participated in a pilot using Duncan and Miller's Session and Outcome Rating Scales. (Miller & Duncan, 2004).
- I proposed and initiated a hospital-based trauma informed care workgroup. This was an interdisciplinary effort with leadership and participation from the psychology department and other disciplines, such as rehabilitation, nursing, and pastoral services. Our accomplishments included the expansion of trauma treatment within the hospital and the development of our own version of a personal safety plan.

While working on these priorities, which were intended to contribute to the hospital's treatment mission, I felt pressured to change our psychologists' roles in ways with which I didn't always agree. For example, as noted above, the hospital's administrative leadership proposed that psychologists take on a greater role in facilitating treatment teams' functioning, due to problems they saw in the manner that the treatment teams functioned. Many administrators perceived the hospital's treatment teams as failing to work together cohesively, even though each team had a 'program coordinator' who served as 'team leader.' Team members from each discipline were perceived as largely carrying out their own components of treatment in compartmentalized ways, with inadequate communication and coordination with other discipline members on the same team. The 'Program Coordinators' were perceived as creating treatment plans largely on their own, although the degree to which that was accurate varied, depending on the manner in which each individual team's leader and members functioned. Hospital administrators' proposed solutions to the problems with team cohesiveness and coordination included changing the treatment plan form and treatment planning process to one that required greater input and interaction. A greater leadership role for psychologists was seen as another part of the solution. Before I took on the leadership of the psychology department, the logic behind the proposed changes in treatment team leadership roles had been discussed and largely determined. However, before this new model was implemented, I voiced my concerns and proposed alternatives. While I thought many psychologists had the skills and intelligence to function well in the integrative and group process skills demanded of team leaders, I knew that not all psychologists would be a good fit for this type of interdisciplinary leadership. Also, I voiced concerns about the impact on psychologists' time and ability to carry out their other professional responsibilities. Ultimately my efforts led to some impact on the way psychologists' treatment team roles were defined. Over time, however, it became clear that my efforts to respectfully express my disagreements at times with agendas advocated by hospital administrators and to suggest alternatives, were not always well received.

During the next 4 years, numerous disagreements relating to psychologists' roles and functions arose. I provided evidence supporting many of my opinions, including the value of psychologists' roles in providing individual therapy services as needed, utilizing a variety of theoretical perspectives, including therapies grounded in psychoanalytic theory. My assertions were supported by current evidence, but were not congruent with the views of my administrators, and were often disregarded. I argued against pressures that ultimately resulted in reducing the provision of individual therapy sessions, and also many of the group therapies psychologists had developed and tailored to specifically address the needs of their patients. Instead, administrators' 'vision' was that psychologists become more focused on implementing a psychoeducational manualized group treatment that was seen as evidence-based.

Decisions made about these and other hospital-wide issues impacted our staff in a variety of ways. A number of experienced psychology department members retired. Several early and mid-career department members, including some who had trained as psychology interns in the facility before taking staff positions, left the hospital for other opportunities. In some cases, staff openly indicated that the changes described above to psychologists' roles and functions contributed to their decisions to leave. At times I was permitted to fill vacated positions. As time progressed, however, at times I was not permitted to fill vacated positions, and instead was told to provide coverage using existing department staff for services on units with psychologist vacancies, encumbering our diminishing staff with more responsibilities.

Moving Through and Moving On

Despite some significant accomplishments, I was replaced as Acting Director after approximately 4 years in that position. Another state hospital had closed, and the psychology director there, who had seniority in the civil service 'Director of Psychology' title, was given the opportunity to relieve me as 'Acting Director.'

Although I was disappointed when I was reassigned from my role as 'acting director' of psychology, there were also positive aspects to my leaving that position. On many occasions, I had expressed disagreement with senior administrators about decisions that were made concerning the functioning and roles of psychology staff. I had advocated points of view that were not always welcomed. I saw my position as an opportunity to voice my perspective in discussions about hospital policies and actions that impacted staff and patients. I frequently persisted, even when I knew administrators disagreed with me about new policies that they initiated, when I thought there was value in ensuring my ideas be heard and considered. However, over time, it appeared that the impact of this approach led to a perception of me as someone who was not as much of a 'team player' as was desired. Perhaps my perceptions and the perceptions of my senior administrators about many aspects of hospital functioning and psychologists' roles were too far apart for me to have ever been a good fit for this administrative team. I always made an effort to be respectful in my interactions but was never able to establish a genuine alliance with some of the hospital's administrative leadership. While at times, my views made some impact, ultimately, I was replaced in my role.

As acting director, it was inescapably evident that my views on how psychologists could best contribute to patient treatment and help the hospital fulfill goals and agendas differed significantly in some ways from those of my administrative leaders. When I took on the position of acting director of the psychology department, I took the assertion seriously by some senior administrators that they wanted honest input and feedback from department leaders and others in comparable positions. I conveyed input even when I knew it might be rejected. I knew my decision to voice my opinions may not have been politically expedient, but I made a conscious decision to do so regardless. I saw a need to advocate for my department members when I thought their time and talents were not being well-utilized. I considered it important to advocate for what I thought was best with regard to treatment. I knew there were legitimate alternate views to mine, but I thought it was important to speak up in support of what I valued, and felt an imperative to do so in order to maintain my own self-respect as well as that of my department members and colleagues.

When I conveyed my perceptions, that at times diverged from those of the senior administrators, they might have seen my communications as an opportunity to consider alternate perspectives to achieve hospital goals, not as a threat to the prevailing views. However, as time passed, it became apparent that I was being seen not only as a critic of aspects of the administration's approach to accomplishing goals but as an obstacle. In fact, while I disagreed with some aspects of the administration's agenda, I agreed with many other aspects.

This administration had initiated a number of steps to transform programming and change the way hospital work was done. I agreed with the 'Recovery,' 'Wellness,' and 'trauma-informed care' concepts generating many of the changes that were being attempted. These were not new ideas, and I had been guided by them throughout much of my career. But I had concerns about the way these concepts and models were now being interpreted and carried out in our hospital. So when I saw implementation as ineffective, contrary to what I understood about these models, or lacking important components such as greater collaboration with patients and respect and realistic expectations of staff, I felt it was important to speak up.

I was open to innovation and transformation in the hospital. I had promoted and initiated important changes in each role I had carried out since working in the hospital. I remodeled many aspects of psychology service in the Travers Complex. I restructured and expanded many components of TPH's pre-doctoral internship program, leading to accolades from the American Psychological Association, and enabling us to attract high-quality interns. As acting director of the psychology department, I successfully initiated and encouraged much new program development within my department to meet emerging and previously unmet needs. Some change taking place within the hospital, and the state in general, represented a break from the way things had been done in the past. But I saw much of the change taking place as a reframing of things that had been done for years, at least by some members of the hospital community, and definitely by many psychologists. I saw what was being called the 'Wellness and Recovery' model as an approach consistent with psychologists' efforts to implement treatment consistent with principles that many psychologists and like-minded colleagues had recognized and carried out for years. The models being introduced by the state into New Jersey's government-led mental health service system were consistent with priorities that had already been recognized by many treatment professionals for many years in the broader treatment world. This approach promoted a philosophy and services with which I agreed and had been influenced by in much of my own work in the hospital. Among these priorities were increasing services addressing the traumatic history of many of our patients, and working with patients in ways that demonstrated recognition that hospitalized individuals could recover. I had advocated and carried out treatment consistent with such principles for decades.

However, despite my agreement with many of the 'new' principles, I had been involved in the functioning of the hospital for many years. It is possible that to the hospital leadership I represented continuity with the past, in contrast to a perception they may have had of themselves as innovators working to make a break from outdated treatment models that needed to be shed and replaced.

I may have been recognized by the administration as an ally in the effort to promote change within the hospital. But for an administration which saw themselves as reformers, and may have truly wanted to advance the hospital for the better, it is not surprising that I was seen as an obstacle. I was part of the hospitals' recent past and linked to a history from which they wanted to diverge. I contradicted some of their perceptions about my department members' functioning and made efforts to maintain some of that which they wanted to change. I openly validated the views of many of those in the clinical leadership, as well as many clinical staff who were in agreement. While I was in accord with the administration regarding some key changes, trends, and models that the hospital was adopting, I frequently disagreed with their implementation. I sometimes proposed alternative approaches to reach goals that I shared with administrators. I was motivated by a belief that an approach that incorporated greater collaboration and valued both staffs' and patients' strengths would lead to better outcomes that could be embraced by staff and administrators. Goals that I shared with the administration included improving patient engagement and ownership of their treatment, implementation of the most effective treatments we could provide, and supporting and motivating hospital staff. After I left the hospital, some of what I argued against was discontinued. Some of my suggestions were adopted. Some ways of doing business have persisted.

I led my department for 4 years as 'acting director.' Ultimately, some kind of change had to occur. The options seemed to be: (1) a change within myself; i.e., I had to be more accepting of much with which I disagreed, (2) a change in the system; i.e., more of what I advocated needed to be understood and genuinely considered, or (3) a change with regard to my role or presence within the prevailing system.

Rebooting

After I was removed from the 'Acting Director' position and replaced by another psychologist, who was civil service 'Director of Psychology' from another New Jersey state hospital that closed, I was then reassigned to the hospital's admissions unit. This was a strong statement, and a reassignment not designed to please me. During my career in the hospital, I had mainly worked in the 'transitional living' cottages which functioned in a manner consistent with a biopsychosocial model. Many patients there were relatively stable, and it was possible to work with many of them in individual and group therapy, psychological interventions I was well trained in, valued and considered to provide great benefit. The way in which the 'transitional living' unit functioned contrasted greatly with that of the admissions units, which more closely followed a medical model. In contrast to the emphasis on psychological and rehabilitation-oriented therapies, and steps directly contributing to transition to the community that were carried out in the cottages, the admissions units were more focused on stabilization and discharge. Each admissions unit housed 40 patients. Each month as many as 20 new patients might be admitted and 20 discharged or transferred to other parts of the hospital. Psychologists were integral to rapid treatment planning, working with patients to develop Personal Safety Plans, and providing documentation of treatment and progress. Most patients in admissions units were more unstable and more violent than those in other units. Mostly short-term psychological therapy and much assessment was carried out by the psychology staff there. I had great respect for the psychologists and other staff working in admissions units but knew it was extremely challenging and saw it as a poor fit for myself in light of the kind of work I had done and enjoyed doing during most of my career, which involved a deeper sense of personal interaction.

As it turned out, I was welcomed and embraced by the other psychologists working in the admissions units. Despite my concerns, and at times fears of how I would manage, things went well. I became part of a treatment team on the unit that included experienced professionals I meshed well with and found myself developing a rhythm to each day that enabled me to carry out the treatment planning, documentation, supervision, and therapy activities. My self-protective instincts were mobilized. This allowed me to maintain my physical safety while working with the often volatile patients in the oftentimes chaotic admissions unit. I provided short-term individual therapy with many patients and ran several therapy groups in which patients could obtain support and provide each other with an understanding of the environment in which they found themselves. I co-led a specialized group for people who had been admitted to the hospital to be treated and evaluated for competency to stand trial. During one treatment team meeting, I served as a physical barrier when a patient was attempting to assault the team's psychiatrist. Occasionally senior administrators would show up at a morning community meeting, usually after some particularly horrific incident had occurred on the ward, but they generally interacted very little with the treatment team, and quickly exited the unit.

When I was transferred to the admissions unit, I had been told by the incoming 'Director of Psychology' that he would 'quickly reassign' me back to the 'transitional cottage' unit. A year and a half later, this had not happened. Despite my successful adaptation to the admissions unit work, the transitional cottage program was still a better fit for my background and clinical skills.

Another path opened, however, that would provide both a degree of continuity and new opportunities. I continued to believe in the mission of working with psychiatric patients, providing the kind of psychological care and services I knew I could offer that would be therapeutic. However, in this hospital, where I had spent most of my career, it had become increasingly difficult to work in ways that I valued and thought were most beneficial for patients. The chance to work in a vastly different role came up at New Jersey's forensic psychiatric hospital, the Ann Klein Forensic Center. In that role, I would be providing therapeutic group work and doing legally related evaluations. Ironically, my work in the admission unit prepared me well for this position. Impeccably timed, the same day I was offered a new position at the forensic psychiatric hospital, I was told that I could be reassigned back to the transitional cottage program. I chose not to go back to the cottages. For both professional and personal reasons, it was time to move on.

Beginning anew, in a job carrying out exclusively forensic psychology work, provided an opportunity to engage in a new organizational system. This work involved greater flexibility, including travel around the state of New Jersey, and performing evaluations with individuals who presented a wide spectrum of legal and psychological problems. This included providing opinions to courts that had direct and sometimes immediate impact, and testifying and defending my opinions under great scrutiny. The groups that I ran were designed to help restore patients' competency to stand trial and were similar to the ones I ran in TPH's admissions unit. Rapport building and interpersonal elements of the groups were crucial in these groups, much as they were with the more clinical treatment oriented groups I had led in the hospital. For a period of time, I also worked on the forensic admissions unit, developed behavior plans, and saw patients individually and in rounds with other team members. My former work on a variety of units helped prepare me for the diverse work that I did at Ann Klein. I also experienced some challenges new to me that were inherent in inpatient forensic work and related to the legal justice system. Working on the interface between the mental health and justice systems brought to light some of the significant problems and imperfections of both of these systems.

After I began working at the Ann Klein Forensic Center, another opportunity materialized. Four years prior, I had been nominated by New Jersey's Chief of Medicine to serve as the state government representative on the New Jersey Board of Psychological Examiners. After silence from the governor's office for 4 years, I no longer expected to be appointed. Receiving a letter in the mail from the governor's office, I wondered if they were returning the paperwork I had submitted to support my nomination. Opening the letter, I was surprised and pleased to read about my appointment to the Board. I was being given a chance to help maintain the integrity of psychology practice on a statewide level, a role and mindset I gladly welcomed. Equally if not more important both personally and professionally, being appointed to the Board provided some additional validation that was welcome in light of all my recent struggles.

In conclusion, I maintain that in any hospital setting, working as a psychologist provides rewards and benefits, and poses many obstacles. It is difficult if not impossible to predict the path one will travel when working in mental health settings. Each time I have taken on new challenges and roles, I have been unsure how things would work out and what the future would hold. It is essential to accept a great deal of uncertainty working in the mental health field. Working as a psychologist provides many opportunities to do things that are personally and professionally meaningful, to apply and expand one's skills, and to have an impact on the field itself. As treatment and systems evolve, psychologists working in inpatient mental health settings will most likely continue to face challenges similar to those described here, as well as unique challenges that are impossible to predict. Described here is one path taken by one psychologist. I am grateful for the chance I have had to follow this path.

References

Beck, A.T., Rector, N.A., Stolar, N., & Grant, P. (2009). *Schizophrenia cognitive theory, research, and therapy*. New York, NY: The Guilford Press.

Chang, N.A., Grant, P.M., Luther, L., & Beck, A.T. (2014). Effects of a recovery-oriented cognitive therapy training program on inpatient staff attitudes and incidents of seclusion and restraint. *Community Mental Health Journal*, *50*(4), 415–421.

Chien, W.T., Leung, S.F., Yeung, F.K., & Wong, W.K. (2013). Current approaches to treatments for schizophrenia spectrum disorders, part II: Psychosocial interventions and patient-focused perspectives in psychiatric care. *Neuropsychiatric Disease and Treatment*, *9*, 1463–1481.

Fallot, R. & Harris, M. (2002). The trauma recovery and empowerment model (TREM): Conceptual and practical issues in a group intervention for women. *Community Mental Health Journal*, *38*(6), 475–485.

Karon, B.P. & Vandenbos, G.R. (1981). *Psychotherapy of schizophrenia treatment of choice*. New York, NY: Jason Aronson.

Lu, W., Mueser, K.T., Shami, A., Siglag, M., Petrides, G., Schoepp, E., & Saltz, J. (2011). Post-traumatic reactions to psychosis in people with multiple psychotic episodes. *Schizophrenia Research*, *127*(1–3), 66–75.

Miller, S.D. & Duncan, B.L. (2004). *The outcome and session rating scales: Administration and scoring manual*. Chicago, IL: Institute for the Study of Therapeutic Change.

Rice, C.A. & Rutan, J.S. (1987). *Inpatient group psychotherapy: A psychodynamic perspective*. New York, NY: Macmillan Publishing Company.

Rosenbaum, B., Harder, S., Knudsen, P., Koster, A., Lindhardt, A., Lajer, M., & Winther, G. (2012). Supportive psychodynamic psychotherapy versus treatment as usual for first-episode psychosis: Two-year outcome. *Psychiatry: Interpersonal & Biological Processes*, *75*(4), 331–341.

Shur, R. (1994). *Countertransference enactment: How institutions and therapists actualize primitive internal worlds*. Northvale, NJ: Jason Aronson, Inc.

Siglag, M.A. (1999). *Psychiatric hospital treatment: Healing versus repetition of trauma* (paper presented at 1999 APA National Convention).
Whitaker, R. (2010). *Anatomy of an epidemic: Magic bullets, psychiatric drugs, and the astonishing rise of mental illness in America*. New York, NY: Crown Publishers.
Yalom, I. (1983). *Inpatient group psychotherapy*. New York, NY: Basic Books.

Part 2

Psychotherapeutic Interventions in the Mental Health Inpatient Setting

Introduction to Part 2

Meidan Turel and Michael Siglag

Psychotherapy is one of the clinical psychologist's most practiced and valuable skills. For the clinical psychologist, psychotherapy is grounded in the systematic and scientific academic study of human psychology and its application in a clinical context, using the rich and sophisticated knowledge and expertise originating from such study to ameliorate mental suffering and psychopathology.

In mental health inpatient settings, psychotherapy with clinical psychologists can directly benefit patients in powerful and significant ways. Additionally, insights and meanings acquired in psychotherapeutic interactions enhance the psychologist's understanding of patients' emotional, mental and behavioral phenomena as observed on the unit. Input provided by the psychologist, who has gained such understanding through therapeutic work with patients, can be used both in the context of the therapeutic relationship and in collaboration with the treatment team, to create a therapeutic space and help shape interventions better aligned with the patient's needs and with the potential for cure.

It is through this meaning-making and relational contact established within the therapeutic relationship that the patient may come to 'find him or herself,' an experience that perhaps explains why survey results repeatedly demonstrate patients' requests for additional therapy sessions during their inpatient stay (Durant & Tolland, 2009; also see Grinshpoon & Kurs in the Introduction of this volume). For the patient, having a therapeutic relationship with a caring other, in which they are 'seen,' recognized and validated, can offer an invaluable supportive experience in the difficult circumstances usually accompanying hospitalization. This relational experience adds to the value of the therapeutic work above and beyond the specifics of the psychologist's therapeutic orientation or technique.

Psychologists' promotion of recognition of the 'person in the patient' contributes to an interplay between two modes of intervention that can take place on inpatient units. The first mode involves the psychologist 'working up' from the intimacy of the therapeutic relationship with the patient toward systemic level work with the multidisciplinary team. In this mode, the psychologist contributes to the psychological mindedness and emotional receptivity of the unit staff, working to ensure that the patient's personal narrative is heard and listened to by the team members. This can come about through initiating interventions on the unit through which the patient can come to speak and express him/herself with an attentive and receptive treatment team. Alternatively, when conditions are not conducive for such patient self- presentation, the psychologist can 'stand in,' and give voice and represent in his own words, something of the patient's subjective experience and narrative, while appropriately safeguarding patient's confidentiality.

In the second mode, the psychologist 'works down,' engaging in systems-level interventions with the multidisciplinary team in work geared toward the patient. Here the psychologist helps the team initiate patient-oriented interventions, using understanding gleaned through the therapeutic relationship while protecting information given within the trust and intimacy of that relationship.

Both of these routes work to enhance the multidisciplinary team members' empathic and supportive stance toward the patient and involve team members as active partners in building and implementing tailored interventions with the patient. Such an involved mode of work creates a satisfying and rewarding experience for the team and benefits the patient who feels better contained and validated.

This necessary interplay between the intimacy of the therapeutic relationship and the social reality of the patient's life within the system of the inpatient unit poses an ongoing challenge for the clinical psychologist practicing psychotherapy in these settings. The psychologist is engaged in repeated efforts to find the optimal balance between appropriate exposure of the therapeutic dyad and the safeguarding of confidentiality and trust within it. On one hand, psychologists incorporate understanding gained from the therapeutic relationship into systemic processes on the unit in order to serve the patient's interests. On the other hand, it is vital to the therapeutic dyad to respect the boundaries of the relationship and to form a 'protective shield' around it, with which to isolate and safeguard the unfolding of the therapeutic process. Over-extending either side of this balance creates a risk of eliciting damaging splits and provoking acting out by all participants in this drama. Finding and maintaining a delicate and workable balance in each situation requires earnest and dedicated involvement on behalf of the psychologist, with a willingness for an element of emotional engagement which when carefully monitored and attended to, can help guide the way. These themes in the clinical psychologist's psychotherapeutic work within the mental health inpatient setting make this work emotionally and professionally challenging in unique ways.

The six chapters in this part of the book each depict these themes. In all of the psychotherapeutic interventions and techniques described in this part, overriding themes of empathic validation, relational support and a meaningful translation of the psychotherapeutic work to a system level dimension are shown to contribute to worthwhile results.

Following is a brief description of the six chapters that make up this part of the book:

In the first chapter (Chapter 10), Manish Parswani and Malcolm Stewart describe the contribution of psychotherapy in short-stay mental health inpatient admissions. Drawing on their experience in the New Zealand public mental health system, the authors explore the role of brief psychological therapy in mental health inpatient settings. They argue that brief therapy has two distinct forms that require radically different skills and most appropriately address different situations. Through case descriptions showing psychologists' involvement in brief therapy in inpatient services, they demonstrate the distinctions between these forms of therapy and the value psychologists contribute to therapeutic endeavors in this setting.

Next (Chapter 11), authors Kim Griffiths, Hannah Green, and Suzie Lemmey describe a model of continuity of clinical psychology service bridging acute inpatient treatment and community mental health care. They developed their model in a unit within the public mental health service in the United Kingdom. This approach to maintaining continuity of care involves the delivery of psychological intervention on an acute inpatient ward and when appropriate, continuation of the intervention with the same psychologist post-discharge in the community service. The model offers an opportunity to complete therapy already in progress, with goals that include reducing the rate of readmission and maximizing recovery. The authors present case studies to illustrate implementation of the model and provide provisional data regarding the model's putative impact on reducing readmission rates and subsequent bed days.

In the following chapter (Chapter 12), Sally Riggs presents a description of Cognitive Behavior Therapy for psychosis (CBTp) – informed interventions in a mental health inpatient unit, emphasizing the role of the psychologist in devising, implementing and disseminating such interventions. The author provides examples from her inpatient work in a public psychiatric facility in the state of New York, illustrating effective strategies and approaches for implementing CBTp practice and techniques addressing a wide spectrum of situations within that setting, including ways in which the unit psychologist can take a leading role in modeling this work for the team.

In the next chapter (Chapter 13), Beatriz Sanchez Curtis describes an approach to the provision of psychoanalytically-informed psychotherapeutic work in a secure inpatient psychiatric unit within the public mental health service in the United Kingdom. The author argues that the depth and sophistication of psychoanalytic thinking can contribute significantly to or even make possible, treatment of hospitalized individuals whose disturbance stems from complex and traumatic experiences and who have often been untouched by other psychological models of interventions. Through case examples, Beatriz demonstrates how psychoanalytic theories can inform the psychologist's formulation of the patients' presentations and pathologies, and how such understanding can crucially influence treatment planning on the ward. She describes the treatment impact on two systemic levels; the first being the direct patient level through the incorporation of psychoanalytic techniques in individual therapy sessions; and second, at the treatment team level, by helping the team understand the patient's unconscious communications of their behaviors and respond to these in helpful ways.

In the fifth chapter of this part of the book (Chapter 14), Dione Johnson-Williams explores the way patients' traumatic attachment histories can result in developmentally-based emotional and behavioral patterns that contribute to their violent behaviors in the inpatient setting. The author explains how violence exhibited by patients with such histories is often the result of impaired mentalization abilities. Threats toward patients and staff, property destruction, self-injurious behaviors, and patient and staff assaults, are often the result of a combination of psychological factors consisting of perceived slights by the patient and inability to appropriately identify and manage their own mental states. Helping patients shift their self-perception, and respond to others via improved mentalization abilities can be a goal of the therapeutic relationship with the unit psychologist. Using a case example from her work in a closed inpatient unit in a New Jersey state psychiatric hospital, Dione examines how improving a violent patient's mentalization abilities via the therapeutic relationship and through work with the team can be an effective intervention helping to reduce patient's symptom presentation, improve unit safety, and increase discharge readiness.

In the sixth and closing chapter of this part of the book (Chapter 15), Hilik Peri describes his experience conducting psychodynamically-oriented psychotherapy with patients confined to a maximum security forensic unit in a public mental health inpatient facility in Israel. Using a case example, Hilik presents the challenges facing the psychologist in the forensic setting, where the patients suffer from complex and severe mental disorders and have exhibited frightening and destructive violence. Many of the patients in this setting present persistent difficulty trusting others, including those who seek to provide help or support and can perceive ward staff as part of a restrictive, rigid, and at times punitive system. In such an atmosphere, the therapist may experience harsh feelings of fear, terror, helplessness, and hopelessness, alongside deep wishes to heal and mend. The author stresses the importance of the clinical psychologist's awareness of these contradictory experiences, both in the therapeutic setting and in work with the team. Hilik describes his continuous struggle to create a transitional space in such a challenging place, where therapeutic work is indeed possible.

This collection of chapters describing the authors' psychotherapeutic work within various psychiatric inpatient settings is an inspiring edifice of their challenging and creative work. The chapters all provide examples of psychologists dedicated to finding the means and developing or applying ways to promote their patients' wellbeing and mental health while facing the difficult circumstances involved in hospitalization.

Originality, innovation and ingenuity, both in thought and in action, are ingredients used by clinical psychologists practicing psychotherapy in these settings, creating better opportunities for patients' treatment and recovery. These 'ingredients' are not necessarily acquired through the methodical studies and training that go into the making of a clinical psychologist. Rather, they are part of the clinical psychologist as a person, ever-motivated to explore and understand human psychology, and through compassion, to connect with fellow human beings' mental misery and plight in a benign and therapeutic manner.

References

Durant, C., & Tolland, A. (2009). Evaluating short-term CBT in an acute inpatient unit. In I. Clarke, & H. Wilson (Eds.) *Cognitive behavior therapy for acute inpatient mental health units: Working with clients, staff and the milieu*. pp. 185–196. New York, NY: Routledge.

10 All Brief Therapy is Not Created Equal

The Contribution of Psychology to Short-Stay Mental Health Inpatient Admissions

Manish Parswani and Malcolm W. Stewart

The role of psychological therapies in the inpatient unit has a long history and well-established utility (Geczy & Sultenfuss, 1994; Nielsen, 2015). The contributions of psychologists in inpatient mental health settings extend well beyond assessment and therapy, and include consultation, behavioral modification, program development, research, staff and student training, management and leadership, and support of other staff and team functions (Geczy & Sultenfuss, 1994; British Psychological Society, 2010; Stein & Jacobo, 2013). This chapter explores the role of brief psychological therapy in the mental health inpatient setting. It argues that brief therapy has two distinct forms which require radically different skills and can address different situations, but which are often treated as the same. Cases showing psychologists' involvement in brief therapy in inpatient services are used to demonstrate this distinction and the value that psychologists add in this setting.

Why Brief Psychological Interventions in the Inpatient Setting?

In many countries, clients identify a lack of access to verbal therapies as a major limitation in the quality of care in mental health inpatient settings (Durant & Tolland, 2009). Despite efforts to improve access (e.g., the UK's Increasing Access to Psychological Therapies (IAPT) program; UK Department of Health, 2012), psychological assistance in the community is limited, often due to financial or service provision constraints. Even when psychological input is available, factors such as client reluctance/avoidance, staff of other discipline's reluctance to refer, and practical constraints (e.g., cost, transport, or organization) may limit community-based access to psychological therapy. Therefore, inpatient settings may provide a rare opportunity for clients to access psychological assessment and intervention (McGowan & Hill, 2009). Sometimes, events that precipitate an inpatient admission may increase motivation to engage with psychological interventions. This motivation may dissipate by the time the client returns to the community.

Arguably, an inpatient admission may indicate that the existing care is not working well for the individual, so the inpatient admission is a useful trigger to review the current interventions. For example, if treatment has been mainly biomedical and supportive, then, while not necessarily abandoning existing treatments, incorporating more psychological or social treatment elements may be indicated. An inpatient psychologist can strongly influence present and future management (often increasing its psychosocial responsiveness) by providing or guiding therapy or by assessment leading to diagnostic/formulation clarification and treatment recommendations.

A continuing trend in many countries is toward shorter duration inpatient stays (Leibenluft, Tasman, & Green, 1993; Lee, Rothbard, & Noll, 2012), with the average length of stay dropping from 13 days in 1995 to 10 days in recent years. In the coming years, the median length of stay will likely decrease more radically. This necessitates increasingly brief interventions in inpatient settings. More generally, there has been a movement toward time- or session-limited psychological interventions, with substantial evidence that these can achieve positive and cost-effective outcomes (e.g., Dath, Sables, Yang Dong, & Stewart, 2014). This trend toward effective briefer psychological interventions suggests that shorter inpatient stays do not discount the utility of psychological interventions in this setting. For example, Bartak et al. (2010) found that outcomes for short-term inpatient psychotherapy compared favorably to long-term inpatient therapy, day hospital therapy, or short- or long-term community-based therapy for treatment of personality disorders.

Another common trend in mental health has been the delivery of psychological therapies by a broader range of health providers (e.g., IAPT: UK Department of Health, 2012). This can be organized as stepped care (Haga, 2000) to ensure that an individual's needs are addressed by interventions of the appropriate intensity to most cost-effectively and least restrictively promote recovery. This allows for consideration of a broad range of interventions, from modifying the social determinants of ill-health, through peer support and social and psychological interventions of varying intensity and sophistication, to acute inpatient admissions. When well organized and operated, this process increases population access to cost-effective interventions including psychological therapies of sufficient intensity and sophistication to meet clients' psychological needs. Interventions, including different psychological interventions, may be competently delivered by a variety of mental health workers. Even within the relatively enclosed mental health inpatient setting, there is typically more psychological work that can usefully be done than there will ever be psychologists to do it, so enhancing the capacity of other staff such as psychiatrists, nurses, occupational therapists, and peer support workers to contribute to this effort is important to optimize patients' wellbeing.

The trends described above combine to create multiple opportunities for psychological practice in the mental health inpatient unit. The provision of skilled psychological assessment and therapy – the psychologist's specialty – within the inpatient setting importantly impacts on care during and beyond the inpatient admission. Safe and effective provision of psychological therapies of various levels of intensity and sophistication by different mental health workers requires good support and supervision. This supervision is often undertaken most effectively by psychologists. Psychologists often develop or adapt group or individual interventions for delivery by psychologists or other staff in the inpatient setting, and undertake formative and outcome evaluations.

Brief Psychological Therapy: Two Distinct Forms

Different types of therapies abound and are used in mental health inpatient settings, including psychodynamic psychotherapies (e.g., Beutel, Hoflich, Kurth, & Reimer, 2005), cognitive-behavior-based therapies (e.g., Bach & Hayes, 2002; Duran & Tolland, 2009), and family therapies (e.g., Lemmens, Eisler, Migerode, Heireman, & Demyttenaere, 2007). Some therapies are predicated on a longer-term engagement between therapist and client, such as Dialectical Behavior Therapy (Linehan, 1993) and many forms of psychodynamic psychotherapy, while others expect a comparatively small number of sessions, such as interpersonal psychotherapy (Stuart & Robertson, 2003). Some long-term therapies have developed brief variants, such as Brief Time Limited Psychodynamic Psychotherapy (Levinson, 1995). However, putting aside the differences between therapeutic models, there are two distinct types of what can be called brief psychological therapy. Both generally involve a relatively small number of sessions over a limited time, but otherwise can be distinguished as follows:

1. **Low-intensity:** Therapy using mid-level psychological techniques, often with a primarily psychoeducational and skills-development focus, frequently based on more-or-less manualized approaches, and not necessarily involving an in-depth psychological understanding of the individual client.
2. **High-intensity:** Highly individualized therapy with the intervention components being tailored to the difficulties, situation, and personal characteristics of the individual client, informed by an in-depth knowledge of psychological theory and therapy and a more nuanced psychological understanding of the client. This may incorporate the psychological and skill components utilized in low-intensity therapy as part of the integrated whole.

The difference between these two forms of brief psychological therapy is often not recognized or acknowledged. Both forms can benefit clients of inpatient services greatly, but the forms are not interchangeable. Many clients will benefit from low-intensity therapy, gaining substantially from what it offers. However, others will require an individualized and integrated approach, such as described by Castonguay, Eubanks, Goldfried, Muran, and Lutz (2015) and Norcross and Goldfried (2005) to maximize their recovery in the inpatient setting. This high-intensity brief therapy involves tailoring interventions to suit clients' psychological needs, their coping resources, psychological mindedness, and cultural beliefs by borrowing effective methods from various therapy approaches. Low-intensity therapy can be usefully provided by a range of suitably trained inpatient staff. High-intensity therapy is most commonly provided primarily by psychologists, although some other health professionals may also receive psychotherapy training to that level.

Psychologists' Skills and Brief Therapy

The difference between these two forms of brief psychological therapy, and its significance for psychologists working in mental health inpatient settings, is underpinned by the "common factors" perspective on therapy and an understanding of the particular added value that psychologists typically provide through their training and model of practice.

"Common factors" research shows that factors that are common to all therapeutic approaches are more important to outcomes than the specific therapy approach used. For example, Hubble, Duncan, and Miller (1999) reported that therapeutic alliance, the approach making sense to the client, and the therapist's efficacy beliefs make more difference to the outcome than the therapeutic approach used. This does not mean that the therapeutic approach is unimportant as it scaffolds the process and likely strongly influences client and therapist belief, which then influences the therapeutic alliance. The common factors perspective suggests a more flexible approach to therapy than is espoused by stricter forms of evidence-based therapy (which demand close adherence to a therapeutic protocol to justify the practice) enabling a better matching of technique to client need. It uses evidence to inform what techniques are likely to be successful ("Evidence-Informed Practice," e.g., Bobart, 2005) while tailoring the specific therapeutic approach to the individual. It emphasizes the importance during formulation of not only considering "what is the situation" (presenting problems, precipitating factors, context, background, perpetuating factors, etc.), but also considering "who is this person" (psychological mindedness, learning style, cognitive ability, etc.), because the "who" question may influence what therapeutic approach, or melding of approaches, are most likely to be successful. However, the decision-making processes required to skilfully integrate these factors, as required for high-intensity brief interventions, takes considerable skill.

The specific value that psychologists add to mental health care is relevant to the delivery of high-intensity therapy. A useful articulation of levels of psychological interventions arose some decades ago from a review of the British National Health Service psychology services, often called the MAS report (Mobray, 1988; Stewart, Bushnell, Hauraki, & Roberts, 2014). This report identified that meeting clients' psychological needs is not solely the role of psychologists – it is actually the responsibility of all staff in health and social services. However, different professions make different contributions. The MAS report identified three levels of expertise in psychological input for health sector staff. These levels are shown in Table 10.1.

In relation to the two types of brief therapy, low-intensity brief therapy often utilizes skill Levels 1 and 2, while high-intensity brief therapy also requires use of Level 3 skills to ensure that optimal outcomes are achieved in the available number of sessions.

In addition to therapy, assessment alone is often an intervention if it informs and influences future treatment. Psychological assessment may indicate types of treatment far broader than psychological interventions. Consultation, in which the psychologist helps other staff to work more effectively with clients, for instance by improving the formulation or by supporting other staff to deliver effective treatments, is also important. Finally, brokering access to other services, such as those addressing the social determinants of ill-health, is often an important result of psychological assessment.

Table 10.1 Levels of Psychological Input (Adapted from the MAS Report)

Level 1:	Establishing, maintaining, and supporting relationships with patients and relatives, and using some simple techniques, such as basic counseling and stress management. These should be within the skill set of, and undertaken by, all health staff.
Level 2:	Undertaking circumscribed psychological activities, such as relatively straightforward (e.g., manualized) therapy approaches. Therapies such as CBT for clients with relatively uncomplicated presentations may fit at this level. These can be undertaken by a variety of professions (e.g., medical practitioners, nurses, occupational therapists, social workers, etc.) with suitable aptitude, training, and support, as well as psychologists.
Level 3:	Psychological interventions in circumstances where complexity or underlying influences require the capacity to devise an advanced and individually tailored therapeutic strategy. This requires a sophisticated understanding of various psychological theories and approaches and flexibility to competently adapt and combine approaches. While not exclusively the case, this level is primarily undertaken by psychologists.

The importance of offering a range of therapies and other interventions to meet the diverse needs and characteristics of people with mental health difficulties is widely recognized (Holmes, 2002; Callan & Fry, 2012). The ability to match interventions to the needs of the individual is also paramount in many situations (Bobart, 2005). Stepped care offers one approach to ensuring that good outcomes are achieved safely and cost-effectively. To do so a broad range of interventions, including both low- and high-intensity brief psychological therapies, need to be available, and the distinction between them needs to be understood to ensure that they are used expeditiously. The remainder of this chapter presents case studies showing primarily high-intensity brief therapy but also discussing the psychologist's role in supporting the provision of interventions by others.

Case Studies

Case Study 1: High-Intensity Brief Psychological Therapy: Psychosis

This case illustrates a psychologist providing relatively brief but sophisticated psychotherapy to a client with long-standing paranoid schizophrenia during an inpatient admission, and providing intermittent follow-up "booster" interventions to support recovery during times of challenge or relapse. This highlights the importance of a flexible and individualized approach, the psychological formulation, and meaning-making in psychosis.

Case Description

Ms. F. was a 44-year-old single woman who was first admitted to an inpatient unit with a psychotic episode at the age of 33 and had multiple inpatient admissions since then despite using antipsychotic medication. Each admission was triggered by intense distress about injustice and the abuse of women and children, distressing religious beliefs (overwhelming thoughts about God and anger toward Jesus), severe agitation, and concern that she may harm herself. She said she had been violated by God and that she would like God to destroy the earth so she could question him about injustice in this world. She felt that she needed to end her life so she could meet God to question him. She described having a companion, a dead opera singer, whom she regarded as her spiritual guide who would help her converse with God. She felt his presence and could talk with him in her head, but denied hearing voices from any external source. She was religious, had read the Bible many times, and frequently cited biblical verses. Prior to her first admission, she was a successful semi-professional person but lost her career due to what she regarded as a minor offense. She was distraught about this and started heavy marijuana use, withdrew from family, lost weight, and was consumed by thoughts of injustice and trauma in the world. Her father was suffering from heart failure, which distressed Ms. F. considerably. Ten years later, she was obese, hypertensive, and had elevated blood sugar levels. She was unemployed and lived with her sister. She spent much of her time using marijuana and listening to music. She reported having experienced the difficulties described above consistently since her first admission 10 years prior.

Intervention

During her admission at this time, she was referred to the inpatient psychologist to assist with her psychotic state, address her spiritually distressing thoughts, and manage her risk of self-harm. She readily engaged in psychotherapy, reporting enthusiasm to feel less hopeless about life. Psychological assessment focused on giving her time to tell her story, with the psychologist helping her to integrate, make meaning, and develop a collaborative formulation involving a different understanding of her situation. This partly involved "de-pathologizing" her psychotic experience and framing it as a coping mechanism; working collaboratively and Socratically toward the formulation; normalizing her distress and anger; and conceptualizing the psychosis with a meaning-making and trauma-focused perspective rather than a biomedical approach. In contrast to most psychosis treatment, the focus was to help her understand the meaning of the symptoms and their relevance to her life rather than on eliminating symptoms (Chadwick, 2006). Assessment indicated that the onset of her mental health issues were closely linked with the trauma of losing her career and the stress of her father's chronic ailment, and the associated losses. Her expression of being violated by God was perhaps a metaphorical expression of her suffering and sense of injustice. She used music, smoking marijuana, and immersing herself in the Bible as coping mechanisms but these proved ineffective for helping her to re-establish wellbeing. Inability to return to her career or sustain work, expressed emotion from her family, and being dependent on her sister were key perpetuating factors. Sustaining themes of loss, shame, and loss of dignity during treatment also exacerbated her condition. Over several sessions of listening, Socratic questioning, and discussion, the psychologist and client collaboratively developed the formulation described in brief above. This formulation was a breakthrough for the client. At one time during its development, she cried without speaking for several minutes and then said: "I never thought this way, it all makes sense." Once the formulation was agreed, and its meaning was explored, the client and psychologist worked toward deriving goals that would empower her and address elements of the formulation. She wanted to work and live independently, lose weight, quit marijuana, stop gambling, pay her debts, and study. In planning to address these issues, therapeutic approaches that helped the client to take the lead were favored. This was partly to enhance her own sense of self-agency, and partly to decrease her reliance on the "spiritual guide" described above. The specific interventions were developed collaboratively with the client. The psychologist continued occasional sessions for 2 years after discharge tapering rapidly from initially fortnightly to approximately every three months.

Outcome

Ms. F. maintained wellness for 2 years after completion of therapy and lived independently. She worked full time and took up part-time study. She had few lapses with gambling and drinking alcohol. She had a mental health relapse (anger at God and not wishing to live) after returning to her hometown, and experiencing strong family-related stress. She had a short hospital admission and re-initiated contact with the psychologist. Her thoughts settled and she was quickly and successfully discharged home. In the following year, she and her psychiatrist agreed that she should stop medication. She had changed remarkably: she had lost weight, normalized her blood pressure and sleep pattern, and reported good energy levels and concentration. She was living a healthy lifestyle and working full time. She had subsequently maintained wellness. She no longer reported distressing thoughts and felt she had resolved the inner meaning of her experiences. She believed she was living life consistent with her values. She reported feeling the presence of her "spiritual guide" once in a while but did not believe this influenced her mood or behavior. The therapy empowered her to seek help earlier, which likely reduced the frequency and duration of hospitalization. Her success also positively impacted on staff attitudes toward psychoses and people with psychosis' ability to recover and live well.

Commentary

This case highlights the importance of developing a therapeutic relationship (the foundation for psychotherapy) and being available to engage during vulnerable crisis periods. Early in therapy, it was very challenging to make sense of her conversations. However, each session provided snippets of insight into her belief system and metaphorical descriptions of experience that allowed both therapist and client to make sense of the confusion. The key to sustaining the conversation was a client-centered approach with a non-judgmental attitude, empathy, and positive regard for the client. This helped to build trust and the therapeutic alliance.

Another key element of this intervention was working with Ms. F. to develop a psychological formulation of her situation that was less "toxic" – less punitive and debilitating – than the formulation she already held. This helped her to develop understanding and optimism and allowed her to marshal and utilize her own resources as well as better utilize the professional and social resources around her.

Case Study 2: High-Intensity Integrative Therapy: Chronic Post-traumatic Stress Disorder

This case highlights the importance of conducting detailed assessment and formulation during the crisis stage and using this to tailor the intervention to the individual's needs and personal characteristics. In this case, the intervention was a relatively high-intensity brief therapy because while it was based on quite straightforward post-traumatic stress disorder (PTSD) work, it integrated many additional therapeutic and self-help components to address particular aspects of the client's presentation. The brief inpatient intervention was backed up with some follow-up sessions to help consolidate and extend progress. Engaging clients with a deep sense of hopelessness and despair requires providing them with a safe therapeutic environment in which to tell their story.

Case History

Mrs. S., a 35-year-old married woman with three children, was admitted after a carefully planned suicide attempt involving overdosing on prescription drugs. Mrs. S. had no previous contact with mental health services and until recently worked full time and supported her family. However, a few weeks before admission she lost her job.

The psychiatrist diagnosed major depression. Psychological assessment revealed more than 20 years of florid and chronic PTSD symptoms following sexual abuse by a close relative from age 7 to 10. She reported disturbing nightmares, flashbacks, intrusive memories from her childhood, and crippling anxiety. She was remorseful that her suicide attempt caused distress to her family. She was grateful to have a loving and supportive husband and children.

Assessment and Intervention

On admission, the psychiatrist prescribed antidepressants and requested psychological assessment and treatment with the expectation of a short inpatient stay. Following a review of the suicide attempt, and development of a safety plan, the psychologist took an emotion-focused approach (Greenberg, 2002) working to create a safe therapeutic environment matching her level of readiness. The initial focus also took a psychoeducational approach to PTSD, its causes, symptoms, and treatment, rather than focusing on her specific trauma history. She was relieved to know that her suffering had a "name" and was a recognized condition. The second inpatient session focused on further developing a safety plan and a post-discharge therapy plan. With her new understanding of her condition, she agreed to engage in therapy and seemed hopeful and curious about it. Her safety plan involved identifying low mood, hopelessness, and negative thoughts and utilizing skills including physical activity and seeking family and professional support from a mental health telephone service if needed. She was discharged from the unit but arranged to return for a series of psychotherapy sessions. These sessions assisted Mrs. S. to return to her family life and deal with the impact of her suicide attempt on the family. Early follow-up sessions focused on psychoeducation and developing new coping strategies through exposure techniques, breathing and grounding exercises, and homework assignments. Functional assessment of her symptom triggers showed two particularly strong classically conditioned triggers (pink violets and specific music songs) associated with the abuse. These were treated with exposure techniques. By the fourth session, she sang along and smiled with the music. She was surprised by these gains and dramatically altered her concept of avoidance. She restarted gardening, which she loved but had avoided due to the triggering effect of some flowers. Homework exercises using exposure and other skills helped her to feel better, but she still expressed a sense of disconnectedness. She felt these changes were helpful but wanted to further process her emotions related to her sexual abuse perpetrator. The empty chair and similar techniques were used to help her process these feelings. This was a very challenging session for client and psychologist. She engaged fully, with tears in her eyes and saying things like "Why would you do this to me?" taking several minutes to regain her composure. The psychologist helped her use grounding skills to bring her attention back to the present. She described a sense of catharsis afterward. Further sessions explored her feelings toward her family and how she could engage well with her children and live in a fulfilling manner. Her children attended one session to express their feelings about her suicide attempt. This helped them to connect and relate better. The final sessions focused on improving her sense of self-efficacy. She was invited to contact the service for further help in the future if needed.

Outcome

Mrs. S.'s mood improved, and she reported feeling a sense of empowerment. She made tremendous progress in terms of her avoidance, anxiety, reduction of flashbacks, and nightmares. She denied ongoing suicidal ideation and made no further suicide attempts. She was discharged to her family physician without needing community mental health care and has not re-presented to inpatient or community services. Toward the end of contact, she reminded the psychologist of a statement made in an early session that she had found particularly meaningful: "The best way to live is to live well."

Commentary

This client's tremendous progress could be attributed to many factors. One significant factor was the psychoeducation that created a platform for psychotherapy. She suffered 20 years of flashbacks and anxiety without knowing these could be treated. Finding this out left her feeling relieved and hopeful. Her psychological mindedness, motivation, courage to engage in therapy with a male therapist, and commitment to homework exercises were all important.

This case highlights the usefulness of an integrative approach using relatively straightforward therapy techniques and tailoring interventions to client needs. The elements of psychoeducation, client-centered approaches, grounding skills, deep breathing, exposure, gestalt techniques, and family involvement in recovery were all valuable tools integrated to meet her various needs.

Case Study 3: Development of Plans to Guide Staff Behavior: Borderline Personality Disorder

This is an example of the psychologist's role in providing consultation to staff to aid management of complex and challenging clients. It emphasizes guiding the staff to implement consistent evidence-informed approaches for clients with personality disorders in inpatient settings and preventing inadvertent reinforcement of problem client behavior by inconsistent staff behavior.

Case Description

Ms. D. was a 32-year-old woman diagnosed with Borderline Personality Disorder (BPD), who was admitted to an acute inpatient mental health unit due to self-harming behaviors. She reported chronic suicidal ideation and had made several previous suicide attempts. She had a past history of sexual abuse. She was unemployed and homeless. She reported having no friends and difficult relationships with her mother and older siblings. She struggled with emotion regulation and engaged in self-harm and other risky behaviors (cutting, burning herself with cigarettes, drug abuse) to attempt to regulate her emotions. These difficulties had started before the age of 17. She was interpersonally sensitive and struggled with the sense of identity, often saying, "I don't even know who I am." She reported having never found anything that helped manage her depressive thoughts or self-harming tendencies.

She had a history of multiple lengthy admissions in different inpatient units but believed little benefit had come from these admissions. She was frequently oppositional, engaged in self-harm on the ward, and absconded from the ward several times. Staff often had difficulties managing her self-harming and oppositional behavior, with some being punitive and/or overprotective. Significant negative counter-transference by staff was evident.

Intervention

Ms. D. initially received general inpatient care, including trials of different antidepressants, but no changes in her mental state or behavior were reported during her lengthy admission. The psychologist was then asked to assess her to develop a different management plan. The psychologist's assessment confirmed the BPD diagnosis and presented to the multidisciplinary team a formulation informed by Dialectical Behavior Therapy (DBT: Linehan, 1993). This formulation was used to develop a management plan (including crisis management plan) to guide intervention in the inpatient and community settings. The plan's rationale was to assist Ms. D. to learn to self-manage her emotions and seek help before self-harming. Some salient points of the management plan were:

- Evidence-based guidelines for BPD suggest inpatient admissions should be short, with management primarily by community services, using techniques such as DBT *and* a consistent crisis management plan between inpatient and community services. This echoed Ms. D. and staff's observation that lengthy hospitalization was counterproductive for her.
- The management plan gave inpatient and community services a consistent approach to her formulation, coping skills, options for seeking help (e.g., via telephone and respite care if necessary) and other supports.
- The approach aimed to encourage verbalizing emotions and asking appropriately for help.
- The management plan allowed for brief hospitalization (up to 72 hours) if needed, to prevent life-threatening self-harm. However, it outlined a number of earlier, increasingly intensive steps that should be taken by the client (with support as needed) to attempt to restore equilibrium prior to hospitalization (e.g., Van Kessel, Lambie, & Stewart, 2003). If admission was necessary, then it should focus on helping her to use crisis and distress management

skills and find practical solutions to the difficulties exacerbating her distress. Staff members were encouraged to avoid being drawn into intervening in issues beyond the immediate focus of the hospitalization. Contact with her community-based DBT therapist was re-established as quickly as possible. It was acknowledged that Ms. D. would still be experiencing a level of risk to safety upon discharge.

- The management plan also allowed for respite care as a step prior to hospitalization. Respite care involved short-term (typically a few days) residential placement in a community-based house with a few clients and on-site monitoring and support by mental health support workers. It provides care that is less intensive and restrictive than the unit while providing additional support during a time of crisis. It provided support and a change of environment to facilitate emotional regulation and engage coping skills and self-care. The plan indicated that hospitalization, respite care, or similar should generally *not* be used after self-injury so as to avoid reinforcing help-seeking by self-harm.
- The plan indicated that if Ms. D. self-harmed in respite then the intended purpose of assisting her in regaining control and not self-injure had failed and her stay should end. This was not intended as a punishment and was communicated to her in a non-punitive way.
- If Ms. D. engaged in self-harm behaviors while an inpatient, staff were requested to respond in a calm fashion, offer her a dressing to clean her wounds and encourage her to talk to staff in the future before self-harming, rather than criticizing her or focusing on the reasons for the behavior. This aimed to decrease social reinforcement of self-harm behavior.
- Ms. D. was encouraged to have day leave with family members to improve her relationships with them, enhance her sense of control, and give her more opportunities to manage her emotions in everyday situations.

As her self-harm improved, she was taken off compulsory legal status.

The inpatient psychologist also engaged her in brief distress tolerance skills (Linehan, 1993) as a first line of defense in managing overwhelming emotions. The skills taught and practiced included:

- Distraction skills, (using a rubber band/wrist band; converting her inner thoughts into drawing and walking).
- Self-soothing skills (visual, such as reading and positive imagery exercises; hearing, such as relaxation music; taste, such as having a really nice coffee; touch, such as stress balls, rubber band; and smell, such as fresh air and coffee).

- Use of a positive affirmation booklet that she liked to read. This was related to the cheerleading concept that is one of the DBT skills (Linehan, 1993).

An appointment was arranged with a psychologist from the community team. The rationale and approach to treatment was, with her consent, explained to her family, and she was discharged to stay with them until ready to find independent accommodations.

Outcome

The management plan decreased her oppositional behavior and cutting on the ward quite quickly. She was easier to manage and quickly showed more settled behavior and positive interactions. It made the ward calmer by eliminating the emotional impact on other clients in response to witnessing her self-harming, aggressive, and oppositional behaviors. The plan was maintained in the community, and she engaged in therapy well, with initial hurdles related to learning to manage self-harm.

She reported considerable improvements in wellbeing and ability to manage her difficulties when in the community. The plan appeared to reduce the frequency and duration of her inpatient admissions. She did not present to the inpatient unit for over a year, and then, consistent with the management plan, required only a short admission offering containment, safety, and a chance to practice her coping skills, followed by re-engagement with her community DBT therapist.

Commentary

This case highlights the effective use of a crisis management plan spanning the inpatient and community settings for BPD clients. Empowering and supporting staff through this plan promoted consistent implementation. The approach was subsequently generalized by staff for other clients. It also reduced the risk of inadvertent harm to the client due to staff counter-transference, secondary gain from unhelpful behaviors, and staff responses that promoted adverse outcomes. Such cases need to be managed sensitively and require a fine balance of effective treatment approaches, skillful engagement of the client, and buy-in and consistency from staff. Psychologists frequently have the best combination of skills to achieve this.

Case Study 4: Guiding Staff in Managing Violence.

In this case, the psychologist contributed brief therapeutic input and assisted staff in understanding and helping the client change patterns of violent behavior that had caused difficulty for many years.

Case History

Ms. R. was a 40-year-old woman with a long history of schizophrenia with paranoid features leading to many inpatient admissions. On this occasion, she was admitted following aggressive and destructive behavior (smashing and damaging property) when responding to delusional beliefs. She did not have contact with her children (now adults), who had been fostered with family members. At admission, she presented as loud and anxious and reported being angry and upset. She said that the upset leading to her destructive behavior resulted from hearing a hallucinated scream that she believed meant her children (who were not present) were in danger. She also reported believing that a child of hers who had died had been reborn and was now alive somewhere. She knew her children were not nearby, but she wanted to check on them. She recalled that some previous admissions had been precipitated by similar concerns. She reported taking her medication as prescribed and denied command hallucinations or any perceptual abnormalities except occasionally hearing the scream. She denied using alcohol or other substances.

Assessment and Intervention

Due to her recurring aggressive acts, frequent hospitalizations, and risk to staff and other clients, a multidisciplinary intervention including psychological input was planned. The psychologist conducted two assessment sessions with Ms. R. while her case manager was present. The resultant formulation identified the emotional impact of the hallucinated screams, signifying a possible danger to her children and her grief about her lack of contact with them, which led to her acting out aggressively. Ms. R. presented as concrete in her thinking and had difficulty explaining her feelings. This may have related to cultural factors, but appeared to be intensified by her psychotic state and possibly the long-term effects of medications. While efforts were made to explore establishing contact between her and her children, interventions to manage problem behaviors (property damage, screaming swearing/talking to herself, intense stare, aggression) were initiated. To achieve this, the psychologist assisted nurses in undertaking a functional analysis by recording the behaviors, their antecedents (hallucinated screams), and the consequences (getting medication or receiving attention from staff who tried de-escalation). As distress triggered the problematic behavior, distress tolerance skills were suggested as a suitable intervention. The psychologist taught the client distress tolerance skills and demonstrated the skills to staff so they could coach her to use skills when needed. The skills and resources included flashcards with self-coping statements; abdominal breathing demonstrated and coached by staff; coping cards with pictures illustrating coping skills she could use such as walking, music, reading, sharing her concerns with others; and sensory modulation (e.g., coloring-in books or squeezing stress-balls). Staff implemented the behavioral management plan, involving encouragement to use the skills and resources whenever behavioral changes suggesting an exacerbation were observed. This helped her learn to de-escalate her own distress and prevent further harm or damage.

Outcome

Ms. R. showed significant improvement in her behaviors. There was no further property damage. When she experienced distress from hearing the hallucinated screams, she asked staff for help. Staff continued to follow the behavioral management plan, which was updated further with the collaboration of the client and her case manager.

Commentary

Ms. R.'s issues needed a broader approach than just reducing problem behaviors. A management plan that helped her and the staff to recognize and address causes for her behavior was critical for success. This differed from years of previous assessments, medication changes, admissions, etc., that had attempted to contain her behavior but with minimal effort applied to understanding the underlying reasons. This approach helped her change her problematic behavior and helped the staff consider the content and context of her symptoms, develop a more empathic view of her, and develop greater willingness to address underlying issues. This approach is useful for many such clients.

Case Study 5: Developing Low-Intensity Interventions: Dealing with Distress Groups for Inpatients

This is an example of psychologists developing and implementing a brief low-intensity emotional regulation group intervention, to be run by psychologists and/or other staff members, with broad applicability to a wide range of inpatients. In addition to learning to facilitate the group, staff frequently learned skills they can use with clients outside the groups.

Case Description

Problems with emotional self-regulation are a central difficulty for many people with mental health problems and are common in inpatient settings. Dialectic Behavioral Therapy (Linehan, 1993) teaches skills that help clients manage distressing emotions. DBT emotional self-regulation skills and related skills from other therapies can be taught in a brief group format and will benefit a wide variety of clients who would not usually be considered for the full DBT program. These are sometimes called "Dealing with Distress" (DWD) programs.

Activity

A manualized DWD group program was established for clients of a community mental health service (CMHS). This involved clients learning and practicing emotional regulation and related skills drawn from DBT, CBT, and other sources in six 90 minute group sessions held over three weeks and attended by up to 15 people. The group was led by mental health professionals, often but not always psychologists. Psychologists from the mental health inpatient unit serving in the same area decided to modify this program for the inpatient setting. Modifications included shortening the sessions and somewhat simplifying the content to suit the shortened attention span, agitation, and medication-related difficulties often faced by people in these settings. It was also modified by making the groups open and rolling so clients could start in any session and attend any subsequent sessions they wished. This made each session a self-contained intervention that did not rely on learnings from previous sessions. Content of the course included goal setting; problem-solving strategies; education about the five-part CBT model; mindfulness; distress tolerance skills (e.g., distraction, self-soothing, improving the moment, pros and cons); and developing a coping plan. Other staff, including occupational therapy and nursing staff, were involved from relatively early in the development process. Any interested staff members were invited to take part in the groups, first as participants alongside the clients, and then as group leaders.

Outcome

In 2 years, 24 groups were held. They were attended by over 200 clients and by 42 staff members, 15 of whom trained as co-facilitators. Outcome rating scales showed positive improvements for client distress tolerance, mindfulness, and confidence, and also improved staff confidence and behavior. Coaching of staff was important to encourage ongoing use of the techniques. Client-completed rating scales indicated that all respondents who attended three or more sessions found the program useful, and 70% reported gaining confidence from the program. Comments from clients and staff indicated that both learned new skills that empowered the clients and helped them self-regulate their behavior while on the ward. Staff also reported finding the skills personally useful. The distress tolerance skills and coping plan development were the most positively rated activities by clients (DuVillier & MacPherson, 2006).

Commentary

In this example, psychologists took a community-based psychological therapy program and translated it into a form usable in the mental health inpatient setting. The approach was designed to allow delivery by other staff so that the impact of its use could spread beyond the direct provision of therapies by psychologists.

Conclusion

Brief therapy is an attractive concept for many reasons. It suggests a relatively quick improvement, reduced cost and inconvenience for clients, cost-effectiveness, and increased access to therapy for more people. While more effective for some difficulties than for others, brief therapy offers hope for healthcare systems that increasingly understand that addressing the psychological and social issues of people with mental or physical health difficulties is an important and often untapped strategy for improving outcomes and reducing the spiraling costs of healthcare (Blount et al., 2007).

However, as argued in this chapter, there are two distinctly different forms of brief therapy that both add considerable value, but which require very different skill sets and expertise. Many people, including those who develop, fund, and direct services, are not aware of this difference, and frequently have only low-intensity brief therapy in mind when making decisions about service design and operation. This limited understanding can affect models of care and operational processes, which then adversely affects the ability of services to optimally respond to the needs of clients. It can also affect staffing decisions. Particularly, the relative invisibility of high-intensity brief therapy can lead to psychologists (as the group often most able to deliver these therapies) being undervalued and under-represented in staff numbers. Increasing understanding of the distinction between high- and low-intensity brief therapies, the different value added by each, and the role of psychologists as the primary professional group who provide high-intensity brief therapy and who can support low-intensity brief therapy provision by others, could be useful for increasing the psychology workforce and improving outcomes and wellbeing for clients.

The case studies above provide examples of some different contributions that psychologists make in the brief therapy field – as providers of high-intensity brief therapy, as providers of nuanced and comprehensive assessments that inform interventions by others, and as developers of low-intensity brief therapies. A hallmark of these case studies is the well-grounded flexibility of approach that comes from a depth and breadth of training in the theory underlying the techniques as well as the techniques themselves. This is one aspect of the particular value that psychologists contribute to the inpatient setting.

No formal definition of brief therapy has been offered in this chapter because what constitutes brief therapy is context-dependent and is impacted by many factors such as the model of care. Some case studies involved several sessions over a short period of time, so engagement was brief. In some instances, the model of care allowed follow-up sessions in the months after discharge, so the period of contact was not brief, but the total therapeutic time was relatively brief. In some situations, there are a fixed number of sessions.

In summary, both high- and low-intensity brief psychological therapy has much to offer in inpatient mental health, and psychologists have much to offer in the delivery of high-intensity (and in sometimes low-intensity) brief therapy, and in supporting others to deliver low-intensity brief therapy.

References

Bach, P., & Hayes, S. (2002). The use of acceptance and commitment therapy to prevent the rehospitalisation of psychotic patients: A randomized controlled trial. *Journal of Consulting and Clinical Psychology*, *70*, 1129–1139.

Bartak, A., Spreeuwenberg, M.D., Andrea, H., Holleman,L., Rinjnierse, P., Rossum, B.V., & Emmelkamp, P.M.G. (2010). Effectiveness of different modalities of psychotherapeutic treatment for patients with cluster C personality disorders: Results of a large prospective multicentre study. *Psychotherapy and Psychosomatics*, *79*, 20–30.

Beutel, M.E., Hoflich, A., Kurth, R.A., & Reimer, C. (2005). Who benefits from inpatient short-term psychotherapy in the long run? Patient's evaluations, outpatient after-care and determinants of outcome. *Psychology and Psychotherapy: Theory, Research and Practice*, *78*, 219–234.

Blount, A., Schoenbaum, M., Kathol, R., Rollman, B.L., Thomas, M., O'Donohue, W., & Peek, C.J. (2007). The economics of behavioural health services in medical settings: A summary of the evidence. *Professional Psychology: Research and Practice*, *38*, 290–297.

Bobart, A.C. (2005). Evidence-based psychotherapy means evidence-informed, not evidence driven. *Journal of Contemporary Psychotherapy*, *35*, 39–53.

British Psychological Society. (2010). *Clinical psychology: The core purpose and philosophy of the profession*. Leicester: Author

Callan, S., & Fry, B. (2012). *Commissioning effective talking therapies*. London: Centre for Social Justice.

Castonguay, L.G., Eubanks, C.F., Goldfried, M.R., Muran, J.C., & Lutz, W. (2015). Research on psychotherapy integration: Building on the past, looking to the future. *Psychotherapy Research*. *25*, 365–382

Chadwick, P. (2006). *Person-based cognitive therapy for distressing psychosis*. Chichester, UK: Wiley.

Dath, S., Sables, E., Yang Dong, C., & Stewart, M.W. (2014) A clinical psychologist in GP-Land: An evaluation of brief psychological interventions in primary care. *New Zealand Medical Journal*, *127* (1391), 62–74.

Durant, C., & Tolland, A. (2009). Evaluating short-term CBT in an acute inpatient unit. In I. Clarke & H. Wilson (Eds.) *Cognitive behavior therapy for acute inpatient mental health units: Working with clients, staff and the milieu.* pp. 185–196. New York, NY: Routledge.

DuVillier, T., & MacPherson, S. (2006, June). Skills groups based on DBT for people with psychosis in hospital and in the community. *International Congress of the International Society for the Psychological Treatment of Schizophrenia and Other Psychoses*, Madrid, Spain.

Geczy, B., & Sultenfuss, J.F. (1994). Contributions of psychologists to inpatient care of persons with chronic mental illness. *Hospital and Community Psychiatry*, 45, 54–57.

Greenberg, L.S. (2002). *Emotion-focused therapy: Coaching clients to work through their feelings*. New York, NY: American Psychological Association.

Haga, D.A.F. (2000). Introduction to the special section on stepped care models in psychotherapy. *Journal of Consulting and Clinical Psychology*, 68, 457–458.

Holmes, J. (2002). Acute wards: Problems and solutions: Creating a therapeutic culture in acute psychiatric wards. *Psychiatric Bulletin*, *26*, 383–385.

Hubble, M.A., Duncan, B.L., & Miller, S.D. (Eds.) (1999). *The heart and soul of change*. New York, NY: American Psychological Association.

Lee, S., Rothbard, A.B., & Noll, E.L., (2012). Length of inpatient stay of persons with serious mental illness: Effects of hospital and regional characteristics. *Psychiatric Services*, *63*, 889–895.

Leibenluft, E., Tasman, A., Green, S.A. (Eds.) (1993). *Less time to do more: Psychotherapy on the short term inpatient unit*. Arlington, VA: American Psychiatric Association.

Lemmens, G.M.D., Eisler, I., Migerode, L., Heireman, M., & Demyttenaere, K. (2007). A brief systemic multi-family group intervention for hospitalised patients and their family members. *Journal of Family Therapy*, *29*, 49–68.

Levinson, H. (1995). *Time limited psychotherapy: A guide to clinical practice.* New York, NY: Basic Books.

Linehan, M.M. (1993). *Skills training manual for treating borderline personality disorder*. New York, NY: Guilford Press.

McGowan, J., & Hill, R. (2009). The role of psychological therapies in acute psychiatric care. *Clinical Psychology Forum*, *196*, 14–17.

Mobray, D. (1988). *MAS review of clinical psychology services* (For the National Health Services/Department of Health Manpower Planning Advisory Group). Cheltenham, UK: Management Advisory Service.

Nielsen, M. (2015). CBT group treatment for depression. *The Cognitive Behaviour Therapist* 8, E8.

Norcross, J.C., & Goldfried, M.R. (Eds.) (2005). *Handbook of psychotherapy integration* (2nd ed.). New York, NY: Oxford University Press.

Stein, M.B., & Jacobo, M.C. (2013). Brief inpatient psychotherapeutic technique. *Psychotherapy*, *50*, 464–468.

Stewart, M.W., Bushnell, J., Hauraki, J., & Roberts, M. (2014). Evidence and wisdom: The role and value of psychologists in healthcare. *Journal of the New Zealand College of Clinical Psychologists*, 24 (1), 3–14

Stuart, S., & Robertson, M. (2003). *Interpersonal psychotherapy: A clinician's guide*. London: Arnold.

UK Department of Health (2012). *IAPT three-year report: The first million patients*. Retrieved from www.dh.gsi.gov.uk.

Van Kessel, K., Lambie, I., & Stewart, M.W. (2003). The impact of brief planned admissions on inpatient mental health unit utilization for people with a diagnosis of borderline personality disorder. *New Zealand Journal of Psychology*, *31*, 93–97.

11 Continuity Model of Care

Working across Acute Inpatient to Community-Based Clinical Psychology

Kim Griffiths, Hannah Green, and Suzie Lemmey

This chapter introduces a novel model of acute inpatient to community clinical psychology service provision which has been developed in our unit, within the United Kingdom (UK) National Health Service (NHS) psychiatric service. This continuity of care method involves the delivery of psychological assessment and intervention on an acute inpatient ward and when appropriate continuation of the intervention post discharge in the community teams to complete therapeutic aims. The model thus offers support through the service users' transition from the ward environment and offers the opportunity to complete therapy and hopefully reduce the rate of readmission and maximize recovery. The associated benefits of continuity of care include avoiding the need for onward referrals, reassessment and unnecessary waiting times. Case studies are presented to illustrate implementation of the model. Provisional data regarding the model's putative impact on readmission rates and subsequent bed days is also presented.

Characteristically, emotional distress lies at the root of many if not all acute mental health admissions (Clarke & Wilson, 2009). Psychological exploration, formulation and intervention offers a valuable and effective vehicle to make sense of and to address such experiences. Indeed, it could be argued that during an acute experience the need for psychological intervention may be most pertinent, given it is likely to be the very time when one has lost connection with one's own "making sense of" and associated meanings, understanding, direction and internal resilience. Thus psychological support during acute episodes of mental distress can be highly meaningful and beneficial for the service user and their loved ones.

Access to psychological therapies on acute inpatient wards has been identified as a requirement in the UK in both local and national service user feedback investigations (Sainsbury's Centre for Mental Health, 2006; NICE, 2011). However, nationwide, provision of psychological services in inpatient settings remains varied and relatively new compared with outpatient work.

The provision of psychological therapy is well integrated and established within community mental health teams (CMHT). Community teams often include several clinical psychologists and psychotherapists working closely with psychiatrists, community mental health nurses, occupational therapists and social workers. In contrast, in the UK acute inpatient systems, there are markedly fewer psychology posts, rarely more than one per ward, or in some cases one post covering an entire unit, which includes several wards. There are still many inpatient services with no direct or "in-house" clinical psychology involvement. This is of course in strong contrast with psychiatry where there is invariably a strong presence of consultant (or consultants) and a team of junior psychiatrists or medics.

This difference between acute and community services can in some ways be understood due to the smaller evidence base for acute care psychological intervention compared with the extensive research and randomized controlled trials of community-based therapies, such as CBT which is an impressive example of this. However, the provision of clinical psychology services on acute wards has been found to have positive outcomes (Donaghey-Spire, McGowan, Griffiths, & Barazzone, 2015) and studies have also found that acute based psychological therapy has been linked with reduced readmission rates (Kerfoot, Bamford, & Jones, 2012).

The Acute Care Pathway

An acute admission can be a frightening, traumatic and often unpleasant experience. As mentioned, one may have lost connection with different forms of self-agency, internal resilience, social and emotional functioning and may require containment, support, safety and direction which at varying levels can or cannot be met in an inpatient setting. Discharge from the containing hospital environment can be a similarly complex emotional process. Service users may find the transition into community services bewildering and anxiety provoking with little time to develop new therapeutic relationships with their newly allocated therapists, or to become familiar with new community teams, systems and care packages.

Some service users find the transition between teams a difficult process. Strong therapeutic relationships can develop during an acute admission; indeed this may be more pronounced in psychotherapeutic relationships given the nature of the psychological work combined with the emotional intensity of the inpatient or crisis experience. Discharge from the ward can feel like an attachment loss; a separation from people who have offered needed support during a complex and distressed period of life. This attachment loss can be further complicated when the transition between the ward-based work and support in the community was not taken into account. Pre-discharge communication with community teams can be important in this respect as it can assist in developing therapeutic relationships that help ease the move back into the community.

Generally, for acute care based work, if a non-brief focused form of psychological therapy had been indicated along the acute care pathway as part of a service user's care package or need, this would ordinarily come via referred assessment into the CMHT and subsequent waiting list allocation. Ordinarily, any psychological work on the ward would be brief or if slightly longer, then fragmented into a referred reassessment and/or significant waiting list delay.

The process of the inpatient care team referring to a community-based care team is a well-founded configuration in the provision of health care services. Often this is beneficial, as different services often require certain skill sets and specialist expertise such as Dialectical Behavior Therapy teams, specialist challenging behavior teams, specific physical condition teams or neuro-rehabilitation teams in the community. However, some disciplines also lend themselves to crossing specialties as they have transferable skills applicable across systems. It is well established that clinical psychology is one such discipline, as it provides transferable expertise and core clinical competencies across different settings. The posts described in this chapter draw upon transferable expertise of clinical psychological assessment, formulation and intervention between acute inpatient and community mental health. Indeed this is not exclusive to the profession of clinical psychology; the same is recognized in other mental health professions including psychiatry and some forms of mental health nursing and occupational therapy.

Continuity of Care

Developing continuity of care between the inpatient and community settings has been central to this model and as a concept is in itself multifaceted. Crawford and colleagues identified a number of factors in the following definition: "the patient remains in contact with services; there are no breaks in service delivery; the patient sees the same member of staff; different components of health and social care are coordinated; and service users experience care as smooth and uninterrupted." (Crawford, de Jonge, Freemand, & Weaver, 2004, p 266).

High readmission rates have been linked with a lack of continuity of care between mental health systems, particularly acute to community care (Durbin, Lin, Layne, & Teed, 2007). Seeing the same member of staff has been identified as a key component reducing personally costly (and at a service level financially) readmissions (Burns et al., 2009; Vandyk et al., 2013). Provision of continuity of care can reduce anxiety, frustration and offer a service user an increased sense of support (Bilderbeck, Saunders, Price, & Goodwin, 2014).

A literature review of continuity work did not find any studies reporting a bridging of psychological interventions (Vigod et al., 2013). However, a report by the British Psychological Society on the provision of inpatient psychological care found that alternatives to inpatient admission require inpatient and community to be "properly connected" (British Psychological Society, 2014).

The model of service provision detailed in this chapter addresses the importance of continuity, detailed above. It has become increasingly recognized that clinical psychology is a necessary component of acute inpatient care. Indeed this covers more than direct inpatient therapy; it includes reflective practice sessions for staff, consultation, training and leadership. Alongside these tasks, the psychology posts described here were introduced to provide psychological support across service systems from the acute inpatient to community team settings, with the intent to deliver a range of benefits for service users, their service journey and the wider system.

Model Overview and Service Context

Locally named the "continuity model," the posts described were split funded between the acute inpatient service (a two ward unit with 20 beds per ward) and the local CMHT. The posts (and model) essentially arose from the vision of our then Head of Psychology, who recognized the need to offer a balance between acute and community work not only to the post holders (reflected on later) but more so for the benefit of the service user's journey. With a focus on providing continuity of care through the transition period of discharge (and beyond if necessary), it was hoped that the process of separation from the ward and engagement with the community team would be improved and short or long term psychotherapeutic goals could be completed without the time and resource consuming need for reassessment, waiting list delay, development of new therapeutic relationships, reformulation and so on.

It was also understood that at that time the acute unit was felt to be somewhat remote and disconnected from the community services. This was in terms of geography (there is a 15-mile cross-city journey) but also with input, particularly with regard to psychological therapy. There had not been a funded clinical psychology post in the acute inpatient service since the unit's inception in the 1990s. Once funding was granted, it provided a bridge between the acute and community services and was viewed as being the most helpful use of this new resource: to bring the acute and community teams closer together, while ensuring that this was done with a psychological approach.

Thus two posts were created: One psychologist per ward working half the week on a ward and half of the week offering continuity sessions in the community teams. This continuity work would focus upon the completion of psychological therapy which had begun on the ward and would assist in engagement liaison or consultation to both acute and community teams and/or completion of extended assessments. The posts were created in 2008. Two of the authors of this chapter are psychologists currently in these roles (KG and HG).

It was hoped that where psychological work on the ward had progressed but felt incomplete upon inpatient discharge, it could subsequently be continued immediately in the community teams. This would likely apply to admissions of at least a few weeks duration, where time would have allowed a certain number of sessions to take place on the ward and at the point of discharge psychological treatment was deemed to be unfinished and if completed recovery could be maximized.

The nature of this work would vary, reflective of the nature of acute service user presentations and length of stay. It may involve brief crisis based work focusing on the nature of the immediate crisis and what may facilitate discharge. In other cases, it may involve longer-term therapeutic goals which naturally would be dependent on the length of stay and the formulation based goals. Locally an average length of stay has been 21 days, thus in some cases three weeks can offer the time required for assessment, formulation and intervention to commence.

Some acute presentations can be too distressed, dissociated or be experiencing complex concurrent social difficulties that would counter-indicate immediate readiness for therapy. However, in our experience, many people are ready to engage with some form of psychological intervention during an admission, and in such cases a waiting list delay would often be highly counter-productive or even detrimental.

We have at times encountered a myth that when in crisis people do not have the internal resources to engage or effectively utilize psychological therapy. We call this a myth specifically as it appears to be based on little research and is indeed counter to our experience and not consistent with what many of the service users we meet are asking for. More often than not, people are admitted to a ward to receive medication, and to experience some form of physical separation from their difficulties, to access associated support and stabilization and talk about their problems. Naturally, the latter does not always mean psychological therapy in one form or another, but in many cases it can.

When assessment on a ward indicated immediate benefits and motivation to engage in the use of talking therapies, whether in terms of a cognitive behavioral approach, a systemic intervention or some of the other paradigms discussed later, such patients would be seen weekly and upon discharge considered for further continuity sessions. This has often felt to be "striking while the iron is hot," immediately looking to address something that has contributed to an emotionally painful and service costly admission without the potentially damaging or destabilizing period of a waiting list delay.

Naturally, the number of people who can be offered continuity sessions would always be influenced by psychologist caseload sizes. We can only hold a certain number of continuity cases open at any given time, and the discharge rate of the wards can be high. When our own capacity does not allow continuity sessions, then the assessment is referred directly onto the waiting list in the CMHT.

However, it should be noted that in some cases a referral to a waiting list may be appropriate particularly in circumstances where patients are not immediately ready for therapy. In such instances, people can be referred directly from the ward to a community waiting list, in order to enable the therapeutic function of time. This can be necessary when there are social problems that would likely interfere with therapy such as homelessness or complex legal proceedings or when there are substance misuse issues which would require primary attention. In some cases, these matters can be addressed while on a waiting list, and if tackled successfully, subsequent therapy could begin at a more suitable time.

In summary, the maintenance of a therapeutic relationship from a ward environment with identified psychotherapeutic goals, during the complex transitional period of discharge and reintegration into home life, aimed to provide stability and improvement to the patient's journey. Essentially therapy would not be punctuated by a waiting list or repeat assessment delays and the therapeutic alliance would not be ruptured. Furthermore, the holding effect of therapy and the stabilizing presence of a secure therapeutic process and relationship was hoped to reduce subsequent readmissions, which can often be a feature of acute discharge, as well as improve patients' engagement with community services.

Indeed, whenever we describe this model to colleagues, commissioners, patients, and caregivers all unanimously respond, "that makes sense!" However, in reality, most services are configured into boxed budgets and the teaming up of the funding for these posts, though not unique, is not commonplace. We expect our service users to move from team to team, yet budgets and job descriptions are less likely to follow suit. This seems contradictory or lacking collaborative parity.

Case Studies and Outcomes

In an attempt to illustrate our work, we have included several clinical case studies as exemplars of this method. The cases presented reveal different complex presentations and diagnoses and include histories of repeat admissions, delayed discharge and high levels of risk to self. The cases vary in therapeutic models, something which is characteristically unique to clinical psychology in comparison with other unimodal psychotherapeutic approaches.

All cases involved actively working with the ward and community multi-disciplinary teams (MDT). In the case of the former, MDT reviews and nursing handovers were meetings where formulation and intervention aims were shared and integrated into the wider inpatient care plan. Consultation and linking with the team in this way are both vital aspects of maintaining and promoting a psychological approach to care. Formulations and interventions were discussed with the wider multi-disciplinary team (psychiatry, nurses, occupational therapy) as well as instructing team-based interventions, e.g., promotion of self-care to manage dependency, spending time off the ward as graded exposure, managing reassurance in the case of anxiety disorders and so on.

Reflective practice sessions are also specific forums where ward based work was discussed, co-created and disseminated with the wider team. Reflective practice is a reserved weekly or fortnightly meeting where the psychologist meets with the team to reflect on the work on the ward, including an impact on staff, as well as discussion and development of individualized formulations or interventions. All team-based work is important in the acute setting given the historical dominance of the medical model and the need to actively promote and emphasize psychological understanding and approaches.

It is of note that the posts described here are ward specific with an identified aim of being a part of the acute multi-disciplinary team. Thus clinical psychology is directly integrated into the ward team culture which can be more of a challenge for unit-wide models or in-reach from outside services.

In terms of team working in the community this would involve liaison with post-discharge services such as crisis teams (who in the UK can offer two week post-discharge support), the CMHT's, co-working or consultation with community allocated professionals (often called care coordinators in the UK, community psychiatric nurses, social workers or occupational therapists).

Following the case studies, we also present some preliminary data on outcomes from the continuity cases. In the absence of routine measures, the outcome was assessed in terms of repeat admissions and subsequent acute inpatient bed days.

Case Studies

Case Study 1: CBT for Psychosis

Beth was a 40-year-old woman who throughout her 20s had worked regularly in a middle-grade administrative post in the city of London. In her early 30s, she started to develop psychotic experiences and received a diagnosis of paranoid schizophrenia. She was in a long term relationship with another service user who had his own issues with anxiety, agoraphobia, and alcohol. Beth was well known to the inpatient service having suffered regular cyclical psychotic relapses involving nearly annual lengthy admissions for the previous 7 years or so. When Beth was not well, she neglected her self-care, developed complex paranoid delusional thoughts (particularly toward her partner and mother) and struggled with hearing voices and some jumbled speech, typical with thought disorders.

Beth had repeatedly declined psychological support from the community psychosis team but had a strong relationship with her community nurse, whom she had seen primarily for medication maintenance for many years. When stable, she maintained a strong oppositional position to her diagnosis and denied and minimized her psychotic experiences. She tended to be admitted against her will, detained under the UK's Mental Health Act. As was part of this near annual cycle, Beth was admitted, and when a clinical psychologist became available on the ward for the first time, she was offered to meet for an assessment. She agreed hoping that if she complied with treatment directives, her discharge would be accelerated. Thus the motivation was not to explore psychological perspectives but rather for the secondary gain of rescinding her mental health detention and returning home.

Though called an assessment the early sessions emphasized engagement, particularly given her past resistance to psychological treatment. This engagement process was parallel to her confusing, distressing and chaotic psychotic experiences and the affect associated with her worries and preoccupations. Many of her psychotic beliefs focused on her belief that her partner and family were imposters and were conspiratorially implicit in her hospital detention.

As some of Beth's more acute psychotic symptoms passed, we continued to meet, having developed a positive therapeutic relationship during the first three months of her admission. She had admitted to hearing voices which drove her beliefs about those close to her and indeed could recall our previous sessions, not always in detail, but in the certainty that they had occurred and had been helpful. This enabled us to speak and openly formulate her psychotic experiences for the first time as we reflected on these sessions. It seemed that having been alongside Beth during such a time of internal chaos gave her trust in therapy, which having borne witness to some of her more delusional beliefs, left her with a lessened drive to deny or minimize them allowing her to reflect more openly. Her sense of her psychotic experiences and comfort in talking about them improved immeasurably. Indeed at times, she was even able to laugh at some of the things she had said.

This process led us to formulate, following a CBT for psychosis model. In exploring aspects of her past and family relationships, Beth started to open up about her long-standing sense of difference with regard to peers and family. She had a higher achieving sister and felt she had struggled more with the loss of her father with whom she likened herself to and had been very close. She perceived her mother to be cold and distant at times, and contrastingly as over-involved and smothering at other times. Her sense of being different, combined with unease in her current relationship and her long-standing low self-esteem, could leave her feeling that people were against her or looked down on her. At times this would develop into delusional thoughts that others would plot against her or that they would not even be whom they say they are.

As we linked her past to her beliefs we could also look at the current influence they could have within her life. Her self-care improved as she was able to reflect more on the beliefs that drove it, namely that people could infect the water to get at her. She could question and disbelieve the voices, which we found were more rumination driven as opposed to voices which had personalities or characteristics. Thus if she could manage her rumination, her voices would reduce as would her distress. She found ways of recognizing her thoughts as cognitive events and thus let go of her rumination. She was also able to slowly spend more time with her partner and mother and manage her avoidance and conflict with them. This eventually enabled her discharge from the hospital to her home.

During her 4–5-month admission, we had 17 sessions on the ward. Given some ongoing tensions in her couple relationship and the potential impact this could have on her recovery process we agreed to continue meeting in the community. With an initial focus on the transition period and the couples' communication issues, which had contributed to the development of some of Beth's delusional beliefs, our community-based work continued to explore the relationship between Beth's psychotic experiences and her self-image and perception of others. Over time, this allowed the therapeutic work to develop a robust relapse prevention plan with acknowledgment that the early warning signs included the development of paranoid thoughts, conflict with her partner and mother, poor sleep, social avoidance and withdrawal and spending more time ruminating. Again, the openness that began on the ward directly informed this process, and Beth could acknowledge different stages of her relapses in a way she had never felt empowered to do before. We had 20 sessions in the community. She continued to receive support from the community mental health team for medication management for a further 2 years and was then discharged from the service. To date, the cycle of admissions has been broken by 8 years.

Case Study 2: Integrative Psychotherapy for EUPD

Amy was a 23-year-old art graduate. In the last 2 years, she was admitted to a private hospital and had a three-month stay in an eating disorder unit, both of which she had absconded. Prior to transfer to our unit she had a 61 day stay in a psychiatric intensive care unit because of her high suicide risk and self-harming behavior. She was admitted under the UK's Mental Health Act.

Amy had a diagnosis of emotionally unstable personality disorder, and much of her damaging eating disorder behavior (vomiting) had been replaced with self-harm by cutting and intense ruminative suicidal ideation. Prior to transfer to our unit Amy's parents had requested psychological therapy for her. Amy was happy to meet for the assessment and though at times highly distressed she was open to talking about her thoughts and feelings and how these related to her self-harm.

Following assessment, brief CBT for managing intense emotions (Bell, 2003) was indicated to help manage Amy's immediate risk and suicidality, and weekly contact was agreed upon. The admission lasted 116 days and was driven by risk and difficulties in finding a placement post discharge as she felt unable to return to the family home. Much of her distress stemmed from a conflict in the family, and it was agreed that moving back home would be counter-therapeutic. In such a lengthy admission the therapeutic relationship, themes, and aims developed. Consequently, the work extended beyond brief self-harm and goal orientated interventions to identify long-term psychotherapeutic aims, which primarily involved exploring attachment issues within the context of a well-educated and striving family system.

Amy received 21 sessions on the ward during which self-harm was managed using behavioral diaries, urge control, mindfulness and a wider formulated understanding of what lay behind her self-directed anger. Much of Amy's self-harm behavior seemed to relate to past difficulties in having felt prevented from expressing her feelings as a child and young adult. Thus the very process of formulation and wider exploration eased this drive as her anger became expressed in a more accessible way. Upon discharge, Amy's risk profile remained high and work continued during her transition from the ward, with which she had become quite attached, to the mental health supported lodging where she received a 1-year placement. It seems fair to hypothesize that the continuity sessions offered some stability to assist Amy in separating from the ward, serving as a transitional object as she moved from the then familiar acute ward to another unfamiliar environment.

Over-time therapy continued to explore attachment issues relating to her two higher achieving younger siblings and complex close and distant parental relationships, often drawing on mentalization principles (Bateman & Fonagy, 2016). Concurrently as particular benefits had been received from mindfulness on the ward, the latter stages also focused on 1:1 Mindfulness-Based Cognitive Therapy (MBCT, Segal, Williams, & Teasdale, 2012). MBCT is ordinarily delivered in a group format, but due to the nature of the therapeutic relationship and the journey thus far it was felt appropriate to do this 1:1. MBCT also has a specific focus on relapse prevention and thus provided an agency and resilience building vehicle for Amy to not only end therapy but also feel confident in maintaining her wellbeing in the future.

Amy was discharged after 45 sessions in the community and has not been readmitted. She continued to receive monitoring support via monthly meetings with a community psychiatric nurse in the Complex Needs team for a further 12 months. At the time of writing, she has remained discharged for 5 years.

Case Study 3: Managing Service Transitions

Emma was 18 when she transferred to the adult psychiatric ward, from a ward for younger people. She came to the ward after losing several of the attachments she had made in Child and Adolescent Mental Health Services, because of her recent transfer to adult services. Building an engagement with Emma was challenging. She would show the ward team her distress by self-harming in cutting and headbanging. An intervention at this early stage tried to engage the part of her that could see a future by inviting her college tutor to the ward. Joint work was undertaken with the ward and college to help Emma continue to study while on the ward. Over time Emma was able to share her experience of hearing voices telling her to self-harm and denigrating herself. She was able to talk a little about her experience of being adopted by the extended family, but what life at home looked like remained unclear and attempts to engage her adopted parents were unsuccessful. We held a hypothesis in mind that Emma's struggle to talk was due to a continued lack of safety at home.

Emma played out a bind on the ward with her discharge. Emma told us she wanted to leave the ward as she felt trapped, but when it came to discharge, would increase her self-harming to the extent that discharge was delayed. Offering continuity work on discharge allowed us to take a positive risk and discharge Emma. She was allocated a skilled senior social worker from the local CMHT, alongside psychological intervention. The bulk of the work was continued together with intensive liaison with Emma's college to help her continue her education, her priority at the time, as well as the initiation of complex adult safeguarding procedures.

Emma continued with psychotherapy sessions for 10 months following discharge and continued to play out the bind expressed on the ward. She would attend psychology appointments regularly but say they weren't useful, would display her self-harm wounds but claim they were an accident, and after several months of meeting in the community, began to dramatically lose weight. Having an overview of the ward together with the community mental health team allowed for continued liaison about the need for a readmission. Conversations were had with Emma about the use of the Mental Health Act given her rapidly decreasing weight. Eventually, Emma was admitted to a general hospital due to her low weight and through liaison with the mental health team in the general hospital, the use of the Mental Health Act transferred Emma back to the acute psychiatric ward. A move to an eating disorder unit was then facilitated from the ward and the psychology continuity role allowed for continued contact with Emma in order to support this transition. Emma spent six months in the eating disorder unit. Since discharge from the eating disorder unit Emma has communicated her gratitude for continued contact despite her inability to talk fully about her experience. She continues to imply that she was not safe at home and could only communicate this through her behavior. Having an ongoing, albeit at times ambivalent attachment through a number of transitions, ensured that Emma was not lost in the system. She has now moved into supported accommodation, has separated from her adopted family and is planning to attend university.

Case Study 4: Working with the Couple

Gemma was in her 50s and admitted to the ward following a number of significant family and social stressors, including the loss of her home through a tenancy dispute. This was her first presentation to mental health services despite a childhood history of continuous neglect and sexual and physical abuse. She had been receiving individual psychological therapy from a community psychologist as she had started to breakdown in the context of her life stressors. However, over time she deteriorated and was admitted to the ward presenting with high suicide risk.

Her individual therapy continued via in-reach to the ward, while concurrently the ward psychologists both worked with immediate coping between sessions. This was assisted by the physical containment of the ward environment and psychological containment, including the use of mindfulness to manage flashbacks and related panic attacks and self-harm behavior. This also included several reflective practice sessions with staff to help formulate and understand her distress on the ward, which was painful to witness.

Several weeks into her admission, ward staff noticed that Gemma seemed to become more distressed following leave with her husband. Despite concerns from the ward team about exacerbating her distress by inviting Keith to the ward, the ward psychologists decided to invite Keith and Gemma to couple sessions on the ward. They both agreed to this, with the goal of managing the transition from home leave to the ward and ultimately, discharge.

Couples sessions allowed a space for Gemma to voice her anger toward Keith in a safe way but also for her to hear Keith's own distress at being made homeless. Gemma noticed her anger was directed at her perceived sense of Keith's passivity and we were able to formulate this as both Keith's way of coping with his own feelings of hopelessness but also his attempt to pacify Gemma in the face of her extreme volatility and distress.

Work was undertaken with the couple as part of the continuity model to help manage the transition from the ward into temporary accommodation. This helped alleviate some of the ward and couple's anxiety about leaving the safety of the ward. Couples work ran alongside Gemma's individual trauma-focused therapy to help them survive periods of distress, including the use of mindfulness as a couple. Since leaving the ward Gemma and Keith were referred to a Mindfulness-Based Cognitive Therapy group for couples in the community (Griffiths & Averbeck, 2016). This was hoped to further their use of mindfulness in managing their own and each-others' distress and was also facilitated by one of us (KG), so continuity was able to continue even further. Gemma has remained out of hospital now for nearly 2 years, and they both report the value of couples therapy in helping them remember and enlist their strengths as a couple to survive periods of adversity.

Initial Service Evaluation

Taking an initial look into the possible influence continuity sessions have had on wider service usage, quantitative analysis has been undertaken of post-intervention readmissions and subsequent bed days over a 1 year period. Across high-income countries, 8% to 18% of clients are readmitted within 30 days of discharge from acute psychiatric wards, with 37% to 50% being readmitted within 1 year (Agency for Health Care Research and Quality, 2012; NHS Benchmarking Network, 2013). Readmissions are viewed as having a negative impact on the client and pose large financial implications for the service and wider NHS (Vigod et al., 2013).

Participants

A period of 5 years, between November 2008 and 2013 was chosen, giving a sufficient length of time post-admission to establish whether service users had been readmitted (N=70). A comparison group was compiled of 70 service users who had been admitted to the inpatient service at the same time but had not received continuity sessions with a psychologist. The groups were matched on certain factors in order to minimize confounding variables namely: Gender, Mental health care cluster data (which is a diagnostic grouping system indicating service needs), Psychiatric Diagnosis, Ethnicity, Age (plus/minus 5 years), Date of admission (within 12 months), Number of previous admissions, Length of stay during the target admission.

The majority of cases had a diagnosis of personality disorder, background history of trauma or abuse and a related affective presentation (depressed and/or anxious). A significant minority had a psychotic presentation of either acute psychotic episode or bipolar mood disorder.

Design

A quasi-experimental, between-group design was used to compare the continuity group with the comparison group. Outcomes were the number of readmissions and length of stay. These variables were collected for the year prior to and after the "target" admission.

Figure 11.1 shows the number of admissions in the previous and subsequent year for each group. In the continuity group, 21 out of 70 (30%; 95% confidence interval 19.26% to 40.74%) were readmitted; shown on the graph as the thatched column, seven having one readmission, nine having two readmissions, two having three readmissions and three having more than three readmissions. In the comparison group, 37 were readmitted in the following 12-month period (53%; 95% confidence interval 41.31% to 64.69%). Via Chi-Square analysis this association was approaching significance, X^2 (2, N = 140) = 5.28, p =0.071. The overall main group effect size was not significant (p = 0.471).

Figure 11.2 shows the average (M) length of stay in the previous and subsequent year for the continuity group (SE = 3.82), compared to the comparison group (SE = 10.31). Looking at the change in the average length of stay between the previous and subsequent year, taking into

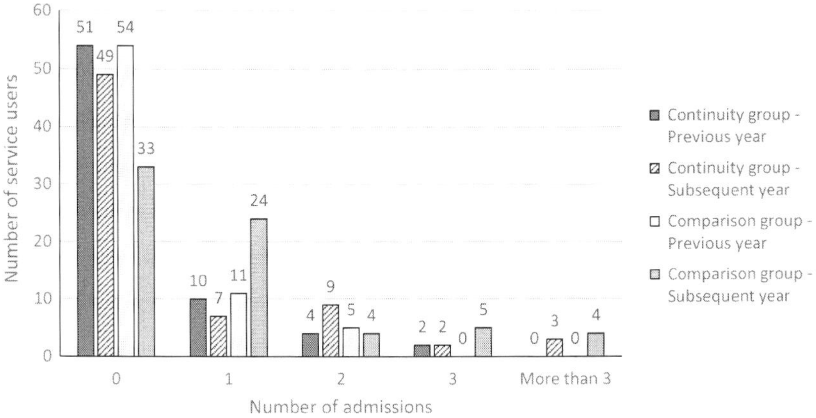

Figure 11.1 Number of admissions over the previous year and subsequent year for each sample.

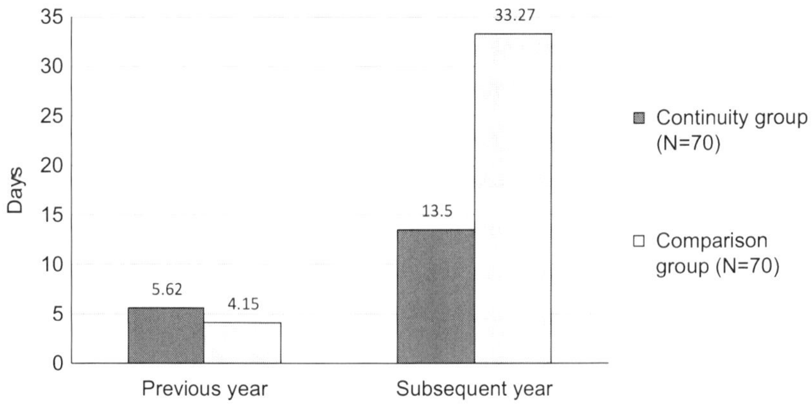

Figure 11.2 Average length of stay on the ward over the previous year and subsequent year for each sample.

account the length of stay at the target admission, the main effect of group was significant, $F(1, 137) = 3.96$, $p = 0.049$, $r = 0.2$. This indicates that the change in the average number of days spent as an inpatient in the subsequent year was lower in the continuity group ($M = 7.88$, $SE = 4.49$) compared to the comparison group ($M = 29.12$, $SE = 9.99$).

Discussion

There was a substantial difference found between subsequent bed days; the matched comparison group had longer subsequent admissions on average than the continuity group. This significant finding took into account the length of stay in the previous year, and during the target admission, thus current and historic acute service usage was accounted for in the matching, essentially an attempt to make the matching process as accurate as possible. This differential in bed days is consistent with previous literature (Omer, Priebe, & Giacco, 2015). The finding suggests that the use of the continuity model may be associated with shorter length of stay in the year following discharge.

The difference in the number of readmissions did not reach statistical significance, though it was approaching significance and perhaps with a larger sample size may have reached significance. The number of readmissions was notably lower in the continuity group (30%) than in the matched comparison group (53%). It is also noteworthy that these figures are respectively lower and higher than the national average range of readmissions of 37% to 50% (Agency for Health Care Research and Quality, 2012). This is encouraging with the continuity group showing lower than the national average of readmission. The comparison group was found to be slightly higher than the national average, which may indicate the complexity of those referred to psychology on the ward, i.e., those who receive psychological input are often the more complex presentations, and thus a matched sample would likely represent a high end or higher than average readmission rate.

Given case complexity, it is to be reasonably expected that such service users would have some form of readmission. However, the lowered number of readmissions and particularly lower number of related bed days is highly encouraging. Further analysis of the data and the nature of the readmitted subgroup of cases would be of interest (i.e., is there a commonality in diagnosis, perhaps personality disorder, or commonality in concurrent social, housing or addiction issues). Looking at the time of the readmission would also be interesting, i.e., perhaps looking at a shorter period of one-month readmission. This would bring the data comparably in line with the published literature reporting a national average of 8–18% of readmissions within a month (Agency for Health Care Research and Quality, 2012).

Reflections

The initial data on the continuity model is promising. Larger samples, a greater sense of the case profiles of those who are readmitted, qualitative and longitudinal data would all be of interest. Anecdotally we receive consistent positive feedback from those we work with in this way. Showing appreciation for all the aspects highlighted throughout this chapter, capturing this qualitatively would be valuable to further the evidence base. However, as noted above, indications that psychological continuity work can reduce readmissions and costly subsequent bed days should be encouraging for clinicians and service providers.

From a clinical psychologists' point of view, this work is stimulating, rewarding, fascinating and enriching. To be alongside people through the intensity of an acute episode and into the phases of transition and recovery is a powerful process. This shared knowledge of the "crisis" is often used therapeutically as part of the work. Being present and developing the therapeutic relationship through an acute crisis seems to add strength to the alliance and offers breadth to what may be possible in the post-crisis phases of the work.

The depth of the therapeutic relationship thus reached is significant, and this is often openly reflected on by those in the process. There is a development of trust in the therapist and the process, often coming at a time when people have lost a sense of hope and trust in themselves. This can only be furthered by the message that you can see them next week instead of "*I will be referring you to a waiting list, for another assessment with someone new.*" This is unsurprisingly positively met by service users and their families.

Having a foot in both camps (community and acute) is also advantageous. Having a systemic overview of services and an awareness of the nuances and characteristics of each side of what can sometimes feel a chasm of a divide is helpful in not only developing treatment formulations and therapeutic goals but also in assisting service users and colleagues in navigating the transition between specialties. This is again borne out in the feedback we get from those we work with. In general, people report that they feel they would have been more likely to be readmitted, struggled to engage with the CMHT or even experience elevated post hospitalization risk without the benefit of such continuity work. Such views are supported by the preliminary data presented here.

When work has begun on the ward, it only seems logical and good practice and therapeutically-wise to have some kind of mechanism to continue and complete treatment aims. Service users, caregivers, colleagues, and commissioners universally all have the same response when the model is described, saying "*that makes sense.*" However, as mentioned, it is flexibility in recruitment processes, job designs and a systemic perspective toward the wider service journey that is required to help create such posts which cross teams.

Indeed in some ways, the continuity posts described could even be viewed as a minimum standard, given the wards have no psychologist on them for half of every week. We are often confronted by unmet need with the high pace and turnover of admissions and discharges from the ward as well as our own caseload capacity restrictions. An increase to two posts per ward would provide comprehensive cover of daily access to psychological support for the whole ward population and significantly more access to direct community follow-up.

Working on psychiatric wards has not been a popular choice for clinical psychologists. Perhaps this may be in part due to the newness of the roles at least here in the UK, despite psychotherapy having had a strong presence back in the days of the larger socially isolated Victorian mental health asylums. Indeed, it may be the echo of the distressing images of those institutions that deter some psychologists. Or it may be the enduring dominance of the psychiatric medical model in inpatient care, with medication and physical containment often seen as the primary interventions. The medical model can be a difficult interface to psychotherapeutically relate to, and this dominance can be off-putting for many psychological or psychotherapeutic clinicians. Clinical psychology's increasing presence in the acute systems has in some ways started to approach this, but not necessarily addressing the dominance; every patient on a ward is likely to be prescribed something, but not everyone will receive psychological treatment. The continuity way of working promotes the existence and relevance of the therapeutic alliance and the necessity to complete psychotherapeutic goals in maintaining or enhancing wellbeing.

Part of the aims of inpatient clinical psychology has been to make wards more psychologically orientated and to try and develop a more truly bio-psycho-social approach to acute work. There is something appealing in the continuity model in allowing scope for short and long term work and in acknowledging the range of work which may be required and the diverse psychological skills we can bring in meeting those needs. We have often reflected how continuity sessions have provided some balance to our work as psychologists, working both on the wards and in the community.

We have also found that working across settings has allowed for welcomed and appreciated variance in the clinical work from a therapist point of view, i.e., the development of longer and deeper therapeutic processes, as well as variety in pace from busy acute crisis work to more explorative longer-term therapy. Acute assessment and brief interventions are valuable and not to be underestimated skills, and they certainly lead to rewarding work. However to have involvement in both short and long term therapy provision has been highly professionally enriching and it has been immensely gratifying to have had the capacity to complete long, complex pieces of therapeutic work spanning the chaotic distressed acute milieu and beyond into the journey of recovery and stability at home.

References

Agency for Health Care Research and Quality. (2012). *Health plan and psychiatric hospitals reduce readmissions by reviewing data and developing strategies to improve postdischarge care*. Retrieved from https://innovations.ahrq.gov/profiles/health-plan-and-psychiatric-hospitals-reduce-readmissions-reviewing-data-and-developing

Bateman, A., & Fonagy, P. (2016). *Mentalisation based treatment for personality disorders: A practical guide*. Oxford: Oxford University Press.

Bell, L. (2003). *Managing intense emotions and overcoming self-destructive habits: A self-help manual*. East Sussex, UK: Routledge.

Bilderbeck, A.C., Saunders, K.E.A., Price, J., & Goodwin, G.M. (2014). Psychiatric assessment of mood instability: qualitative study of patient experience. *British Journal of Psychiatry, 204*, 234–239.

British Psychological Society. (2014). The commission to review the provision of inpatient psychiatric care for adults in England, Wales and Northern Ireland. Commission response document. Retrieved from www1.bps.org.uk/sites/default/files/BPS-response-CAAPC_Call_for_Evidence-Approved.pdf

Burns, T., Catty, J., White, S., Clemenet, S., Ellis, G., Jones, I.R., & Wykes, T., for the ECHO Group. (2009). Continuity of care in mental health: Understanding and measuring a complex phenomenon. *Psychological Medicine, 39*, 313–323.

Clarke, I., & Wilson, H. (2009). *Cognitive behaviour therapy for acute inpatient mental health units: Working with clients, staff and the milieu*. East Sussex, UK: Taylor & Francis.

Crawford, M.J., de Jonge, E., Freemand, G.K., & Weaver, T. (2004). Providing continuity of care for people with severe mental illness: a narrative review. *Social Psychiatry and Psychiatris Epidemiology, 39*, 265–272.

Donaghay-Spire, E., McGowan, J., Griffiths, K., & Barazzone, N. (2015). Exploring narratives of psychological input in the acute inpatient setting. *Psychology and Psychotherapy: Theory, Research and Practice, 89*, 464–482.

Durbin, J., Lin, E., Layne, C., & Teed, M. (2007). Is readmission a valid indicator of the quality of inpatient psychiatric care? *Journal of Behavioural Health Services & Research, 34*, 137–150.

Griffiths, K., & Averbeck, M. (2016). Mindfulness-Based Cognitive Therapy for Couples. In S.J. Eisendrath (Ed.) *Mindfulness-Based Cognitive Therapy Innovative Approaches* (pp. 123–131). Switzerland: Springer International Publishing.

Kerfoot, G., Bamford, Z., & Jones, S.A. (2012). Evaluation of psychological provision into an acute inpatient unit. *Mental Health Review Journal, 17*, 26–38.

NHS Benchmarking Network. (2013). *Mental health benchmarking report 2013*. London: NHS Benchmarking Network.

NICE. (2011). *Service user experience in adult mental health: improving the experience of care for people using adult NHS mental health services*. CG136. Retrieved from www.nice.org.uk/guidance/cg136/resources/service-user-experience-in-adult-mental-health-improving-the-experience-of-care-for-people-using-adult-nhs-mental-health-services-35109513728197

Omer, S., Priebe, S., & Giacco, D. (2015). Continuity across inpatient and outpatient mental health care or specialisation of teams? A systematic review. *European Psychiatry, 30*, 258–270.

Sainsbury Centre for Mental Health. (2006). *The Future of Mental Health: A Vision for 2015*. London: The Sainsbury Centre for Mental Health.

Segal, Z.V., Williams, J.M.G., & Teasdale, J.D. (2012). *Mindfulness-based cognitive therapy for depression*. New York, NY: Guilford Press.

Vandyk, A.D., Graham, I.D., Van Den Kerkhof, E.G., Ross-White, A., & Harrison, M.B. (2013). Towards a conceptual consensus of continuity in mental healthcare: focused literature search and theory analysis. *International Journal of Evidence-Based Healthcare, 11*, 94–109.

Vigod, S.N., Kurdyak, P.A., Dennis, C-L., Leszcz, T., Taylor, V.H., Blumberger, D.M., & Seitz, D.P. (2013). Transitional interventions to reduce early psychiatric readmissions in adults: systematic review. *British Journal of Psychiatry, 202*, 187–194.

12 Cognitive Behavioral Therapy for Psychosis on the Inpatient Unit

The Role of the Clinical Psychologist

Sally E. Riggs

Approximately 2.4 million American adults, or about 1.1% of the population age 18 and older in a given year experience a psychotic disorder (Robins & Regier, 1991). Large numbers of these individuals receive inpatient psychological treatment; in 2010, there were approximately 397,200 hospitalizations for psychosis nationwide, and about 88,600 (22.3%) were readmitted within 30 days (Elixhauser & Steiner, 2013). Although not all units have their own Ph.D. level psychologist, many have at least access to one. And we also have a rigorous, evidence-based treatment that works for psychosis: Cognitive Behavioral Therapy for psychosis (CBTp) (Mueser & Glyn, 2014; Pilling et al., 2002). But somewhere there is a disconnect: psychologists who work on inpatient units are not trained in CBTp. Administrators responsible for inpatient programming and staff training are not aware that a therapy designed for 45-minute individual sessions can also be relevant to a milieu setting, and other staff working in inpatient settings see their role in a patient's treatment as being something different (medication modification; diagnosis; boundary and structure oriented).

General Role of the Psychologist

It is the firm belief of this writer, supported by her years of experience working on inpatient units, and corroborated by numerous psychology colleagues in similar positions, that the primary role of the psychologist on the inpatient unit is that of "modeling." Modeling empathy and respect for patients, modeling advocacy for patients, modeling best practice therapeutic interventions. To do this, one cannot be the clinician who sits in their office all day, coming onto the unit briefly to run a group, see a patient or attend a meeting. You have to sit in the day room and interact with patients, gaining their trust and showing that you are approachable. You have to be willing to assist patients with whatever they need: getting their clean laundry out of the dryer; a cup of juice; toothpaste; a clean towel. You have to be willing to assist other staff with whatever they need: spending time in the nursing station;

interacting with the psych techs in the hallway; learning the names of the janitor, unit clerk, and students on rotation. In treatment teams; in community meetings; in the dining room; modeling how to ask questions, phrase things, set up the lunch line, decide who gets to watch what on the television, all of these interactions count and are amazingly powerful. You will be respected as a staff member, and slowly, over time, other people's interactions will change too, and for the better. In this context, it naturally follows that evidence-based psychological interventions, in this case CBT for psychosis, would also be modeled by the inpatient psychologist as a powerful tool for therapeutic milieu change, even in the absence of specific or explicit training and dissemination endeavors.

Of course, the Ph.D. level clinical psychologist has more to offer the unit than just being an additional pair of hands. Once integrated into and respected by the unit, the psychologist brings unique qualities that are not available from any other team member. The most important of these is the formulation driven consideration of patients. Through their graduate school training, the psychologist becomes highly skilled in understanding patients' difficulties from multiple theoretical perspectives. People are not simply their diagnosis and so-called prognosis. They are a combination of their social, cultural and environmental histories and present lives. Psychologists are very good at conceptualizing psychological difficulties in this multi-factorial way, and tailoring person-centered interventions to these individual experiences. They are also very good at explaining these things to others, both professionals and treatment participants. A key "added-value" role for the psychologist is formulation, explanation of formulation to team members, including the patient and their family members, and modeling of formulation to their colleagues. This is certainly central to CBTp on the inpatient unit.

What is CBTp?

CBTp is based on the "basic" cognitive model, which states that our perceptions of our experience shape our feelings and resulting behavior (Beck, 2011). Certain techniques for engagement and forming a therapeutic alliance are used, which include making modifications to "traditional" session structure and settings, talking about delusional beliefs empathically and without colluding, normalizing the symptoms of psychosis, and understanding psychotic symptoms as part of a spectrum exacerbated by stress, rather than as normal versus abnormal (Sivec & Montesano, 2012). In addition, CBTp aims to instill hope, reduce distress caused by psychotic experience and improve quality of life. It uses the ABC model (activating event – belief – consequence) to assess beliefs about psychotic experiences, and uses formulation, Socratic questioning and guided discovery, cognitive behavioral change strategies and homework to bring about change (Morrison & Barratt, 2010). CBTp skills and strategies have been successfully delivered in group settings (Granholm, McQuaid, & Holden, 2015; Hill, Clarke, & Wilson, 2009; Landa, Silverstein, Schwartz, & Savitz, 2006; Romme & Escher, 1989; Wright et al., 2014), and by non-therapists in brief format in milieu settings (Chang, Grant, Luther, & Beck, 2014; Perry, Murakami-Brundage, Grant, & Beck, 2013; Sivec, Montesano, Skubby, Knepp, & Muntez, 2017; Turkington, Kingdon, & Turner, 2002; Turkington et al., 2006, 2014; Waller et al., 2013). In this chapter, I will discuss specific elements of the CBTp model and how they have been applied effectively in these milieu settings. I will also describe ways in which the unit psychologist can take a lead role in implementing this work on the inpatient unit.

Therapeutic Stance

It has been stressed time and again that the therapeutic relationship is central to any psychotherapeutic work (Lazarus, 1992). More recently in the case of CBTp, however, it has been shown that when therapeutic alliance is low, the more treatment sessions the person has the worse the outcome (Goldsmith, Lewis, Dunn, & Bentall, 2015). So if the therapeutic relationship is not good, we can actually do harm. Empathy has been highlighted repeatedly to be of central importance to therapeutic engagement (Reynolds, Scott, & Jessiman, 1999) and is routinely cited as being crucial in the psychological treatment of psychosis (Kingdon & Turkington, 1994; Nelson, 2005). However, a key difference in working with persons experiencing psychosis is that empathy may not be profuse. McLeod, Deane, and Hogbin (2002) suggest that attitudinal factors (such as beliefs that psychosis cannot be successfully treated or that working with people with psychosis will impede career prospects and job satisfaction), could inhibit empathy. This research also highlights the potential for a lack of empathy due to clinicians' lack of personal experience of psychotic symptoms (Chadwick, Birchwood, & Trower, 1996; Fowler, Garety, & Kuipers, 1995). When learning CBT for psychosis, but more importantly in applying it to a milieu setting, empathy is the key starting point, coupled with an awareness that we may have to work even harder than usual to generate this empathy.

Another important aspect of therapeutic relationship building, and key to CBT, is the concept of being collaborative. Again, in CBTp this is a little different than with regular CBT. Chadwick (2006) talks about "radical collaboration," which he defines as "a process of allowing clients to find their own goals within a supportive collaborative relationship that is free from therapist demands about how therapy should progress." (p. 26.) This can certainly be difficult to achieve on an inpatient unit where the patient is not free to come and go, and certain goals and demands may be placed upon him or her by the unit. But for hospitals that are using the recovery model (SAMHSA, 2006) this fits well, and with support, staff can learn the key elements of this process: active listening; negotiating a common language; guided discovery; a commitment to openness; and the floating of ideas in a detached manner.

A third fundamental skill for working with psychosis from a cognitive-behavioral perspective, which also supports the above two mentioned concepts, is that of "suspending disbelief" or "working within the patient's belief system" (Nelson, 2005). Again, this is subtly different to standard CBT, and clinicians who have some previous knowledge of CBT often misunderstand the cognitive aspect of intervention in relation to psychosis, thinking that the primary objective is to *change* or *challenge* the person's delusional beliefs. Others who have been trained that one must not *collude* with delusions to avoid strengthening them, often extrapolate that one cannot talk about delusions at all. Helping clinicians to understand the concept of working within a delusional belief system, as a middle ground between these two alternatives, is vital. How these three elements of the therapeutic stance are used in the milieu setting is elaborated below.

Brief Therapeutic Conversations

The most important mindset to consider shifting in the provision of treatment for psychosis in inpatient settings is that every conversation has powerful therapeutic value. Interventions do not just happen in groups, treatment team meetings or an individual staff member's office; rather every interaction has the potential for contributing to the maintenance of psychosis, or the facilitation of its improvement. When a person comes to the nursing station and asks for a cup of juice, there is an opportunity for engagement and empathy; when a person paces in the hallway, talking out loud to their voices, there is an opportunity for engagement, assessment of voices and facilitation of coping strategies; when a person walks up to a member of staff and spontaneously elaborates on their delusional belief systems, there is an opportunity to work within this system to engage, assess and intervene. CBTp is subtly different from standard CBT (Riggs, Stirman, & Beck, 2012). As a staff member, I can challenge a person's beliefs or tell them not to listen to their voices, and by invalidating their emotional experience or pushing them to find more evidence to support their beliefs, am contributing in just five minutes to the perpetuation of their psychosis. Or in about the same amount of time, I can provide a therapeutic interaction that does the opposite. The unit psychologist specifically can take the lead by modeling such interactions routinely throughout her day on the unit.

This not only provides access to a therapeutic environment that actually works but also reduces staff burnout by increasing a sense of efficacy and competence. Helping so-called non-clinical staff to realize the clinical utility of their five-minute conversations is an important part of CBTp for the inpatient unit, and the psychologist plays a big role in conveying and maintaining this. This utility is three-fold: facilitating engagement; gaining useful information about the person's psychotic experience (which they often withhold from clinical staff due to fears of longer detention, treatment etc.); and reinforcing other specific clinical interventions initiated on a different ward shift or tour with a primary therapist, in a group, etc. (to be described in more detail below).

Coping Skills Enhancement

Helping people to identify and utilize strategies to manage their distressing experiences has long been a part of cognitive therapy. Even for those not trained in CBTp, facilitating the development of specific skills for dealing with voices or other hallucinations has been an important focus of good practice in treating serious mental illness. These strategies can be broken down into several categories: physiological strategies such as relaxation; cognitive strategies such as self-instruction or attentional switching; behavioral strategies such as increasing or decreasing activity; sensory strategies such as listening to music (Breier & Strauss, 1983; Tarrier, 1992).

Unfortunately, coping skills enhancement rarely goes beyond "do you listen to headphones when the voices are bad?" We can do so much more than this. On initial discussion, a useful starting point begins by asking what coping skills a person has attempted to utilize in the past and to what effect. Next comes ranking strategies in order of effectiveness and troubleshooting for roadblocks, and considering whether existing strategies can be refined, or whether new ones might be added. Then perhaps the most crucial part of the process is to make a plan, have the person carry it out, get feedback and adjust. All of us, at one time or another, are guilty of having suggested a strategy for homework and then never checking in with the person about it. It is important to remember that success is in the feedback and adjustment, not in the prescription.

Chadwick et al. (1996) suggest that the first and most important step in coping skills enhancement is to congratulate the person on what a great job they have been doing so far in surviving the distress incurred by the psychotic experience for so long. Much like in motivational interviewing (Rollnick & Miller, 1995) it is important to empower the person first by affirming their strengths. Fowler et al. (1995) depict these strategies as those that help to "self-regulate distressing psychotic symptomatology" (p. 106). That is, they are more than just distraction techniques but actually important in reducing psychotic experiences. They stress the importance of determining the antecedent to the psychotic experience first as a means of selecting the most likely effective strategy. For example, if the person notices that their voices are preceded by a failure in a certain task and a reduction in self-esteem, the coping strategy offered is going to be different (catching and checking the negative thoughts) than for those whose voices are preceded by the sun going down in the evening and an increase in anxiety (anxiety management techniques such as relaxation, mindfulness etc.)

The most effective way to utilize coping skills enhancement in the inpatient setting is to have the psychologist meet with the person individually or in a group for assessment that informs an action plan. This can be then detailed on a coping card that the person carries and can be referred to by other staff throughout the day or night. Staff can be alerted to and prompted to ask about the existence of coping cards by information disseminated by the psychologist at shift change, and by leaving a copy of the card in the shift change report or patient's chart. For example:

> when the voices say really mean things over and over, sometimes it's because I'm anxious or stressed. If this happens, I can take my stress ball from the cabinet and play with it for a while or listen to soothing music or talk to a member of staff about what's stressing me out.

However, if this detailed assessment work is not possible, general coping strategies can also be referred to on an ad hoc basis by all staff throughout the unit. For example: "I can see the voices are pretty bad right now. What do you think might help: some relaxing music; the Look-Point-Name game; or maybe we could just walk and talk for a bit?" Then successes should be shared with the rest of the team, including non-clinical staff, during a team meeting or equivalent, again in order to maximize the continuity of care and the efficacy of strategies identified.

Relaxation and Sensory-Modulation

Most inpatient settings have access to materials and staff trained to facilitate relaxation and/or sensory-modulation. Distressing psychotic experiences often happen at times of either heightened or diminished arousal. Deep breathing techniques, progressive muscle relaxation, and guided imagery can all be used to reduce arousal. In addition to anxiety, other intense emotions can also be a trigger for psychosis. Putting together a specific music playlist to lift a person's mood, help them relax, or help them be more focused and energized can all be helpful in dealing with specific experiences. If a person is experiencing a particular sensory hallucination, helping them to focus on a different sensory experience by having them describe it out loud, can also be grounding. Many clinicians on the inpatient unit may have expertise in relaxation and sensory-modulation, and this may not necessarily be the preserve of the inpatient psychologist. However, the psychologist can take the lead in the treatment team in connecting a person's psychotic experiences to their emotional state, and in facilitating their access to a group or specific staff member who can carry out this work.

Voices

It is important to make the distinction here between strategies that help patients *cope* with voices and those that actually have the potential to *diminish* them in volume or intensity. Many people who hear voices learn to deal with their voices by listening to loud music, by answering back, or shouting profanities. At worst, this serves to make them louder, and at best it just serves to drown them out. There are a number of strategies, however, that can bring immediate improvement in the voices. This, in turn, has the effect of increasing the person's sense of control, thereby working to change the belief that the voices are all powerful and breaking the cycle of maintenance (Chadwick & Birchwood, 1994). These include focusing or concentrating on the voices, sub-vocal speech, singing, humming, reading aloud or just talking to someone. In particular, a strategy that combines elements of these and can be taught to people who hear voices as a very simple game is described in Box 12.1. It is often referred to as "Look-Point-Name." The practice of these strategies can be made even more effective by having the person bring the voices on first, by thinking about particular things that they commonly say (Fowler & Morley, 1989). In addition, people who hear voices can find relief from their distress by setting a particular, limited time of the day when they are going to interact with the voices.

The psychologist on the unit can trail blaze here by talking about strategies for voices openly and often, and by using them frequently with patients individually throughout the unit or in groups. By doing so, over time, all other staff will come to know about Look-Point-Name, sub-vocal speech, or any of the other effective strategies, and may feel confident to suggest these to people newly admitted or during the evenings and weekends when the psychologist is not present.

Box 12.1 Look-Point-Name Strategy For Voices

- Rate the loudness of the voices (0–10)
- Look at an object, point to it and name it out loud
- Keep going until you run out of objects
- Rate the loudness of the voices again (0–10)

Delusions

Delusions can be much more diverse, so it is harder to list specific strategies that might be helpful to a person without first assessing the details of their unique belief system. Certainly, showing "natural curiosity" (Nelson, 2005) through questions can be an intervention in itself, and all staff can be taught to do this by the unit psychologist. Hazel Nelson (2005) lists specific questions that might be useful in this situation, stressing the importance of a neutral tone of voice. Furthermore, if a person's belief system includes elements of paranoia or suspiciousness, then stress reduction or relaxation (see above) would be indicated. Staff members can also help the person pick out an activity to reduce their preoccupation with ruminative thoughts making suggestions such as: "I can see that you have a lot on your mind right now, which is causing you distress. Is there something else you might enjoy doing to take your mind off it? How about a game of checkers?"

For the many people who experience complex beliefs concerning being followed, having their life interfered with by a particular agency, "sabotage," or other concerns of this nature, it can be extremely validating and empowering to have this experience conceptualized as a form of "bullying." Comments like "I am so sorry this is happening to you," "this is really not acceptable," and "I wish there was something I could do to stop this, but unfortunately I'm not really important enough in these circles" can be extremely supportive. In addition, urging the person not to let the bullies win, and supporting them to continue making steps toward achieving their goals anyway, can be very powerful. Clinicians often fear that engaging in the delusional content in this manner serves as colluding with it and therefore increases conviction in delusional beliefs; however, this assumption has not been borne out in clinical practice. Instead, these interventions can be strongly therapeutic for facilitating recovery. Typically, the role for the psychologist here is that of modeling, validating the person's experiences, and talking about the bully analogy in treatment planning meetings and ward rounds, such that other staff may pick up on and utilize a similar approach.

Negative Symptoms

Over the years, negative symptoms of psychosis have been a source of major difficulty for staff on the inpatient unit. As systems become more person-centered and federal bodies require hospitals to show evidence of active treatment (not just "warehousing") patients lying in bed during the 9am to 5pm "programming" time is not received well. It is common for staff to knock on doors and loudly encourage patients to attend programming. However, we now have studies that support a cognitive therapy approach for the treatment of negative symptoms as well (Grant, Huh, Perivoliotis, Stolar, & Beck, 2012; Perivoliotis, Grant, & Beck, in press), which is extremely simple for all unit staff to carry out, and more effective than knocking on doors.

Activity is the backbone of negative symptom treatment. According to the cognitive model of negative symptoms, people with negative symptoms experience a diminished capacity to anticipate pleasure from previously enjoyed activities, as well as impaired reward learning when actually engaged in such activities. Coupled with the effects of cognitive limitations, aversive life experiences (e.g., failures in school, work, relationships), positive symptoms, and societal messages about psychosis and its prognosis, they come to believe that it is not worth engaging in productive or pleasurable activities and that they cannot enjoy or succeed in anything again (Perivoliotis, Grant & Beck, in press). Supporting someone while they engage in activity, enhancing their enjoyment of it through praise and reward, and helping them to notice and build on the enjoyment and success they do experience helps to correct these maladaptive and recovery-interfering defeatist beliefs.

Determining an activity that a person used to like or enjoy, encouraging them to engage with it again, perhaps bringing it to their bedside or to where they are, and providing ample praise when there is even a flicker of a smile or enjoyment: this could be described as the "cheerleader" intervention. This can be as simple as playing a game of cards or checkers, watching funny clips on YouTube, listening to music, or taking a walk up and down the unit together. The unit psychologist may initiate this intervention himself, or he or she may work with identified nursing or support staff that have connected with the person or those assigned to work near the patient's bed area, to do this work. Regardless, it is important that the staff members have the patient rate their anticipation of enjoyment or sense of achievement on a 0–10 scale before and then again after the activity, with much praise and reinforcement for even one point of difference.

Building upon this work would be activity monitoring/scheduling, again using ratings for enjoyment and sense of achievement, as well as closeness to other people. This can be related to the daily programming schedule. Having someone monitor how their mood and experience changes as a result of different items in the program, and modifying their schedule the following week in order to capitalize on positive outcomes can be extremely powerful. It not only facilitates recovery and hence discharge, but also helps someone learn their own self-efficacy in this process. In addition simply helping someone reduce the amount of time spent on minimally pleasurable activities (e.g., lying in bed, sitting in the day room staring at the TV), and maximize pleasurable activities (e.g., a favorite group, time in the gym, a favorite game or conversation with a particular staff member) in their daily schedule can also positively impact negative symptoms. Again, this might be the work of the unit psychologist, or of the primary nurse with the support of the psychologist.

This leads to goal setting, which again fits with the recovery driven model toward which many inpatient units are now reorienting their programs. Here the key is assisting the person to break down every goal (however unrealistic) into tiny, daily achievable steps, and then having them celebrate the achievement of every single step along the way. For a person with the ultimate goal of having a girlfriend, shorter-term goals might be to learn how to speak to people more effectively, to have more confidence, and to improve personal hygiene. Hence, steps toward these goals taken on the unit could be going to groups that focus on interpersonal effectiveness and increasing self-esteem, giving a compliment to someone each day, taking a shower and changing clothes once per day, doing laundry regularly, etc. The unit psychologist can make sure that staff members are aware of these goals and steps and helping participants applaud these steps. By doing so, the staff are investing in a strategy that the person can continue to utilize post discharge and which can be shared with their next provider(s) to facilitate continuity of care.

Coping Cards

Although many people have access to smart technology devices these days, traditional pen and paper coping cards still have strong value. In the majority of inpatient units, phones or other devices are not allowed and, in many neighborhoods, it may not be prudent to pull out devices on the street. A simple flashcard with handwritten items on the front and back can be taken almost anywhere and used easily to reorient someone during a time of distressing psychosis. Specific strategies that have been determined to be effective in specific moments can be briefly detailed, providing cues for a particular cognition, behavior or technique. In addition, they help large teams of staff to know specific interventions relevant to each individual: the unit psychologist can initiate the creation of coping cards, potentially in conjunction with other licensed clinicians on the unit who may be primary to the person with psychosis. Then any staff member can simply say "I can see you are having difficulty with your voices right now. Is there anything on your coping card (see Box 12.2) that I can help you with so that you will feel better?" Coping cards can also be used for daily goals, and again to facilitate the sharing of information between staff specific to each individual in the program. For example, copies of the coping cards can be kept in the shift log, and updates can be discussed with staff at shift handover, team meetings or during ward rounds, etc.

Box 12.2 Sample Coping Card

When the voices are really bad, I can:

1. Check my emotion and my thoughts to see what made them start
2. Do "Look-Point-Name"
3. Remind myself that the voices don't know what they are talking about "they are only 10% wise"
4. If I'm feeling stressed, my soothing activities are:

    a. Drawing and art
    b. Writing in my journal
    c. Listening to music from the 1980s
    d. Reading about animals on the internet

Group Interventions

Groups are a wonderful modality for inpatient units and commonly cited by the administration as the key part of an inpatient psychologist's role. Although people experiencing psychosis typically avoid social interaction and can struggle to attend groups on an outpatient basis due to suspiciousness, social anxiety and a host of logistical factors, on the inpatient unit it is often a required part of treatment. If patients do not show up, staff can easily go to their bedside and gently encourage and help motivate. Some units even use group attendance as a road to discharge. As such, groups can be a way to provide much-needed psychotherapy in these settings, and CBTp is no exception to this.

There are a number of evidence-based CBTp groups that are appropriate for inpatient settings and have successfully been taught to group therapists. The most well-known of these, albeit still outside the US, are the Hearing Voices groups pioneered by Romme and Escher (1989). Consistent with principles of the CBTp model and traditionally peer-led, these groups encourage patients to share experiences, beliefs about their voices, coping strategies for dealing with voices and to promote normalization. This, in turn, helps facilitate improved self-esteem. Pennings and Romme (1997) found that participants who could recognize their own experiences in others' narratives became more accepting of their voices with attendance in the group, and were better able to cope with them. Downs (2005) found that these groups also reduced stigma and isolation and facilitated coping.

The "what is real and what is not" group (Hill et al., 2009) is a four-session group using third wave CBT techniques such as mindfulness

(Chadwick, Newman Taylor, & Abba, 2005) normalization principles (Romme & Escher, 1989) and a dialectical behavioral approach (Linehan, 1993). This group has been enjoyably and helpfully taught to staff using role-play (i.e., the trainer takes the role of the group facilitator, and the staff role-play individual patients in the group). In particular, it can be helpful to include all clinical staff in such a role-play, even those who will not specifically be facilitating the group. This helps promote general CBTp principles, gives a greater understanding for staff who may be asked to encourage program participants to attend, promotes empathy for those taking the role of the program participants, and helps with continuity of care and consolidation of therapeutic interventions. Nicola Wright's group has a similar focus (Wright et al., 2014); adding positive psychotherapy (Seligman, 2002) Acceptance and Commitment Therapy (Hayes, Stohsal, & Wilson, 2012) and Compassion Focused Therapy (Gilbert, 2009) elements to the CBTp model as applied to psychosis in a group context. This group intervention has evidenced great success in Canada, as per Wright and colleagues. Both of these groups are entirely appropriate for inpatient settings and have been used flexibly by this writer with good face validity.

Another evidence-based group that has been gaining use in community mental health settings is Landa and colleague's CBT for paranoia group (2006). This is a longer 15-week closed group that utilizes the ABC model of CBTp via patient workbooks in group exercises and between-session homework to treat paranoia in a group setting. For clinicians to be trained in how to facilitate this group, a basic working knowledge of cognitive behavioral concepts and the ABC model are required. It may be useful to co-facilitate with trainee facilitators in pairs, with brief targeted and specific feedback after the session. This allows for both modeling of good practice and facilitation as well as live practice that can be observed and shaped. This group may only be appropriate for long-term inpatient settings where patients can be present consistently for 15 weeks.

Granholm and colleagues' Cognitive Behavioral Social Skills Training group (Granholm et al., 2015) is another skills-driven, manualized CBT group for people experiencing psychosis, designed specifically to be facilitated by people with a master's level education or less with little or no background in CBT or other group therapies. Groups run for 24 to 36 weeks of weekly two-hour group sessions and are split into three modules: thought challenging; social skills training; and problems solving. Participants can join at the beginning of any particular module and modules repeat on a rolling schedule. This group has been effectively taught to over 150 staff in assertive community treatment teams, yielding good to excellent CTS-Psy (Haddock et al., 2001) scores after a one-day workshop and weekly 30-minute group consultation provided over a six month period (Granholm, Loh, & Link, in press). Although this published data relates primarily to community-based clinicians, the material and structure of the groups would lend itself well to longer stay inpatient settings such as state hospitals or units whose programming enables daily scheduled groups, allowing patients to complete at least one module during their admission. The most recent addition to the group CBT for psychosis repertoire is also the most comprehensive and relevant to inpatient settings. Group CBTp (Lecomte, Leclerc & Wykes, 2016) is a 24-session group protocol, which includes a workbook for participants, that utilizes both the recovery (Noordsy et al., 2002) and stress-vulnerability-competence models (Liberman, 1982) in addition to Beck's (2011) basic cognitive model, and more specific cognitive-behavioral models for psychosis (Chadwick, 2006; Chadwick et al., 1996; Fowler et al., 1995; Kingdon & Turkington, 1994; Morrison, Renton, Dunn, Williams, & Bentall, 2004). This group protocol has been utilized with individuals with early psychosis (Lecomte et al., 2008) and with participants with more long-term experiences of psychosis. It was found that those receiving the CBT for psychosis group showed fewer positive, general and negative symptoms at post-treatment and six-month follow up, compared with wait-list controls, as well as improvements in self-esteem, coping skills and social support (Lecomte et al., 2008, Lecomte, Leclerc, & Wykes 2012). The group treatment also showed a higher retention rate than anticipated, suggesting that it was enjoyed by participants. It is also worth noting that this group protocol was designed to be delivered by therapists with knowledge of CBT for psychosis, but with minimal training or experience (two days intensive). Four modules of six sessions each include: Stress, how it affects me; Testing hypotheses and looking for alternatives; Drugs, alcohol and how I feel; Coping and competence.

Brief CBTp-Informed Interventions Plus Full CBTp

All of the CBTp interventions described above are what consensus opinion in the field has recently come to refer to as "CBT informed interventions", with "full CBTp" defined as the formulation driven, transdiagnostic, comprehensive CBTp that is typically provided by a licensed clinician in an individual, weekly one-to-one therapy format (Riggs & Creed, 2017). For milieu programs that have both licensed clinicians (in addition to the unit psychologist) and support staff, an emphasis is placed on specialized formulation driven CBTp work taking place during clinical "therapy" sessions, with plans then written and shared with all staff so they can support and encourage no matter what time of day or night. In order for this to take place, an emphasis is placed on a coordinated team approach for an inter-disciplinary treatment team, with all staff regardless of their training background given a working knowledge of specific skills based strategies such as coping skills for voices and behavioral interventions for paranoia and negative symptoms. This knowledge can be imparted by specific "in service" training, through role-plays in team meetings, or more informally by the psychologist modeling specific interventions and then coaching unit staff live in their interactions with patients. Licensed clinicians may then take the lead in developing and sharing the case conceptualization, and support staff help extend the clinical interventions into the milieu. Many inpatient units already use such an inter-disciplinary approach, and so this fits nicely onto an already functional model of intervention.

A description of full CBTp is beyond the scope of this chapter, and there are many treatment manuals and summary articles that this writer would recommend (Chadwick, 2006; Chadwick et al., 1996; Fowler et al., 1995; Kingdon & Turkington, 1994; Morrison et al., 2004; Sivec & Montesano, 2012). However, it is important to highlight a key element that fits with the inpatient model of CBTp delivery outlined here, namely the detailed voices assessment. The psychologist often has the opportunity to meet with a newly admitted patient shortly after their arrival onto the unit. Using the model of Chadwick et al. (1996), a comprehensive voices assessment can give much more information to inform formulation and treatment planning, than simply asking if voices are present or absent and whether these are commands. The person is asked about the qualitative sound of the voice: whether it sounds male, female; how many are talking; whether the voices talk to or about the person; whether they use his or her name; the specific content of what is said, with examples; whether or not the voice gives commands, advice, criticism, abuse or hostility. The person is also asked about any antecedents they have noticed, their affect when they hear the voice, and their behaviors. They are also asked whether they have a sense of who the voice is; their inferred meaning about its presence; and their perception of its power and/or control. A voice diary can be used to collect additional information about this. The Beliefs about Voices Questionnaire (BAV-Q) (Chadwick, Lees, & Birchwood, 2000) can also be used to ascertain information about the inferred meaning, sense of omnipotence, omniscience, malevolence and benevolence, all of which can inform treatment. This information helps the psychologist build up the cognitive behavioral formulation of the person's voice hearing experience, but it also helps the voice hearer become aware of and gain more understanding about his/her voices; what they can and cannot do; what they do and do not know etc. In addition, this important information can be utilized in the tailoring of specific coping strategies, that in turn are shared with all unit staff.

Case Examples

Voices and Paranoia

Douglas was a 19-year-old man from the Caribbean, brought to the hospital by the police department after repeated calls to 911 complaining about his neighbors. He described concerns that his neighbors had implanted a chip in his brain and were following him. This was his first admission to a psychiatric facility, and he did not agree with the diagnosis being given or the offer of medications. During a treatment team meeting, the staff endeavored to explain to him that he was in a psychiatric hospital and that in order to be eligible for discharge he should get up and dress in the morning, attend groups and take his medication. Of course, this did not fit with his explanation of what was going on. He wanted to talk about his concerns about his neighbors and how to get law enforcement involved. He was a young man with a lot of energy and would run up and down the unit, especially when asked to do something that did not make sense to him, which of course caused alarm to the unit. The staff were encouraged to work within his delusional belief system in order to build therapeutic alliance and engagement.

When the psychologist met with him individually, she attempted to gain a more thorough understanding of his experiences from a CBTp perspective. She asked about what was happening with his neighbors and how he had come to know about the surveillance and the chip. It became apparent that he had been hearing voices (undisclosed to the team) commenting on what he was doing frequently throughout the day, which made him feel anxious and fearful. The young man had recently moved to the neighborhood from the Caribbean, did not know his neighbors well and had few friends. The psychologist hypothesized that he often felt fearful and uneasy in his new surroundings, and was connecting the two emotions to conclude that the neighbors were surveilling him.

Given his medication refusal, he was also asked about his experiences with the medication given on the unit: what bad things he noticed about it as well as what good things. He voiced that he did notice that at times it made him feel less anxious. The psychologist was able to float the idea "ok so it's not that the meds will make your neighbors stop interfering with you, but if you take them perhaps they could help you deal with the situation better," to which he was receptive. This formulation was shared with the treatment team so that they might approach his treatment from a perspective that made more sense to him and was more likely to allow him to engage. In the treatment team meetings, the psychologist was also present to model and coach staff through using this patient-centered approach and language.

The team was worried about relapse prevention, and in fact when the patient was initially discharged, he did call 911 again the next day and was readmitted. This time the psychologist discussed with him the function of the behavior of calling 911 and some alternative ways to manage the "situation with his neighbors." The young man was coached to identify when he was feeling anxious, and through individual and group work on the unit was able to increase his repertoire of anxiety management and relaxation techniques. This particular hospital had licensed creative arts therapists at the center of its therapeutic group programming, and through a variety of groups based in music, visual arts, sensory-modulation and relaxation, he identified a list of strategies that he detailed on a coping card and later entered into his phone when he left the unit. When discharged the second time, he was given a coping card of things to do instead of calling 911 when he was concerned about his neighbors. Ultimately, he was able to manage his experiences and was not readmitted to the hospital.

Extreme Negative Symptoms

A patient was admitted in the dead of winter having been found by the police after sleeping in the park in subzero temperatures for several days in a row. Hospital records showed a history of diagnosis of schizophrenia. On this admission, he presented as mute and could not engage in the assessment process. He lay in bed for weeks, un-showered and undressed, only coming out for meals and refusing medication. Some of the staff on the unit began to hypothesize that he was just taking advantage of the free bed, warmth and food in the cold seasonal weather.

However, the psychology intern on the unit took a CBTp for negative symptoms approach with him, hypothesizing that his inactivity and inertia was caused and maintained by defeatist beliefs. She started going by his bedroom to introduce herself and to take interesting materials to comment on (books, magazines etc.). She was rotating on the unit every morning, and for at least 10 minutes every day, she would go by and talk to him in an animated fashion (no questions) and bring him materials on which she would comment. For weeks, there was no response, or his only response was to pull the covers over his head. With time, however, he slowly began to engage, taking an interest in the magazine or other materials she brought by, such as games. The trainee responded with praise and reinforcement, commenting on the differences she noticed in his reactions in a positive way. She also asked him, when he did engage, to rate how much fun he had on a 10-point scale. Whatever number he gave she used a cheerleading style response, commenting on improvements or changes from his assumption of how much fun he might have. With encouragement, he was able to leave his room and play a short game of checkers with her alone in the group room. Again, this rating system and cheerleading style were used before and after the activity in order to help disconfirm inaccurate and maladaptive beliefs regarding his ability to partake in such activities and the pleasure that can be experienced from them.

By the time the trainee was almost finished with her four-month rotation he was meeting with her daily to play checkers, smiling and laughing as he won, and engaging with her in brief conversation. As staff came to notice this interaction, others also began to invite the patient to play board games, in either the afternoon or the evening hours. As the patient's negative symptoms improved, he was also better able to interact with his treatment team, giving more information about his other psychotic experiences (delusional beliefs). With this information, the unit staff as a whole were able to understand more about how he came to be admitted, better able to empathize with his experiences and change their original perceptions that he was taking advantage of the free food and accommodation.

Conclusion

CBTp is an evidence-based therapy that can be utilized on the inpatient unit; championed by the psychologist, but with support and consistency from all unit staff. Many of these strategies may be recognized as classic CBT interventions, just applied in a more specialized way. It is critical to engage all staff on an inpatient unit to consider how their interactions can impact the experience of psychosis and to give them the tools to contribute to treatment through brief interventions and interactions. Not only does this facilitate faster and more lasting recovery for clients, but it also empowers and validates staff, reducing burnout for those who perform some of the most valuable roles in the treatment of mental illness in the US.

References

Beck, J.S. (2011). *Cognitive behavior therapy: Basics and beyond.* (2nd Ed.). New York, NY: Guilford.

Beck, A.T., Perivoliotis, D., Brinen, A., Inverso, E., & Grant, P.M., (in press). *Recovery oriented cognitive therapy for schizophrenia: a treatment manual*. New York, NY: Guilford.

Breier, A., & Strauss, J.S. (1983). Self-control in psychotic disorders. *Archives of General Psychiatry*, *40*, 1141–1145.

Chadwick, P. (2006). *Person-based cognitive therapy for distressing psychosis*. Chichester, UK: Wiley.

Chadwick, P., Lees, S., & Birchwood, M. (2000). The revised Beliefs about Voices Questionnaire (BAVQ-R). *The British Journal of Psychiatry*, *177*, 229–232.

Chadwick, P.D.J., & Birchwood, M. (1994). The omnipotence of voices: A cognitive approach to hallucinations. *British Journal of Psychiatry*, *164*, 190–201.

Chadwick, P.D.J., Birchwood, M., & Trower, P. (1996). *Cognitive therapy for delusions, voices and paranoia*. Chichester, UK: Wiley.

Chadwick, P.D.J., Newman Taylor, K., & Abba, N. (2005). Mindfulness groups for people with distressing psychosis. *Behavioral and Cognitive Psychotherapy*, *33*, 351–359.

Chang, N. A., Grant, P.M., Luther, L., & Beck, A.T. (2014). Effects of a recovery-oriented cognitive therapy training program on inpatient staff attitudes and incidents of seclusion and restraint. *Community Mental Health Journal*, *50*(4), 415–421.

Downs, J. (2005). *Coping with voices and visions*. Manchester, UK: The Hearing Voices Network.

Elixhauser, A., & Steiner, C. (2013). *Readmissions to U.S. hospitals by diagnosis, 2010. HCUP Statistical Brief #153*. Rockville, MD: Agency for Healthcare Research and Quality. Retrieved from www.hcup-us.ahrq.gov/reports/statbriefs/sb153.pdf.

Fowler, D., Garety, P., & Kuipers, E. (1995). *Cognitive behavior therapy for psychosis: theory and practice*. Chichester, UK: Wiley.

Fowler, D., & Morley, S. (1989). The cognitive-behavioral treatment of hallucinations and delusions: A preliminary study. *Behavioral Psychotherapy, 17*, 267–282.

Gilbert, P. (2009). *The compassionate mind: A new approach to life's challenges*. London, UK: Constable & Robinson.

Goldsmith, L.P., Lewis, S.W., Dunn, G., & Bentall, R.P. (2015). Psychological treatments for early psychosis can be beneficial or harmful, depending on the therapeutic alliance: an instrumental variable analysis. *Psychological Medicine, 45*, 2365–2373.

Granholm, E., Loh, C., & Link, P. C. (2010). Feasibility of implementing cognitive behavioral therapy for psychosis on assertive community treatment teams: A controlled pilot study. *International Journal of Cognitive Therapy, 3* (Special section: Cognitive processes in anxiety), 295–303.

Granholm, E., McQuaid, J.R., & Holden, J. (2015). *Cognitive behavioral social skills training: A practical guide and consumer workbook*. New York, NY: Guilford.

Grant, P.M., Huh, G.A., Perivoliotis, D., Stolar, N.M., & Beck, A.T. (2012). Randomized trial to evaluatie the efficacy of cognitive therapy for low-funcionting patients with schizophrenia. *Archives of General Psychiatry, 69* (2), 121–127.

Haddock, G., Devane, S., Bradshaw, T., McGovern, J., Tarrier, N., Kinderman, P., & Harris, N. (2001). An investigation into the psychometric properties of the Cognitive Therapy Scale for Psychosis (CTSPsy). *Behavior and Cognitive Psychotherapy, 29*(2), 221–233.

Hayes, S.C., Stohsal, K.D., & Wilson, K.G. (2012). *Acceptance and commitment therapy: The process and practice of mindful change*. (2nd Ed.). New York, NY: Guilford.

Hill, G., Clarke, I., & Wilson, H. (2009). The "making friends with yourself" and "what is real and what is not" groups. In I. Clarke & H. Wilson (Eds.), *Cognitive behavior therapy for acute inpatient mental health units* (pp. 161–172). London: Routledge.

Kingdon, D.G., & Turkington, D. (1994). *Cognitive-behavioral therapy of schizophrenia*. New York, NY: Guilford.

Landa, Y., Silverstein, S.M., Schwartz, F., & Savitz, A. (2006). Group cognitive behavioral therapy for delusions: helping patients improve reality testing. *Journal of Contemporary Psychotherapy, 36*(1), 9–17.

Lazarus, A.A. (1992). Clinical/therapeutic effectivness. In J. Zeig (Ed.), *The evolution of psychotherapy* (pp. 100–109). New York, NY: Brunner/Mazel.

Lecomte, T., Leclerc, C., Corbiere, M., Wykes, T., Wallace, C.J., & Spidel, A. (2008). Group cognitive behavioral therapy or social skills training for individuals with recent onset of psychosis? Results of a randomized controlled trial. *Journal of Nervous and Mental Disease, 196*, 866–875.

Lecomte, T., Leclerc, C., & Wykes, T. (2012). Group CBT for early psychosis: Are there still benefits one year? *International Journal of Group Psychotherapy*, *62*, 309–321.

Lecomte, T., Leclerc, C., & Wykes, T. (2016). *Group CBT for psychosis: A guidebook for clinicians*. New York, NY: Oxford University Press.

Liberman, R.P. (1982). What is schizophrenia? *Schizophrenia Bulletin*, *8*, 435–437.

Linehan, M.M. (1993). *Cognitive-behavioral treatment of borderline personality disorder*. New York, NY: Guilford.

McLeod, H.J., Deane, F.P., & Hogbin, B. (2002). Changing staff attitudes and empathy for working with people with psychosis. *Behavioral and Cognitive Psychotherapy*, *30*(04), 459–470.

Morrison, A.P., & Barratt, S. (2010). What are the components of CBT for psychosis? A delphi study. *Schizophrenia Bulletin*, *36*(1), 136–142.

Morrison, A.P., Renton, J.C., Dunn, H., Williams, S., & Bentall, R.P. (2004). *Cognitive therapy for psychosis: A formulation based approach*. New York, NY: Routledge.

Mueser, K.T., & Glyn, S.M. (2014). Have the potential benefits of CBT for severe mental disorders been undersold? *World Psychiatiry*, *13*(3), 253–256.

Nelson, H. (2005). *Cognitive behavioral therapy with schizophrenia: A practice manual*. Cheltenham, UK: Stanley Thornes Ltd.

Noordsy, D.L., Torrey, W.C., Mueser, K.T., Mead, S., O'Keefe, C., & Fox, L. (2002). Recovery from severe mental illness: An intrapersonal and functional outcome definition. *International Review of Psychiatry*, *14*, 318–326.

Pennings, M., & Romme, M. (1997). *Gesprek groepen voor mensen die stemmen horen*. Utrectht: Stichting Weeklank.

Perry, Y., Murakami-Brundage, J., Grant., P.M., & Beck, A.T. (2013). Training peer specialisits in cogntive therapy strategies for recovery. *Psychiatric Services*, *64*(9), 929–930.

Pilling, S., Bebbington, P., Kuipers, E., Garety, P., Geddes, J., Orbach, G., & Morgan, C. (2002). Psychological treatments in schizophrenia: I. Meta-analysis of family intervention and cognitive behavior therapy. *Psychological Medicine*, *32*(5), 763–782.

Reynolds, W.J., Scott, B., & Jessiman, W.C. (1999). Empathy has not been measured in clients' terms or effectively taught: A review of the literature. *Journal of Advanced Nursing*, *30*, 1177–1185.

Riggs, S.E., & Creed, T.A. (2017). A model to transform treatment for psychosis using CBT informed interventions for the mental health milieu. *Cognitive and Behavioral Practice*, *24*, 353–362.

Riggs, S.E., Stirman, S.W., & Beck, A.T. (2012). Training community mental health agencies in cognitive therapy for schizophrenia. *The Behavior Therapist*, *35*(2), 34–39.

Robins, L.N., & Regier, D.A. (1991). *Psychiatric disorders in America: The epidemiologic catchment area study*. New York, NY: The Free Press.

Rollnick, S., & Miller, W.R. (1995). What is motivational interviewing? *Behavioral and Cognitive Psychotherapy*, *23*(4), 325–334.

Romme, M., & Escher, S. (1989). *Accepting voices*. London: Mind Publications.

SAMHSA. (2006). National consensus statement on mental health recovery. U. D. O. H. A. H. Services (Ed.). Washington, DC: Center for Mental Health Services.

Seligman, M.E. (2002). *Authentic happiness: using the new positive psychology to realize your potential for lasting fulfilment*. New York, NY: The Free Press, Simon & Schuster.

Sivec, H.J., & Montesano, V.L. (2012). Cognitive behavioral therapy for psychosis in clinical practice. *Psychotherapy*, *49*(2), 258–270.

Sivec, H.J., Montesano, V.L., Skubby, D., Knepp, K.A., & Muntez, M.R. (2017). Cognitive behavioral therapy for psychosis (CBT-p) delivered in a community mental health setting: A case comparison of clients receiving CBT informed strategies by case managers prior to therapy. *Community Mental Health Journal*, *53*(2), 134–142.

Tarrier, N. (1992). Management and modification of residual positive psychotic symptoms. In M. Birchwood & N. Tarrier (Eds.), *Innovations in the psychological management of schizophrenia* (pp. 147–170). Chichester, UK: Wiley.

Turkington, D., Kingdon, D., Rathod, S., Hammond, K., Pelton, J., & Mehta, R. (2006). Outcomes of an effectiveness trial of cognitive-behavioral intervention by mental health nurses in schizophrenia. *British Journal of Psychiatry*, *189*, 36–40.

Turkington, D., Kingdon, D., & Turner, T. (2002). Effectiveness of a brief cognitive-behavioral therapy intervention in the treatment of schizophrenia. *British Journal of Psychiatry*, *180*, 523–527.

Turkington, D., Muntz, M., Pelton, J., Montesano, V., Sivec, H., Nausheen, B., & Kingdon, D. (2014). High-yield cognitive behavioral techniques for psychosis delivered by case managers to their clients with persistent psychotic symptoms: An exploratory trial. *The Journal of Nervous and Mental Disease*, *202*(1), 30–34.

Waller, H., Garety, P.A., Jolley, S., Fornells-Ambrojo, M., Kuipers, E., Onwumere, J., & Craig, T. (2013). Low intensity cognitive behavioral therapy for psychosis: A pilot study. *Journal of Behavioral Therapy and Experimental Psychiatry*, *44*(1), 98–104.

Wright, N.P., Turkington, D., Kelly, O.P., Davies, D., Jacobs, A.M., & Hopton, J. (2014). *Treating psychosis: A clinician's guide to integrating acceptance & commitment therapy, compassion-focused therapy & mindfulness approaches within the cognitive behavioral tradition*. Oakland, CA: New Harbinger Publications, Inc.

13 Psychotherapy in an Inpatient Ward

A Clinical Psychologist's Use of Psychoanalytic Informed Work with Adult Survivors of Childhood Trauma

Beatriz S. Curtis

Clinical psychologists are trained to formulate a psychological-based understanding of the issues and problems presented by patients, as an alternative or to complement the use of diagnostic categories. It is this capacity to formulate that makes the clinical psychologist's role in the mental health inpatient setting most valuable.

Formulations provide a narrative intended to explain the difficulties that a person is dealing with, unique to that individual. They attempt to define what the problem is for the patient and/or others around him and what the causes might be, considering bio-psycho-social factors holistically. As an important component of the therapeutic process, formulations are constructed together with the patient, and reviewed and expanded as long as the treatment lasts. In formulations, we attempt to capture the person as a whole, with his/her weaknesses and strengths. We identify what the patient might gain from treatment, and the formulations inform our intervention plan (Johnstone & Dallos, 2013).

As part of our role in a multidisciplinary team (MDT), psychologists need to discuss and be cognizant of the ways in which our interventions are in line with and complement what the rest of the team is doing. We can, with our formulation, influence the team's understanding of the patient's presentation. This helps to ensure a level of empathy within the team, which at times is difficult to sustain because of the complexity of the cases we treat and the emotional disturbances they can bring upon us. A formulation has a function of containment not just for the patient but also for the professionals working with the patients. A clinical psychologist has the potential to provide such containment for the team.

In this chapter, I attempt to illustrate with two composite examples the benefits of formulating and intervening using a psychoanalytic body of theory and principles. The therapist's role as an emotional container

(Bion, 1967) and the process of identification with the aggressor (Ferenczi, 1949; Freud, 1992) provided the basis for my formulations and therefore have shaped my interventions as well as those of the MDT.

The treatment of these two patients, Kevin and Peter, took place in a secure inpatient psychiatric unit. These units followed a multidisciplinary approach, in which mental health professionals of different disciplines, namely psychiatrists, nurses, social workers, occupational therapists, and clinical psychologists, worked together. As a team, we provided specialist assessments, and delivered bio-psycho-social care, and developed treatment plans for patients. It was common practice to regularly discuss individual patients in MDT review meetings. A patient's first few weeks on the ward comprised the assessment period. Once an assessment was completed, an MDT treatment plan was designed to meet the patient's needs, covering all areas of care. In the review meetings, interventions were discussed, and the treatment plan was amended when deemed necessary. Knowing about and understanding the interventions carried out by the other MDT members was as important as reviewing one's own interventions. The review meeting offered an opportunity to gain a more holistic picture of each patient. Risk assessments and management plans were continuously revisited and updated. As most patients were hospitalized against their will, there were strict protocols to follow to protect their rights and everyone's safety. For example, a common theme discussed at every review for each patient was the level of supervision required for that patient when they left the unit's grounds. The more stable a patient's presentation, the less supervision was required. After a period of stability, the team would begin to consider the patient's move to a less secure and less supervised environment. Incidents of violence and the use of illicit substances were often indications that the risk presented by a particular patient was increasing; therefore, level of supervision and restrictions would be increased to ensure that the risk was being managed. The role of the clinical psychologist consisted of (1) providing specialist assessment, using structured and semi-structured assessment tools, and psychometric batteries when necessary, and (2) delivering treatment, in the form of psychotherapy. Treatment was delivered through individual and group sessions.

Kevin had a diagnosis of Borderline Personality Disorder (*DSM-IV*) and Peter a diagnosis of Antisocial Personality Disorder (*DSM-IV*). While Kevin was seen as someone who presented a risk to himself, Peter was seen as primarily presenting a serious risk to the public. The MDT interventions were aimed at both assessing and managing these risks in order to enable moving them to a less secure environment. However, developing formulations to help guide interventions and treatment of these patients involved more than the assessment and management of risks. An initial task was to try to understand the meaning and function of their risk-posing behaviors so that we could begin to build a detailed narrative of their personal and unique histories as well as develop an understanding of their conscious and unconscious minds. Albeit different in presentation, the similarities at the root of their pathologies became apparent.

Identification with the Aggressor

The psychoanalytic frame of long-term psychotherapeutic work with frequent set sessions, with generally no specific agenda to follow but free association, and adherence to the principle of offering a safe and protected space to think and reflect upon oneself in the presence of another, has been the backdrop of these two cases. Bringing past experiences into the room to throw light into the present and together, patient and therapist, building up a narrative of who the person is and what his struggles are about, was part of the method. Psychoanalytic theories and ideas which helped make sense of ways the patient has found for mental survival, made it possible to develop our understanding, and most important, to enable patient and therapist to tolerate the psychological pain involved in the therapeutic process.

The concept of containment developed by Wilfred Bion has underpinned the therapeutic work done with these patients. Bion (1967) used this term to describe the mother's function to contain the infant's mental state in her mind. In the psychotherapy, it was this 'thinking' activity that served to hold the patients' anxieties in mind and to make sense of them. Both Balint (1979) and Winnicott (1960a, 1960b) stress the containing function of the analyst, also emphasizing non-verbal acceptance and the management of regression (Davies & Frawley, 1994).

Another theoretical concept that was particularly relevant with these two patients was identification with the aggressor. Identification with the aggressor was first developed by Sándor Ferenczi in 1932 (Ferenczi, 1949) to help understand early trauma. It was used in a slightly different way by Anna Freud 4 years later (Freud, 1992) and consequently taken forward by numerous psychoanalysts, including those who have studied the treatment of trauma (Frankel, 2002).

Anna Freud used the terminology 'identification with the aggressor' to describe a defense mechanism applied to the normal development of the super-ego in children and involved in the pathology of paranoia. However, Ferenczi's understanding of the concept is related directly to the psychological response to early sexual trauma and was broader, as he emphasized 'the pervasive change in someone's perceptual world' (Frankel, 2002, p. 102) which is often found at the root of severe personality disorders.

Sándor Ferenczi was one of the first psychoanalysts to identify trauma, more specifically the sexual trauma, as the pathogenic factor in many of his neurotic patients. He considered sexual abuse of central importance when trying to understand the origin of the pathologies he often faced in his clinical practice (Frankel, 2002).

Ferenczi (1949) identified several consequences of early sexual trauma, some of which are pertinent to the cases discussed in this chapter. For example; identification with the aggressor, pervasive guilt and shame, perversion and sexual dysfunction, and a profound splitting of the ego associated with dissociation.

When describing the phenomena that he calls 'identification with the aggressor,' Ferenczi described it as it follows:

> The children feel physically and morally helpless, their personalities are not sufficiently consolidated in order to be able to protest, even if only in thought, for the overpowering force and authority of the adult makes them dumb and can rob them of their senses. The same anxiety, however, if it reaches a certain maximum, compels them to subordinate themselves like automata to the will of the aggressor, to divine each one of his desires and to gratify these completely oblivious of themselves, they identify themselves with the aggressor [...] The weak and undeveloped personality reacts to sudden unpleasure not by defense, but by anxiety-ridden identification and by introjection of the menacing person or aggressor.
>
> (p. 228)

In his theory of identification with the aggressor, Ferenczi described three mechanisms, namely identification, introjection, and dissociation. These facilitate the victim's ability to assess the environment and calculate the best way to survive. Identification involves the victim 'getting into' the aggressor's head to feel what the aggressor is feeling. This is followed by the victim feeling the way he thinks the aggressor expects him to feel. Identification is used to cope with an actual threatening person, i.e., by the victim knowing what the aggressor feels and thinks and expects the victim to do; the victim increases chances for survival. In introjection, the aggressor becomes intra- rather than extra-psychic. Fairbairn (1943) called this internalization of the bad object (Frankel, 2002). The abuser becomes part of the victim's self. In dissociation, there is a split from the immediate perception of experience that is intolerable.

Introjection perpetuates the experience of trauma. It is through the process of introjection that personality distortions can take place, when identification with the aggressor becomes habitual, a way of life (Frankel, 2002). Introjection is used to manage vulnerable feelings by providing the victim with a sense of control and a feeling of becoming powerful as opposed to passive and powerless, namely, by the victim becoming an aggressor himself.

Frankel (2002) understood Ferenczi's concept of introjection as similar to Anna Freud's concept of identification with the aggressor. Anna

Freud (1992) described introjection as a defense mechanism employed by the ego to deal with external objects that raise anxiety.

In her paper, Anna Freud illustrated her understanding of this process by describing how some children's games involve children becoming the very same thing that makes them anxious. For example, the ghost they fear is hidden in a dark corridor or the dentist who performed a painful procedure on them; i.e., they become the ghost and the dentist in their play, making others or their toys, become the passive victim. She explained how this process provides them with pleasurable security. 'By impersonating the aggressor, assuming his attributes or imitating his aggression, the child transforms himself from the person threatened into the person who makes the threat' (Freud, 1992, p. 113).

Kevin, a Victim of Abuse Who Became a Perpetrator to Himself

Kevin was a young man diagnosed with Borderline Personality Disorder. He engaged in self-harming behaviors and was highly suicidal. However, he functioned well when not in distress. Unlike many of the other patients treated in that unit, who presented complex needs and displayed apparent difficulties in social and living skills, Kevin had all the necessary living and social skills. Kevin reported that he had not found cognitive behavioral therapy helpful during previous admissions; therefore, I decided that an exploratory and psychoanalytically informed approach was perhaps necessary to understand how to best try to help him.

I knew little about his personal history before I started to work with him. It was over the course of our 2-year psychotherapy sessions that he spoke with me about his upbringing and significant events in his life. In our work together, we were able to reflect upon how his current struggles were related to his past, particularly to traumatic events in which he had been victimized.

Kevin was raised by both his parents. There was nothing in his preteen history that would suggest that his psychological development was compromised, and this was a protective factor for Kevin. The fact that he had grown up in what according to all indications was a safe and loving environment seemed to have given Kevin a significant degree of resilience, and the ability to engage in treatment with much benefit. During the course of our work together, Kevin disclosed for the first time, that he had been the victim of violent sexual assault in his teens. Kevin had previously not talked to anyone about this in any detail.

My first impression of Kevin was of a withdrawn young man who was unable to verbalize his thoughts and feelings, apart from the fact that he wanted to die. He had no hope for his future, and it appeared he struggled to accept any help. When discussing his case in the weekly

MDT meetings, incidents of self-harm including cutting, swallowing sharp objects, and overdosing were repeatedly reported. He continuously expressed a wish to die. Kevin also often experienced hearing voices which, however, as became clear over the course of the treatment, were trauma-related and did not indicate an underlying psychotic illness.

Self-harming behavior can be a way of dealing with distressing feelings, painful memories, or overwhelming situations and experiences that feel out of control. Such behaviors can be an indication of emotional distress and do not necessarily indicate an attempt to commit suicide; in fact, they are often an act of self-preservation (Royal College of Psychiatrists, 2010). Self-harm can be seen as a defense mechanism that aims at bringing relief, but often it also brings other sets of complex feelings, such as shame and disgust (Skegg, 2005; Chapman et al., 2006). Self-harming as a behavior has the potential of communicating something that can be more productively articulated through words. While the boundaries and practices on the unit aimed at managing such behavior by minimizing chances for patients to self-harm, our work also consisted of developing a thorough understanding of the meanings and functions of this behavior for each specific patient. Motives for self-harm can differ on each occasion and can even evolve over time (Royal College of Psychiatrist, 2010). By understanding the function and meanings of Kevin's self-harming behaviors, we as a team could respond in the best possible way to help him find alternative ways of communicating and dealing with his struggles.

Kevin's self-harming behavior was an assault on his body and a self-inflicted punishment. Using Ferenczi's theory of identification with the aggressor, it could be said that Kevin had identified with and introjected the aggressor. He re-enacted the assaults on his body, perpetrated by the aggressors in his past, through insertions and cuts into his skin. His repeated threats to take his life could also be seen as re-enactments of the life threats from his aggressors. By being the one who inflicted the pain during his self-harming episodes, he moved from being the passive victim to being powerful and in control. Becoming the agent of aggression aimed toward himself had become a habitual way of life. It was the psychological mechanism he had developed to deal with the consequences of trauma. He had become the perpetrator as much as the victim. The danger resided in him, as a part of him; the introjected aggressor was the one he needed to gain protection from. Identifying with the aggressor had become a perpetuating disruptive process to combat the helplessness and shame he experienced and from which he protected himself. Helping Kevin face the shame he felt, and to accept his helpless, vulnerable and injured self, was necessary in order to help him stop this identification and self-aggression.

This understanding of his disruptive behavior helped alter the MDT's orientation and treatment approach toward Kevin. Before this formulation was introduced, it was difficult for team members to empathize with him. Unlike many other similarly diagnosed patients who demonstrate vulnerability in many aspects of their personality, Kevin's ability to function well in many other aspects of his life made it difficult for the team to understand his self-harming behavior. It was difficult for the MDT to realize how much distress he often experienced. The team often interpreted his disruptive behaviors as being manipulative and controlling, and this interfered with their ability to empathize with him. For this reason, I found it important to share with the team some of the details of his trauma, and explain how injured and distressed this patient was deep down, despite his ability to disguise it at surface level. Kevin gave his consent for me to speak regularly with the team members about his treatment and accepted my judgment on the matter of how much I shared. Communicating with the MDT members about Kevin in the review meetings was important but challenging. There was a need to balance between sharing information about treatment progression and with keeping confidentiality as much as possible, particularly regarding sensitive details. I shared with him any legal documents I wrote that concerned him, in order to involve him in the formulation as well as to protect our therapeutic alliance.

After several months of working together, Kevin began to share some details of the sexual assaults in which he had been a victim. The guilt and shame he felt made it extremely difficult for him to talk about these events and to allow us to think about them. However, I think that a key to his recovery was my readiness to listen and stay with his pain, to be with the vulnerable, helpless part of him, without my defending against it.

Kevin showed increasing signs of progress the more we were able to explain his behavior and feelings in light of his experiences of abuse. We began to develop a more elaborated insight into the complexities of his mind. We identified several parts of his self. There were primarily the violent part and the vulnerable part. Kevin's violent part wished him to suffer and inflicted pain through self-harming behaviors. This violent part also wished him dead, explaining his suicidal state of mind. It was through introjection and identification with the abusers that this side of him had developed, a mechanism adopted in order to defend against feeling the helplessness and powerlessness of the vulnerable victim.

In contrast, there was a vulnerable or injured part of his self. This was the most difficult side of him to think about and accept. For that to happen, he had to cease identifying with the abusers and begin identifying with the victim. This was a more painful position to accept. We spoke about the injured part of himself that came up when he felt distressed, often prior to self-harming, before taking control by becoming his self-abuser, inflicting pain and causing physical injury. These were the times when he felt vulnerable and anxious. This part of himself was difficult for Kevin to think about and embrace, but the more we talked about it by reflecting on daily situations that fueled his anxiety, the less often his self-harming episodes occurred.

We also explored his anger. He was vindictive and hurtful toward others as well as toward himself. It was quite astonishing to see how Kevin was unable to feel anger toward his abusers and yet he was full of anger when directing it toward himself and those who cared about him. Being angry with the aggressors would have meant acknowledging the abusers' overbearing power and his helplessness at the time. He had identified so deeply with the abuser that he truly believed he was not a victim. His abusers had blamed him for what they did to him. Sex offenders, as we will see in Peter's case, find ways of justifying their actions, giving themselves permission to offend and evade feeling guilt. In our sessions, we spoke about how Kevin's self-harm was sometimes an angry communication through actions. What he could not talk about, he acted out. The nursing team and I were also targets, as the levels of anxiety in caring for a suicidal patient can get very high, as their behavior could potentially cause death.

Over the course of our 2-year treatment, Kevin improved as he was better able to manage periods of distress and his incidents of self-harm reduced significantly. His wish to die was at bay for longer periods of time. After 2 years of treatment, the MDT decided that he could be discharged to sheltered housing in the community.

Kevin had found within our therapeutic relationship an emotionally available and containing figure at a time when he felt capable of taking the risk to trust someone and face his disturbed mind. The crucial intervention was through the therapeutic relationship. This relationship provided a platform, allowing Kevin to explore and integrate different parts of his self, his split ego (Ferenczi, 1949), i.e., the violent and the vulnerable, the victim and the perpetrator. His emotional maturity allowed him to tolerate the challenge and pain that this work entailed.

This work was made possible by the continuity of the inpatient unit's holding environment as well as the MDT members' work conducted in-between sessions. The nursing team made sure Kevin was safe at all times. The consultant psychiatrist and the rest of the team were aware that our therapeutic work would make Kevin feel more vulnerable and therefore at risk, and they responded accordingly, helping him get through those difficult times by giving him more space and support. Had it not been for the continuity and consistency provided by the unit, such therapeutic work would not have been possible.

Peter, a Perpetrator Who Also Was a Victim of Abuse

Peter was a young man referred to the unit for assessment and treatment. He was a sex offender detained in the hospital with special restrictions in order to protect the public.

Peter suffered a disturbing upbringing as he was severely neglected by his drug-addicted mother. As a child, he suffered physical abuse as well as a violent assault and rape. From an early age, Peter displayed aggressive and sexualized behaviors that led to his expulsion from school. At the time of his expulsion, Peter disclosed, he was sexually assaulted, although the police did not charge the perpetrator owing to lack of sufficient evidence. Later, as an adolescent, Peter sexually assaulted a much younger child.

Peter had been both a victim and a perpetrator of sexual abuse. His experience of sexual and violent assault had left significant sequela, i.e., anxiety, resentment, shame, and sexual interest in minors.

Unlike Kevin who directed his aggression inward and was unable to feel anger toward his aggressors, Peter externalized his anger. He was an angry man and his anger was easily triggered. Peter was aware of his rage, particularly toward the person who assaulted him. He was also angry with the professionals who had been involved with him since he was a child. He was very resentful that his perpetrator had not been brought to justice, while he himself was detained and forced to receive treatment.

Peter's therapeutic plan included long-term twice weekly individual psychotherapy sessions. The aim of these sessions was twofold: (1) to address his antisocial traits and sexual interest in minors in order to reduce the risk he posed to the public, and (2) to address his psychological problems of anxiety, resentment, and shame. For psychotherapy with Peter to succeed, it had to address, hold together, and integrate his perpetrator and victim sides. The psychotherapy sessions aimed at providing him with a steady space in which to reflect upon ways in which his current state was related to his previous experiences of neglect and abuse. A psychoanalytically informed understanding made this possible and provided a holding experience that enabled him to question his thinking and actions and experiment with new ways of being. The theories that informed my practice provided me and subsequently the MDT, a holding platform, which enabled bringing together what looked like two sides of a coin: his perpetrator and victim sides.

Peter was often talkative and would speak about stories related to his past. He called them his 'happy memories.' He spoke about jobs he had held, places he had been, girlfriends he had. There was an element of confabulation in his stories, as they lacked consistency. Much that he reported did not seem to be factually true. He often portrayed himself as a successful and brave young man. However, in a way, this was true of him. He had survived severe abuse and rape in his childhood. Perhaps it was important for Peter to make up for the scarcity of good experiences during his early years, adding on to them through his confabulated stories.

It took Peter six months before he began talking about what he called his 'bad memories.' He spoke about some of his most traumatic stories involving physical abuse, sexual abuse, and neglect. At times, these stories lacked consistency as well. However, regardless of the inconsistency of the details, it was clear that this young man was seriously psychologically traumatized from an early age. Peter now found our relationship safe enough to talk about and explore how his mother's neglect had affected him. He also talked in more detail about having been sexually abused as well as his own sexual abuse offensive action. At first, he expressed little understanding about the relationship between his experiences of being abused, and his offense. It was important to clarify to Peter that by linking these, one was not excusing his offensive behavior, that understanding the factors that led him to commit such an offense was not the same as accepting the behavior. It was also important to emphasize the sole responsibility of his abusers for their abusive actions. Gradually, Peter developed a more sophisticated understanding of what led to his offense, and how having been neglected and sexually abused were key factors related to his behavior. He had defended against feeling vulnerable by identifying with his abusers, in an attempt to move from a position of powerlessness to that of overpowering another person. Through his psychotherapy, Peter began to understand himself and feel understood by another.

By the end of his 2-year placement, Peter had gained insight and connected his damaged and revengeful sides in a way that allowed him to begin to forgive and care for himself and others.

In work with the MDT for this patient, my role consisted of highlighting his victim side. Peter was known and recognized as the patient who sexually abused a child, referred to our unit to address his index offense. However, through our intensive work with Peter, we were able to find a narrative about his past, which linked his experiences of neglect and abuse with his later offensive actions. The gradual progress made with these understandings enabled the team to respond to him in more helpful and empathic ways. For example, when Peter asked to attend various events in the community, the team was able to see his request as an opportunity for him to grow and build his future, rather than as a strategy for finding another victim. Likewise, the work and input of the other MDT members allowed me to learn about Peter in ways that I could not have done through our sessions. For example, Peter would not tell me about incidents on the ward in which he was involved, but as I learned about them through the nurse handovers and review meetings, I invited him to talk about them, so that we could reflect together on these events. Unlike in outpatient practice where a clinician needs to rely purely on what the patient says, in inpatient work as part of the MDT, one has the opportunity to hear different stories about patients and become aware of their various behaviors in a variety of settings and situations. This is especially helpful in work with patients who present complex needs.

In this chapter I attempted to demonstrate the added value of the clinical psychologist's work on an inpatient unit, illustrating the way in which psychological formulations can explain the underlying causes of disturbing behaviors, informing the MDT treatment plan and interventions. Psychoanalytic theories can be used to enhance and deepen understanding of the pathological presentations of patients. Psychoanalytic principles of practice can offer a non-threatening and non-prescriptive framework for patients who have found it difficult to engage in other types of psychological treatment, and who are willing and able within the therapeutic relationship to look back at their personal experiences in order to develop an insight into the present. Through the two composite cases of Kevin and Peter, I have illustrated how underlying their different presentations lay similar psychological defense mechanisms, awareness of which informed their treatment in the psychotherapeutic relationship and with the MDT on the unit. For members of the MDT, understanding the psychological basis for their patients' disturbed behavior, contributed to their empathy and support for a psychological treatment that aimed to facilitate change in behavior through psychological growth.

References

Balint, M. (1979). *The basic fault*. New York, NY: Brunner/Mazel.

Bion, W. R. (1967). *Second thoughts: Selected papers on psychonalysis*. Bath, UK: Heinemann.

Chapman, A. L., Gratz, K. L., & Brown, M. Z. (2006). Solving the puzzle of deliberate self-harm: The experiential avoidance model. *Behaviour Research and Therapy*, 44(3), 371–394.

Davies, J. M., & Frawley, M. G. (1994). *Treating the adult survivor of childhood sexual abuse: A psychoanalytic perspective*. New York, NY: Basic Books.

Fairbairn, W. R. D. (1943). The repression and the return of bad objects (with special reference to the 'war neuroses'). *British Journal of Medical Psychology, 19* (3–4), 327–341.

Ferenczi, S. (1949). Confusion of the tongues between the adults and the child. *The International Journal of Psycho-Analysis, 30*, 225–230.

Frankel, J. (2002). Exploring Ferenczi's concept of identification with the aggressor: Its role in trauma, everyday life, and the therapeutic relationship. *Psychoanalytic Dialogues, 12*, 101–139.

Freud, A. (1992). *The ego and the mechanisms of defence*. London: Karnac.

Johnstone, L., & Dallos, R. (2013). *Formulation in psychology and psychotherapy: Making sense of people's problems*. London: Routledge.

Royal College of Psychiatrist. (2010). Self-harm, suicide and risk: Helping people who self-harm. Retrieved from www.rcpsych.ac.uk/files/pdfversion/CR158xx.pdf.

Skegg, K. (2005). Self-harm. *The Lancet*, 366(9495), 1471–1483.

Winnicott, D. W. (1960a). Ego distortion in terms of true and false self. In D. W. Winnicott (Ed.), *The maturational process and the facilitating environment* (pp. 140–152). Madison, CT: International University Press, 1965.

Winnicott, D. W. (1960b). Counter-transference. In D. W. Winnicott (Ed.), *The maturational process and the facilitating environment* (pp. 158–165). Madison, CT: International University Press, 1965.

14 Mentalization and Psychotherapy

A Way to Understand Patient Violence on the Psychiatric Inpatient Unit

Dione Johnson-Williams

Violent and aggressive behavior, directed toward both self and others, are problems that exist on many psychiatric units. In this chapter, an explanation of psychological etiology and treatment addressing this violence is provided, based on theories relating to attachment and mentalization. The psychologist led treatment interventions described address attachment and mentalization issues with a patient diagnosed with personality disorder and mood disturbance who presented violent and aggressive behaviors on the ward.

Among the many aspects of treatment within the inpatient setting, the staff-patient dynamic can help facilitate a paradigm shift in which the patient's intra- and interpersonal deficits are ameliorated. This is a challenging task for the clinical staff and for the unit in general, particularly when patients' aggressive and violent behaviors evoke negative countertransference. Yet, it is crucial that ward staff work to help patients develop more reality-based and prosocial modes of relating via engaging therapeutic relationships.

Negative countertransference reactions among staff members in response to patients' violence can increase problematic communication patterns between staff and patients, ultimately reinforcing the likelihood of a repetitive pattern of violent behavior (Nijman, aCampo, Ravelli, & Mercekelbach, 1999). Avoidance of and lack of assertion with aggressive patients, inconsistent limit setting regarding hospital policies/rules and ward routine (Nijman, aCampo, Ravelli, & Merckelbach, 1999), and deficient treatment team cohesion and decision-making, are among the problematic patterns that may emerge (Rossberg & Friis, 2003).

In a study that examined the relationship between inpatient characteristics and staff members' emotional reactions, staff characteristics such as guardedness and lack of confidence were associated with aggressive and volatile behavior among patients (Rossberg & Friis, 2003). These results suggest that when staff members feel ill-equipped and unprepared to clinically intervene, patients are more likely to become violent toward themselves and others. This dynamic between patients and staff compromises both the safety and integrity of the treatment milieu.

In the psychiatric unit, clinical staff often implicitly assume the role of a caregiver and may elicit attachment needs within the patient (Ma, 2007). For many patients, efforts to satisfy these needs occur within the context of unresolved and maladaptive attachment patterns from early childhood and impaired mentalization abilities. It was found (Adshead et al., 2013) that in both clinical and forensic inpatient samples, individuals classified as having insecure attachments have poor mentalizing abilities and are more likely to exhibit violence when unable to manage negative affect and emotional states.

Furthermore, Fonagy, Target, and Gergely (2000) suggested that early childhood experiences of abuse and neglect become the template for problems in subsequent attachment relationships. These include fears of being abandoned, judged or neglected within an interpersonal context.

Case Example

David had been hospitalized at various points in his life, since age 11. David was adopted at an early age, and prior to that he resided in various orphanages and residential placements. As an adult, David did not have much contact with his adopted family. David indicated that he had been physically abused by his adoptive parents for his many "misbehaviors" as a child, and he no longer wished to communicate with them. On the unit, David admitted that whenever he felt scolded or rejected by a clinical team member (typically when limits and boundaries were imposed in response to his behaviors and in accordance with hospital protocol), he would cut himself and would recall instances of physical abuse from his childhood.

On a Monday morning when the treatment team met to review the weekend events, David paced at the team room door. As the nurses read the morning report, David repeatedly interjected with his comments from the other side of the door. He yelled and insisted that the team listen to his commentary on the report. When it was reported that various contraband items were found on his person and in his room during a search, David's verbal protests became physical. He banged and kicked the team room door threatening to spit on or kick the nurse who "was lying" about him. When the team members ignored him or warned him that an emergency code would be called if his behavior did not stop, David went to his room and cut his wrist. This resulted in an emergency code, and the team members responded to his self-injurious behaviors in crisis.

This interaction between David and the team is an example of what Fraley (2010) described as triggers to the faulty attachment behavior system. Developmental research and literature indicate that attachment related patterns of behaviors are relatively persistent and consistent across the lifespan. That is, ways of relating to others in childhood are shown to endure in adulthood (e.g., Harder, 2014). For David, this meant that he experienced a pervasive and foreboding worry that clinical staff would reject him. His ability to recognize adaptive caregiving was hindered. He displayed anger readily when he felt judged, rejected, or neglected. Aggression and volatile outbursts were means he used to communicate his protest to clinical care decisions and responses to his behavior. And, when David would attempt to directly force clinicians to bend to his will and demands vis-à-vis self-injury, he felt a sense of relief. In David's view, the setting of limits and boundaries to help him regulate his behavior(s) was perceived as rejection or failure on the part of the clinician to understand and respond to his needs. David would readily blame his treatment team, including this author, for provoking his anger and violence, much in the same way he experienced his foster parents provoking his anger during his childhood.

The development of mentalizing capacities is relationally bound. Fonagy and Bateman (2008) explored the concept of mentalization as a crucial aspect of attachment relationships. Secure attachment relationships facilitate the ability to mentalize vis-à-vis reflective functioning (Fonagy, Gergely, Jurist, & Target, 2002). This reflective capacity assists in the development of mentalization abilities in the child and helps to create an "internal working model" enabling the child to think about the mental states of self and others. Originally described by John Bowlby, the internal working model is a cognitive schema, consisting of mental representations a child uses to understand himself and the world around him (Bowlby, 1969). When there are strong and healthy attachment bonds, an individual can more accurately infer the mental states of himself and others, in addition to recognizing the impact of such mental states on his cognitions, affect, and behaviors (MaBeth, Gumley, Schwannaeur, & Fisher, 2011). The internal working models among those described as securely attached are often flexible and contribute to more regulated behaviors. The internal working models of those with avoidant or ambivalent insecure attachments often entail individuals minimizing their experiences. Internal working models among those classified with disorganized insecure attachment styles are characterized by a breakdown in, or lack of strategies to regulate emotional experiences (MaBeth, Gumley, Schwannaeur, & Fisher, 2011).

Fonagy and Target (2000) suggested that a perceived lack of security and trust in primary attachment relationships that lead to insecure attachment is a core feature of many later forms of psychopathology. Interpersonal deficits are likely to emerge as a result of sustained traumatic histories with primary attachment figures and to contribute to compromised mentalization abilities (Fonagy & Bateman, 2008). Pathways and manifestations of these disruptions are well described by Fonagy and others. Such disruptions contribute to attachment patterns characterized by emotional dysregulation, self-harming behavior, emotional lability, cognitive distortions, suspiciousness, confusion, and anxiety (Crawford et al., 2007).

Research has indicated that compared to a control group, psychiatric inpatients were more likely to be preoccupied with past trauma and were classified as having more disorganized and unresolved attachments (Fonagy et al., 1996).

> David became angry with the treatment team after they met with him to discuss a recent interaction he had with another patient. David was confronted about his bullying and threatening behaviors toward the other patient. David was reminded of the consequences of such actions, primarily a decrease in the behavioral level system and loss of privileges. He was advised that the team would meet with him later in the day after they had a chance to further discuss the recent events. David stood on the outside of the meeting room and eavesdropped on the team's discussion. He overheard the psychiatrist summarize the team's decision. David followed the psychiatrist off the unit into the hallway and violently attacked him, causing him serious injury.

There are numerous challenges within the psychiatric inpatient setting that make it difficult to manage patient violence and aggression. Practical limitations include limited resources, high staff turnover, un-filled positions or shifts due to staff injury, and scheduling conflicts for staff and patients which impact access to treatment. In addition, there are often various policies and procedures within institutions that limit patient movements within the setting, such as group attendance to treatment(s) that are not on the patient's unit (Adshead et al., 2013).

Ma (2006) suggested that the use of interpersonal approaches is indicated in response to "maladaptive expressions of attachment needs, in circumstances where the attachment system is activated" (Ma, 2006, p. 444). Such approaches transition treatment beyond symptom management (e.g., decreasing the number and frequency of violent behaviors), adding the important dimension of helping the patient resolve stagnating transference experiences. A targeted and holistic examination of attachment patterns vis-à-vis treatment interactions with clinical staff stands to evoke a change in how the patient understands his life experiences and current symptoms. Clinical staff members such as psychiatric nurses and mental health technicians are able to form relationships with patients that are caregiving and show characteristics of attachment bonds (Ma, 2007). Psychologists, with a theoretical understanding of developmental influences on current behavior, are uniquely positioned to provide clinical leadership that can facilitate a transition from treatment with an emphasis on symptom management to an integration of interpersonally informed interventions. Both interpersonally oriented treatment team interventions and individual psychotherapeutic interventions can contribute to such a treatment shift.

The development of patients' mentalization abilities in psychotherapy can occur when the therapeutic relationship with the psychologist forms the foundation for treating and understanding symptoms. This dynamic becomes the primary context through which the individual understands himself and other relational exchanges. During this process, the clinician should be prepared for some symptoms to increase. As part of patients' re-enactments, violence and aggression may be directed toward the clinician. When the clinician comes to represent an attachment figure in the treatment process, targeted violence can be viewed as reactions to perceived slights (Adshead, 1998). Here, the therapist must remember to respond to any threats to safety seriously and proceed with caution and care. A plausible and expected response is to implement some physical boundary and distance. But, it would be a mistake to not see beyond the explicit behavior manifestations and understand the larger implications of such re-enactments. Failure to consider the patient's internal reality, however distorted, is shortsighted and premature. In addition to the violence that stems from the re-enactment of earlier traumatic experiences of abuse and rejection within the attachment relationship, emotional outbursts and volatility directed toward staff can be a way for patients to manage any anxiety that is evoked during interactions with the clinician. Fonagy and Target (2000) explained that our patients will "push" us to respond in the transference in a way that confirms their negative expectations and experiences.

> When angry, David would assault other patients so severely at times that they would require off-site medical services. However, when David became emotionally overwhelmed and dysregulated in response to his interactions with staff, his aggression was different. In response to frustrating staff interactions, David would typically self-injure. In these instances, self-injurious behaviors were often triggered by the inconsistent setting of limits and boundaries by the treatment team. This unpredictability would confuse and further frustrate David. David's self-injury in many ways was "a show of protest." David punished the treatment team by injuring himself. Both before and after he would self-injure, David would tell the psychologist, "You made me do it."

A lack of consistent and clear clinical team responses likely mimicked insecure attachment patterns from David's early childhood. Erskine (2011) identified the resolution of such patterns as a seminal treatment goal. Understanding this resolution as a process rather than an event, the therapist's own mentalization of the patient can arise from and further elicit an empathic stance.

The ability to better represent or "hold" the client's experiences vis-à-vis affective attunement, explanation, and validation extends beyond treatment sessions. Psychologists are particularly well-equipped to bring to bear a holistic approach in conceptualizing the patient and his or her symptoms. In addition to adeptness at considering and integrating the various biological, psychological, and behavioral factors that inform symptoms, the psychologist is trained to understand the developmental impact of early caregiver experiences on current patient interactions. Using this knowledge, the psychologist can provide a secure base from which clinical staff members' countertransference reactions to the patients' maladaptive behaviors can be reflected upon. Discussions with staff concerning reasons for inconsistent treatment team responses to his behaviors were an important aspect of David's treatment.

As efforts were made to maintain consistent limits and boundaries with David, ever-present concerns for staff, including this author, centered on safety. Staff had particular concerns about David engaging in retaliatory aggression. Helping David identify less pathological responses to feeling slighted vs. his tendency to exhibit familiar problematic responses from early caregiving exchanges when he felt triggered or aroused was a primary function of our therapeutic relationship.

The psychologist's mentalization of the patient can also be useful in other treatment dimensions of the inpatient milieu. Participants in group treatments are noted to have improved outcomes, such as symptom reduction, decrease in re-admission rates, and after-care follow up (e.g., Bateman & Fonagy, 2001; Combs et al., 2007; Talbot et al., 1999). In a pilot study assessing the efficacy of interventions aimed at enhancing mentalizing to decrease violence in an inpatient forensic sample of men diagnosed with co-occurring personality disorder and a primary diagnosis of paranoid schizophrenia, Adshead et al. (2013) found that a group activity was effective at improving mentalizing abilities. However, Adshead (2015) also suggested that attachment-related behaviors are likely evoked in one-to-one sessions with a clinician in ways that are not triggered in group interactions.

The dynamic and fluid aspect of the relationship between the psychologist and patient in treatment increases the psychologist's ability to accurately perceive and empathically respond to patient's constructs of reality (Rogers, 1959). The success of therapy is embedded within the psychologist's capacity to avail varying aspects of his/her person to be impacted by the patient's relational patterns. The therapist forms a holding and a "good-enough" relationship with the patient vis-à-vis the "therapist's use of self." It is through this empathic presence and involvement that the psychologist's mentalization of the patient can expand. The patient identifies with and is grounded within the clinician's mentalization of himself and may use such mentalization to integrate his own self-image and self-concepts (Fonagy & Target, 2008). Thus, the psychotherapist's mentalization practically frames various aspects of the "here-and-now" context of the therapeutic relationship. In this way, mentalization "acts as a buffer" through which the patient's assumptions and expectations are treated as working hypotheses (Fonagy & Target, 2008, p. 1139). The clinician's ability to mentalize alternative forms of reality often brings to bear painful and split off memories and experiences for the patient.

> Whenever a new staff member came onto the unit, David made every effort to let that staff member know who he was and conveyed to the new staff member the expectation that the new staff member would leave the hospital (e.g., quit/resign) before David was discharged. David often expressed this point together with threats to injure and assault staff. During one of my first days on the unit, David followed me as I made rounds. When I advised him that following me made me feel uncomfortable, David insisted that if he wanted to harm me he would purposefully do so and that I need not be concerned. He insisted, "You don't have to be afraid of me. I won't hurt you." For the next several days, I ignored David's efforts to interact. One day, when I entered the unit, I asked David if he knew any alternative ways to engage me, besides intimidation. David was struck by my inquiry. He was speechless. Among many other treatment goals, helping David to identify responses to my question facilitated the beginning of individual therapy that we engaged in over the next year.

My initial reactions to David's stalking me on the ward included both a sense of curiosity and avoidance. To say that I was trepid in directly confronting David about his behavior is an understatement. David had a way of evoking anxiety and nervousness in others when they interacted with him. However, in that moment, I felt – almost intuited – that there was something David wanted to express to me. I sensed that he struggled in knowing how to communicate without using intimidation, bullying, or other manipulative behaviors. There was something very visceral and primal about how David was trying to connect with me and gain my attention. In addition to testing my boundaries in order to see just how far I would let him go, David was trying to gauge whether or not he could trust me. David trusted no one. His interpretation of his life experiences inside and outside of the hospital reinforced that belief. In certain situations, David was keenly aware of just how disrespectful and inappropriate he was and could be when interacting with others. If David saw that others would allow him to violate their boundaries, David's insolence would escalate and persist. For him, it was better not to talk to and to ignore some folks than to engage and disrespect them. At least in his mind, David knew exactly what the limits were for those with whom he did not speak. While with caregivers and those in authority positions David resented limits and boundaries being set, at the same time there was something very calming and containing for him when he knew what the expectations were. Both consciously and unconsciously, he looked to the environment to provide the structure and containment that he lacked internally. As his psychologist, my ability to recognize, reflect, and subsequently facilitate this dynamic, and process it in treatment was the hallmark of mentalization in my work with him.

The vignette presented above illustrates how the clinician can help provide a corrective experience addressing likely early childhood attachment needs. The recognition of one's own and others' mental states, known as intersubjectivity (Larsson, 2012), is a dynamic which has developmental implications that relate to both the mother-child dyad and the therapy context (Mills, 2005). In its basic and simplest form, intersubjectivity is a form of interconnectedness – social exchange – between two people whose relational interactions occur within a specific social context (Owen, 2006). The clinician develops her own mental space to hold those of the patient. Such mentalization illustrates to the patient an awareness of a caring and attuned other who considers and allows the patient's dynamics to impact him. It is hoped that when the clinician's mentalization is part of the clinical process, it will create opportunities in treatment in which experiences of trauma can be addressed (Larsson, 2012).

There were instances throughout the course of treatment where I would prompt David in and out of session to consider his tendency to threaten and intimidate others and self-injure when he felt frustrated. David would yell, argue, and demand that the team (myself included) modify our team decisions that involved imposing consequences in order to hold him accountable for his behaviors. Helping David manage his volatile impulses and reactions in the moment, while not giving in to his threats and remaining consistent in our position, was crucial. However, it was equally and perhaps more important for him to understand the paradoxical effect of his behaviors on himself and on those with whom he interacted. What others saw and what David expressed were visceral reactions to his emotions. This, in turn, would lead to David's feeling increasingly agitated because of what and how he truly felt was often not expressed. In addition to feeling angry, David often felt rejected, ignored, dismissed, and powerless. In those instances, I would cautiously prompt David to consider how he was feeling (other than angry), and communicate to him my perceptions of his behaviors and any of his unexpressed emotions in the moment. David's ability to recognize and express feelings such as frustration and anxiety improved. It was crucial for David to begin utilizing alternative ways to understand and express his affective feeling states which were evoked during interpersonal encounters.

The psychologist's mentalization leads the way in every aspect of treatment. Such a framework helps the patient connect differently to the surrounding milieu. In the psychiatric hospital setting, it can be helpful for treatment to explore the ways in which the patient understands his stay and symptoms vis-à-vis maladaptive attachment patterns. Many individuals who are hospitalized on a closed ward are disconnected from society and themselves. The clinician and patient both benefit when they recognize and remember that what happens on the unit, and the patient's responses, are not always direct consequences of recent interactions. This is especially noteworthy for those diagnosed with characterological issues. The clinician must hone his ability to recognize, recall and utilize representational images and nonverbal behaviors that patients may rely on to communicate. Doing this will enhance the conceptualization of patients' symptoms and behaviors, improve treatment planning and goal-setting, and help implement more practical and developmentally-relevant interventions.

The psychologist's mentalization of the patient can impact the entire system throughout the course of the patient's hospital stay. What becomes most salient on the unit are the day-to-day interactions and decisions regarding patient care which require a more accurate understanding of and response to the patient's behaviors. In the midst of ongoing activity on the units and the numerous duties of clinicians and nursing staff, it can be challenging for caregivers to consistently take the time necessary to consider alternative explanations of patients' problem behaviors beyond the often negative connotations given at shift change, nursing and clinical incident reports, etc. The psychologist continuously acts as a mediator between the patient and the hospital milieu. The psychologist draws upon his clinical encounters with the patient to communicate and inform treatment planning at every level of care for the patient in the hospital system.

> Several months into individual therapy, the team and I agreed that we would re-visit the topic of discharge planning with David. We each agreed that David would benefit most from a highly structured, forensic, group home setting, one in which staff was available 24 hours/7 days per week, and were skilled at managing very volatile behaviors often displayed by residents. In our individual sessions, David and I discussed his discharge from the hospital and the significance of community re-entry. As part of discharge planning, a meeting was scheduled with a housing provider, to meet with David and the team. Five minutes into the meeting, David became angry and started cursing at the provider before walking out

of the meeting. With my encouragement and redirection, David was able to return to the meeting. Both David and I discussed his propensity to become emotionally explosive and volatile toward others when he feared that they were going to judge or dismiss him.

At the conclusion of the meeting, David returned to the unit, and the housing provider finished meeting with the team. She admitted that David's behavior was off-putting, provocative, and potentially unsafe. Aside from his disconcerting inpatient hospital and criminal records, David's episode put him at risk of not being considered for the placement. Each of the provider's concerns were realistic and valid. The reality was that, at times, David's fear and insecurities about being rejected would become so pronounced that he would become extremely aggressive. When that happened, it was quite the task to de-escalate him. In response to his outbursts, staff members, would usually disconnect from him and be more inclined to keep their interactions with him to a minimum. This dynamic would reinforce his feelings of rejection and his view of how others perceived and interacted with him, which further validated his manipulative and reactive behaviors toward others.

Attachment relationships with clinicians and systems of care can provide a secure base with a sense of safety and positive regard, and facilitate the development of psychological resources for inpatients to manage distress (Mikulincer & Shaver, 2011). The psychologist allows his mentalization to inform every aspect of his role in the provision of clinical intervention, assessment, and administrative duties regarding the patient. Ideally, this mentalization becomes a mediator through which other staff members can identify and better respond to the mental states of the patient and their own reactions to the patient's behaviors. In this way, the psychologist also models other ways of more appropriately responding to their own countertransference evoked by the patient.

For the hospital to be a secure base in which the patient's symptoms are ameliorated, and level of functioning is increased, it is important that key staff at every level of patient care are able to recognize when patients evoke pathological interactions. Skilled staff can then help to defuse those interactions. One pathway that can help facilitate this process is for clinical staff to have an understanding and familiarity with mentalization theory and then incorporate it in their therapeutic interactions with the patient.

The stressful and rapid pace of the psychiatric ward often demands that decisions be made in an instant. Consistency of staff responses and provision of feedback helps to reduce patients' emotional dysregulation and patient violence (Adshead, 1998). However, such consistency in responding, either as an individual staff member or as part of a team or unit collective, is often challenging. Either the over-identification with or dismissal of patient feelings, both forms of maladaptive caring in the psychiatric setting, can evoke violence, further exacerbate symptoms (Adshead, 1998), and lead to increased anger by not addressing dependency needs (Bowlby, 1984). Occasions such as 24 hour-report, shift handovers, and incident debriefings avail the psychologist opportunities to communicate her understanding of the patient to others and help others to enhance their understandings as well. The psychologist not only models such an engagement to staff but also intervenes when situations present themselves. Interventions such as modeling/rehearsal, providing alternative explanations of the patient's behaviors when they occur, and helping staff develop skills which will enable them to more accurately assess and respond to the patients' needs are foundational.

> The treatment team, which consisted of the psychiatrist, social worker, rehabilitation therapist, substance abuse counselor, nurse, and myself conducted routine clinical rounds. A unit-based direct care staff member was also present during rounds. David would frequently try to intrude into other patients' time with the team. His negative attention-seeking behaviors persisted as he called out to the team, walked alongside the team for brief moments down the unit, and gestured me to come to meet with him. The week prior to the current rounds, David and I discussed this behavior, including how he felt when neither my, nor the team's attention were fully focused on him, and different ways that he could respond. As I expected, David put to the "test" what we reviewed in the session and my response – or lack thereof – to his behaviors. During rounds one day, there was a moment in which David diverted his attention from me and baited the direct care staff member. The staff member was in the process of walking away from the team with David when I interrupted the staff member from leaving during rounds. I discussed with the staff – in David's presence – more adaptive and developmentally-appropriate ways to communicate and maintain boundaries with him. David got angry with me and cursed the staff member for not doing what he wanted. The next week in our session, David chuckled while telling me that his behavior during rounds was a test for me. He advised me that he wanted to check to see if I was going to follow through with what we discussed. In addition, he found it amusing that other staff were so easily "spun in circles" (i.e., confused, manipulated) by him.

While the psychologist is equipped to provide in-service training and closer supervision to improve staff clinical competencies, such formal training is probably not the best use of hospital and staff resources. To add additional activities for the clinicians and staff in the inpatient setting will produce further strain on already tight schedules and job demands. Instead, Daffern, Howells, and Ogloff (2007) suggested that incorporating additional interventions and staff training into routine clinical activities such as was described above, is more timely and effective. For example, clinical encounters between staff and patients, such as during ward rounds or treatment team meetings, are timely and apt occasions for the psychologist to model and rehearse mentalization with staff. Rather than describing mentalization as an abstract concept and way of understanding patient behaviors via an in-service or staff training, "real-time" encounters increase the salience and understanding of the process more efficiently.

Staff on the inpatient unit contribute to important and discipline-specific aspects of patient care. The goal and expectation is that the various duties performed by staff will coalesce and form an integrated care approach for the patient. However, systemic barriers related to large numbers of patient loads for clinicians, and disagreements among staff compromise the efficacy of treatment interventions in general, particularly in enhancing others' abilities to utilize mentalization. The lack of consistency between staff and their responses to patients is an ongoing barrier.

Another obstacle is that the feedback and clinical suggestions that the psychologist presents may be minimized and/or dismissed. Treatment based on a medical model is often the preferred framework guiding inpatient psychiatric care. Some psychologists have felt frustrated that their knowledge and clinical suggestions are not valued and or incorporated into inpatient care (Geczy & Sultenfuss, 1994). Concerns remain around the use of psychotropic interventions as the primary way to treat illness with little to no parity given to psychological interventions (Anthony & Liberman, 1986). This tension must be addressed and considered, particularly in light of empirical findings, which suggest that the use of psychotropic medications alone is insufficient in maximizing patient functioning subsequent to community discharge (Bellack & Mueser, 1986). Arguments over the treatment of psychiatric illness in a dichotomous way either as a medical or as a psychological process are futile and distracting. Such contention, coupled with issues related to staff competence, creates divisiveness among staff.

When the psychologist's mentalization of the patient has the desired impact, it can help the patient to explore the ways in which he engages with others beyond his current psychiatric admission. Adshead (1998) suggested that the ways in which the patient thinks about his relationship to the psychiatric hospital is an important aspect of discharge planning. A regression or increase in psychiatric symptoms is not uncommon, reflecting patients' efforts to stall termination or separation from the therapy. Similar to other therapeutic relationships and encounters, the resolution of the treatment goals often signals the end of the professional relationship. However, at this juncture, the psychologist's mentalization of the patient and the clinical relationship needs to evolve in a unique way. As the patient becomes more psychiatrically stable, the expectation is that he can begin to draw on clinical encounters and healthy attachment experiences with the psychologist to develop a more integrated awareness of self in relationships inside and outside of the institution. However, for individuals who have a history of fractured and insecure attachments, the thought of intentionally ending a relationship in which there is trust and acceptance can be daunting. In a secure relationship between the caregiver and child, there is often a developmental shift in the caregiver's own mentalization of the child as the child matures toward adulthood. The dynamic changes as the caregiver is able to contain and approximate responses in light of whatever the developing child presents. This process is often continuous and lifelong. On the psychiatric unit, the interaction can and must evolve with more than one caregiver. Interventions that are focused on helping the patient feel understood and to engage with others will allow him to slowly transition through and beyond the individual therapy. Fostering nurturing relationships with other staff who are able to utilize mentalization to some degree in their interactions with the patient are essential. These relationships can help to increase the patient's commitment to his change and to safely feel connected to others.

> David and I had individual sessions twice per week for eight months. He insisted, one day before each scheduled session, that he was not sure if he would be available to meet for the session. Yet, David was always waiting promptly for my arrival to the unit to begin each session. For the last several weeks following his meeting with a housing provider, David continued to discuss his relationship with a former paramour. At the end of one of our sessions, David discussed the impact of their relational distress on his decision to engage in a particularly severe (and almost lethal) act of self-injury. David then indicated that he no longer wanted to continue our sessions. He noted how emotionally overwhelming our therapy was for him and how he was struggling with the reality that our work would terminate once he was discharged. Prior to our last session together, David was able to identify some of the ways a female clinical staff member on the unit was helping him rehearse some of the self-regulation strategies and alternatives to self-injury we identified throughout his individual therapy.

The ability to mentalize and become better attuned to one's own and others' internal feeling states is grounding. That is, an awakening occurs among many who are either oblivious to or overwhelmed by their cognitions and emotions, once their ability to form healthy interpersonal relationships improves. Some might suggest that the work that

David and I did was incomplete. I do not think that any psychologist or therapist purposefully wants to end treatment as abruptly as it initially felt between David and myself. However, perhaps one of the most seminal treatment goals and adaptive skills had already been accomplished in David's self-disclosure to me. That goal was his awareness of and responsiveness toward his own limitations and needs in our relationship. David's ability to safely communicate his feelings to me and for such an assertion to be both heard and responded to is the epitome of mentalization.

Mentalization within the therapeutic context and in its essence is truly about enhancing attachments and correcting self-perceptions. Mentalization helps the patient shift from a reactive position in relationships to one which is more assertive and less rigid. The patient is able to explore varying realities and mental states, which he was previously unable or unwilling to explore. This process is supported by the psychologist within the safety of the psychiatric unit. For many patients requiring psychiatric inpatient treatment, the opportunity and willingness to engage in such a therapeutic process in any other setting is unlikely. Mentalizing within therapeutic encounters helps the patient to explore, recognize, and shift his self-perceptions and those of others. This connection becomes the psychological space and support the patient needs in order to expand his repertoire beyond violent and aggressive behaviors as primary methods to cope with his psychic states. While the most significant benefit of mentalization is to the patient, potential benefits are felt by staff and other inpatients, and ultimately by those the patient may interact with outside of the hospital when the patient proceeds toward discharge and life outside the containing inpatient environment.

References

Adshead, G. (1998). Psychiatric staff as attachment figures: Understanding management problems in psychiatric services in light of attachment theory. *The British Journal of Psychiatry*, *172*, 64–69.

Adshead, G. (2015). Security and the social mind: Attachment and therapeutic communities. *International Journal for Therapeutic and Supportive Organizations*, *36*(1), 12–20.

Adshead, G., Moore, E., Humphrey, M., Wilson, C., & Tapp, J. (2013). The role of mentalizing in the management of violence. *Advances in Psychiatric Treatment*, *19*(1), 67–76.

Anthony, W.A. & Liberman, R.P. (1986). The practice of psychiatric rehabilitation: Historical, conceptual, and research base. *Schizophrenia Bulletin*, *12*(4), 542–549.

Bateman, A., & Fonagy, P. (2001). Treatment of borderline personality disorder with psychoanalytically oriented partial hospitalization: An 18-month follow up. *American Journal of Psychiatry*, *158*(1), 36–42.

Bellack, A.S., & Mueser, K.T. (1986). A comprehensive treatment program for schizophrenia and chronic mental illness. *Community Mental Health Journal, 22*, 175–189.

Bowlby, J. (1969). *Attachment and loss, Volume 1*. New York, NY: Basic Books.

Bowlby, J. (1984). *Attachment and loss: Attachment, Volume 1*. London: Penguin Books.

Combs, D.R., Adams, S.D., Penn, D.L., Roberts, D., Tiegreen, J., & Stem, P. (2007). Social Cognition and Interaction Training (SCIT) for inpatients with schizophrenia spectrum disorders: Preliminary findings. *Schizophrenia Research, 91*, 112–116.

Crawford, T.N., Livesley, W.J., Jang, K.L., Shaver, P.R., Cohen, P., & Ganiban, J. (2007). Insecure attachment and personality disorder: A twin study of adults. *European Journal of Personality, 21*, 191–208.

Daffern, M., Howells, K., & Ogloff, J. (2007). Interaction between individual characteristic and the function of aggression in forensic psychiatric inpatients. *Psychiatry, Psychology, and Law, 14*(1), 17–25.

Erskine, R.G. (2011). Attachment, relational needs, and psychotherapeutic presence. Keynote address at International Integrative Psychotherapy Association Conference, Vichy, France.

Fonagy, P., & Bateman, A.W. (2008). The development of borderline personality disorder: A mentalizing model. *Journal of Personality Disorder, 22*, 4–21.

Fonagy, P., Gergely, G., Jurist, E.L., & Target, M. (2002). *Affect regulation, mentalization, and the development of the self*. New York, NY: Other Press.

Fonagy, P., Leigh, T., Steele, M., Steele, H., Kennedy, R. Mattoon, G., & Gerber, A. (1996). The relation of attachment status, psychiatric classification, and response to psychotherapy. *Journal of Consulting and Clinical Psychology, 63*(1), 22–31.

Fonagy, P., & Target, M. (2000). Playing with reality III: The persistence of dual psychic reality in borderline patients. *International Journal of Psychoanalysis, 81*(5), 853–874.

Fonagy, P., & Target, M. (2008). Attachment, trauma, and psychoanalysis. In Jurist, E.L., Slade, A., & Bergner, S. (Eds.), *Mind to mind: Infant research, neuroscience, and psychoanalysis*. New York, NY: Other Press, 15–49.

Fonagy, P., Target, M., & Gergely, G. (2000). Attachment and borderline personality disorder: A theory and some evidence. *The Psychiatric Clinics of North America, 23*(1), 103–122.

Fraley, C.F. (2010). *A brief overview of adult attachment theory and research*. Chicago, IL: University of Illinois.

Geczy, B., & Sultenfuss, J.F. (1994). Contributions of psychologists to inpatient care of persons with chronic mental illness. *Hospital and Community Psychiatry, 45*(1), 54–57.

Harder, S. (2014). Attachment in schizophrenia: Implications for research, prevention, and treatment. *Schizophrenia Bulletin, 40*, 1189–1193.

Larsson, P. (2012). How important is an understanding of the client's early attachment experience to the psychodynamic practice of counseling psychology? *Counseling Psychology Review, 27*(1), 10–21.

Ma, K. (2006). Attachment theory in adult psychiatry. Part 1: Conceptualisations, measurement, and clinical research findings. *Advances in Psychiatric Treatment, 12*, 440–449.

Ma, K. (2007). Attachment theory in adult psychiatry. Part 2: Importance to the therapeutic relationship. *Advances in Psychiatric Treatment, 13*, 10–16.

MaBeth, A., Gumley, A., Schwannaeur, M., & Fisher, R. (2011). Attachment states of mind, mentalization, and their correlates in a first-episode psychosis sample. *Psychology and Psychotherapy, 84*(1), 42–57.

Mikulincer, M., & Shaver, P.R. (2011). The attachment behavioral system in adulthood: Activation, psychodynamics, and inter-personal processes. *Advances in Experimental Social Psychology, 35*, 53–152.

Mills, J. (2005). *Treating attachment pathology*. Toronto, Canada: Jason Aronson.

Nijman, H.M., aCampo, J.L., Ravelli, D.P., & Mercekelbach, H.L. (1999). A tentative model of aggression on inpatient psychiatric wards. *Psychiatric Services, 50*(8), 832–834.

Owen, I.R. (2006). *Psychotherapy and phenomenology: On Freud, Husserl, and Heidegger*. Bloomington, IN: Indiana University Press.

Rogers, C. (1959). A theory of therapy, personality and interpersonal relationships as developed in the client-centered framework. In S. Koch (Ed.), *Psychology: A study of a science, Volume 3: Formulations of the person and the social context*, pp. 184–256 . New York, NY: McGraw Hill.

Rossberg, J.I., & Friis, S. (2003). Patients and staffs' perceptions of the psychiatric ward environment. *Psychiatric Services, 55*(7), 798–803.

Talbot, N.L., Houghtalen, R.P., Duberstein, P.R., Cox, C., Giles, D.E., et al. (1999). Effects of group treatment for women with a history of childhood sexual abuse. *Psychiatric Services, 50*, 686–692.

15 The Clinical Psychologist's Work in a Forensic Psychiatry Ward

Building a Transitional Space for Individuals with Mental Disorders Who Committed Crimes

Hilik Peri[1]

Aggression, destruction, fear and danger. These are the charged, crucial words in the therapeutic work in the psychiatric hospital's forensic maximum security ward. The patients in that ward, a closed men's unit, crossed the line between fantasy and reality and acted on their raw impulses, causing harm, destruction, loss and distress in their lives and for others in their environment. Most are considered dangerous to themselves and to others, impulsive and unpredictable, with severe mental disorders. They are characterized by maladaptive personality traits, with only a loose connection to the limitations of reality and the expectations of society. These patients usually meet criteria that contra-indicate psychotherapeutic treatment: they experience the world as a dangerous and arbitrary place, and their lives are geared toward survival. They experience interpersonal relationships as harmful and disappointing, and usually have weak ego strength with rigid and maladaptive defenses. The patients, for the most part, are not psychologically minded, and their motivation for treatment is very low. Most patients have committed crimes of varying severity: threats, physical or sexual assault, or murder. Sometimes their crime involved harming a familiar person, a family member, sometimes a complete stranger. Other patients were admitted to the ward as transfer patients from other hospitals across the country, after attacking staff and patients, or after escape attempts.

The space I will describe was built in the face of violence that could not be contained within the space of everyday reality: it includes a strict set of procedures, inspections and searches, fences, cameras, mobile distress devices, and many locked doors. The descriptions presented thus far, of patient characteristics and the physical conditions that surround the staff, may evoke unrest in the reader. It is certainly difficult to imagine that under these conditions that a sensitive and empathic observation of the patient's world is possible. Many factors reduce the therapeutic space. In this treatment context, maintaining a professional stance based on recognition and belief in the existence of psychological and developmental processes tapped by creating contact and building trust in a containing and enabling relationship, is very complex. The tension among these diverse factors lies at the heart of the work of the clinical psychologist in the forensic psychiatric ward.

On the ward, there is a convergence of crime, delinquency and complex and severe mental disorders, mostly schizophrenia. It is of utmost importance to recognize the social and cultural context of this encounter. Human society has always coped with manifestations of violent, destructive and harmful behaviors of individuals. This is a complex human phenomenon, for which there are various practical responses, primarily punishment and exclusion, in an attempt to reduce and even eliminate aggression and destruction from the world, though without significant success. An individual who crosses the boundaries of the social norm and harms others often elicits anger and revulsion. Until a century ago, in most cases, no space was allotted for the subjective experience of the assailant, who embodied impulses and destructiveness that were seen as needing to be eliminated or removed. Ostensibly, the entire being of the individual was manifested in the crime he committed, and he was attributed characteristics of evil and wickedness. Through the process of splitting, the other, "the deviant" or "the sinner" embodied these impulses for the community at large. Society thus seemingly relieved itself of the need to take ownership over such content, and of the need to contain and process the impulses. Thus, it may be possible to understand how vengeful and murderous practices, such as stoning, were created.

Individuals treated in the forensic ward are viewed much in the same way as persons who committed a crime and had to be removed from society. However, here the individual is part of an additional group that is excluded from society, individuals who suffer mental illness; a multiplied complexity that further burdens society's ability to see their human needs (Kahr, 2003; Maruna, Matravers & King, 2004). It seems that the way to deter society's drive for vengeance, exclusion and harm toward those accused of harmful deeds is by creating a space. A created space allows society to delay raw emotional responses, and exchange split and partiality with an integrated and deeper understanding of the person. The forensic ward aims to create a space of this sort, in a complex institution, where the residents, both employees and patients, have unsettling emotional experiences; moving between the most primal feelings and the attempt to create a containing therapeutic space.

Sometimes, as I walk into the forensic ward, the image of the biblical "city of refuge," first mentioned in the Bible (Numbers 35, 9–12) comes to my mind, an asylum built to enable a similar type of protective space. Individuals who had killed others escaped to those cities of refuge in order to save their lives from the revenge of the families of the deceased, who would have certainly consumed the killer to death with their anger. At the entrance to the city of refuge, there was a group of "elders and wise men." This was a select group that dealt with weighty questions, gathering details and evidence and finally determining the fate of the killer. It is possible to imagine the meeting at the city gates where the killer tells his life story and the series of events that led him to seek refuge. The listeners fluctuated between identifying with the killer's painful plight, and trying to evaluate the credibility of his words, while also identifying with the pain and loss of the deceased person's family. Between compassion and rage, between belief and doubt. If the select group ruled that the killer did not intentionally kill, they would allow him to enter the city of refuge, and protect his life. I wonder if they would have been able to assess the mental fitness of the killer who was standing before them. How were they affected by harsh depictions of manslaughter and loss? Were they able to consider and give room to the various contents that arose, facing those they had to judge?

Many questions resonate in my meetings with those arriving at the forensic unit. Today, we are working toward an in-depth understanding of the internal world of the perpetrator, who for us is the patient, trying to contain a variety of insights regarding his mental state and needs, both in the evaluation and in the treatment processes. The psychological perspective allows us to observe the individual in a different way, to recognize underlying layers that do not necessarily respond to orderly, available rules of logic. The clinical psychologist is a partner in the evaluation and the diagnostic process of the individuals that enter the ward, assisting in the decision-making processes that carry great legal weight. Is the patient's place in the therapeutically oriented psychiatric ward, or alternatively, does he belong in prison, as a punishing and distancing act? Such decision-making in the ward regarding the patient's status is ongoing and continuous throughout his stay, as part of the monitoring and assessment of his mental state.

The clinical psychologist is a partner in the ward's multi-disciplinary team of mental health professionals responsible for creating a therapeutic space: psychiatrists, nurses, social workers, criminologists, and occupational therapists. The interpersonal space on the ward is a world saturated with massive projections, where raw aggression and fear are present, a world dominated by powerful unconscious schizoid-paranoid processes (Klein, 1946). At one moment, it seems that the staff are viewed by the patients as a source for consolation and nourishment, and then in an instant, can suddenly be conceived of as part of a malignant and evil system. These processes can be viewed as part of a projective identification mechanism, where negative and aggressive mental parts are split and projected toward the staff so that the team can unknowingly be activated and may respond according to the set of projections it has absorbed (Ogden, 1980). Here, one of the main roles of the clinical psychologist on the ward is to help the multi-disciplinary staff with empathic observation and processing of the various emotions in an attempt to transform the massive projections into a conscious and insightful communication.

Staff members' ongoing acquaintance with the patients on the ward and the exposure to their worlds creates close ties with the patients and does not permit a judgmental, indifferent and distant attitude. It is often possible to "forget" that a terrible act has been committed and to feel empathy for the person suffering. These fluctuations in the emotional experiences vis-a-vis the patients in the ward must be monitored and supervised, so that the split, which may be necessary to enable empathy for the patient, will not hinder the therapeutic process as well as bring potential for actual harm to the patient and staff. Such a split may reduce the level of alertness among the caregivers and expose the close and intimate therapeutic encounter to a dangerous destructiveness that has already proven to be possible. There must be a constant effort to hold the tension between these parts, between the illusion of security and real security, between excessive caution that does not permit emotional encounter, and a correct and well-measured vigilance. This requires great alertness to external and internal signs, the most intimate knowledge of body language and facial expression, quality of eye contact and more. In view of the patients' fragile mental states, close teamwork is required with regular updates regarding any change in patients' situations and an endless and complex decision-making process where security and safety concerns can take precedence over maintaining the therapeutic setting. Still, there remains an unsettling question: "can we really anticipate what will happen?" Based on our experience on the ward, despite our skills and efforts, severe cases of violence can erupt that result in serious injury to patients and staff (Minne, 2009).

The psychologist's involvement on the forensic ward has a profound and positive effect on the systemic processes encompassing the patient. Additionally, unique and central aspects of the psychologist's work here, are individual and group psychotherapeutic processes with patients. These are undertaken in an attempt to promote patients' emotional development and wellbeing and to help patients deal more effectively with life inside the ward and subsequently with the processes of rehabilitation. In the professional literature, caution is expressed regarding the ability of these patients to benefit from psychotherapeutic treatment. It seems that any therapeutic progress, such as providing space for the patient's inner world and history, raising awareness and exploring projections and identifications, as well as recognition of the act of violence and the consequences for the offender and the victim, may lead to further regression and risk. This is the defense of the maimed personality from exposure to dangerous internal links that trigger anxiety (Yakeley, 2009).

Many of the patients on the ward carry mental complexities that make it difficult for them to view psychotherapeutic treatment as a source of growth and development, as a place where a regressive process can exist and from which they can grow. We witness many patients with traumatic histories who find it difficult to build trusting relationships, a basic and necessary ingredient for forming a benign therapeutic relationship. Most of the patients on the forensic ward experience psychotic states over extended periods of time, and improvements in their conditions are partial, at best. There are those who remain in internal stormy dialogs, which the external observer experiences as meaningless. Other patients, introverted and quiet, remain unreachable. Some continue to engage in disturbed attachment patterns and relational dynamics that are intensely re-enacted with various figures on the ward. There are also patients who, in a delusional way, hold beliefs concerning a complex and intricate set of facts, details and interpretations that serve as a reality that exists alongside our reality. The latter are rigid paranoid thinkers, who eagerly absorb any hint from the environment to further tighten their complicated world and deluded reality. In the mental spaces where we meet, we can observe blurred self – other boundaries, rigid defensive structures, projective identification, control, denial, splitting and fragmentation. In psychotic transference, it is difficult to distinguish between the experience of the therapist and the patient, the container and the contained (Bion, 1962). Moreover, when there is degraded reality testing, it becomes difficult to reflect in a thoughtful and symbolic manner on the transference relations that develop in therapy.

The process of establishing a relationship with patients on the ward is a complex and significant achievement. The therapeutic relationships can vacillate between periods charged with aggression, abysmal sadness and destructive anxiety; experiences of closeness alongside distancing, detachment and indifference; connection and finding meaning together with loss of way and confusion (Kernberg, 1986). As an example of these moving experiences, I present a psychotherapeutic case that reflects aspects of the psychodynamic therapeutic encounter in the ward. The encounter described is a composite case example, in order to maintain patient confidentiality, while preserving the essence and complexity of the situation. I emphasize the process of building confidence and establishing a therapeutic relationship, describe the initial achievements of the therapeutic work and highlight the need for systemic work with the multi-disciplinary team.

D., in his 40s, has been hospitalized on the ward for over a decade following a murder that he committed. He is diagnosed with paranoid schizophrenia; his cognitive abilities are preserved and he does not exhibit any violent behavior in the ward.

In his past, D. was not known to have had any serious adjustment difficulties. He achieved some professional success at work and married in his early 30s with the understanding that it was the appropriate thing to do. The birth of his eldest son coincided with his being fired from work due to a failed project there. For the first time, D. found himself without a clear and holding framework. During the first months of his son's life, D. turned to various clinics seeking help. He asked for someone to calm the baby's incessant crying and unrest. He distanced his spouse from caring for the child, as well as other members of the extended family. Various doctors examined the baby and dismissed D. by saying that the child was healthy. One physician referred D. to a psychiatrist, who recognized D.'s high level of anxiety but attributed it to his transition to fatherhood. D. relentlessly continued to investigate and inquire and turned to doctors throughout the country. Slowly but surely he developed a delusional understanding that there was an attempt at a "cover-up." He understood that various elements accused him of failure of the project at work and believed they had decided to take revenge on him through his son. In this way, he was being persecuted by them. Why are the answers always the same? Why is no one prepared to write a letter to ensure the safety and welfare of his child? How did they harm his son? D. approached his former workplace, sent angry letters in an attempt to get some type of clue, and turned to various government agencies. He began to feel that all of the doors were closing and that he needed to do something drastic, to shock the system and create an opening. D. came to the emergency room with his son, this time equipped with a lethal weapon. When again he was faced with what he experienced as a wall, he violently attacked and critically injured a nurse who later died from her wounds. A security guard, who rushed to the scene, rescued his son.

On the ward, he tended to stay away from the rest of the patients, looking at them with a perplexed and perhaps even a patronizing look. During the ward community groups, he covered his eyes with his hands and refused to participate. He usually kept himself busy with reading; his senses were sharp, and he kept up to date with current events. He considered himself the focus of the activity in the ward, and that all the others served different purposes in some scheme concerning his hospitalization: simple workers who followed instructions from state agencies to keep him out of the public eye so as not to expose the complicit array of ties and interests built around him.

During our first session, D. clarified that he did not want to find himself "treading water" in discussions about the "incident" and focused his counseling needs on how he could see his son again, despite the objections of his spouse and her parents. D. emotionally described his relationship with his son, during the first months of his life, and it was evident that the loss of contact with him caused great distress. However, before the meeting ended, D. regained composure, and made it clear that he was not interested in a prolonged treatment, but rather wanted only a few sessions. I experienced a sharp transition between empathy for the distress that came forth in his story and his creation of emotional distance; his regaining control and of being in charge. The dramatic transition challenged my ability to organize my thoughts and find an integrative place within myself, and in facing D. I managed to find a flexible and enabling position that would also help coordinate expectations for the future: I reflected his distress and difficulties as expressed thus far, and the need for treatment and guidance in the process of coping with the distance from his son. In parallel, I emphasized that our therapeutic work was a process and that in order to contribute and promote the process it must be done with his cooperation and through his willingness to understand himself.

"We are at the start of a process, and questions naturally arise: where are we going? Who is leading? Is it possible to choose to stop?"

During this stage of our work, we held weekly sessions for approximately a year. Early sessions consisted largely of descriptions of his attempts to renew a relationship with his son, and his concern for his son's welfare. After about four months, descriptions of the murder, and the delusional system intertwined with it, began to appear: his experiences with all the institutions that imprisoned and persecuted him and did not allow him the freedom to get on with his life. D. described his various attempts to continue to struggle with his inner truth, truth that made it difficult for him to appear before the psychiatric committee and to tell them what he knew was the right thing to say: "I am ill, my son is not sick, now I am taking medication, and I am stable." This struggle became the center of his life. It seemed he was trapped within the story he spun for himself. Without the narrative he had created, his son's difficulties seemed meaningless and the murder of the nurse irrelevant. I revealed deep empathy for the processes that D. described. Through his descriptions, I was able to see quite clearly something of the reality that he experienced. In those moments, I could imagine the anxiety that gripped him as he saw his son, who according to his interpretation, was destined to die in agony. From that observation, I could appreciate, in a way that I did not expect prior to the therapeutic process, his fatherly devotion to his son, and I told him in our session that it was understandable that he was under significant pressure, was worried, anxious and felt helpless. From D.'s reaction, it seemed that he was quite surprised, and a bit shaken. Possibly, because the humane dimension of his worry during that period found its place; seeing not only the monstrous and cruel aspects of his murderous behavior, but as distorted as it was, the aspects of a person who found himself in a distress that he could not contain.

At this point in the therapy, D. raised many questions in an attempt to place me in the complicated system of his world: am I a psychologist from the Ministry of Health, or from some other organization? What was I sent to clarify and to reveal about him? Many questions fraught with anxiety and suspicion colored the process of creating a relationship and building the foundation for treatment. Alongside these, other expressions surfaced: "I am sure that you believe me, I see it in your eyes, but you are forbidden to say that out loud because you are part of the system." D. looked at me piercingly, and tried to extract hidden information from my verbal and especially non-verbal reactions. Every nod of the head became saturated with meaning for him, and I became aware of even my slightest movements. Quickly, it seemed that on whichever side D. tried to place me I felt bound, and with no way out. I felt my anxiety rising, and I became alert and vigilant. These intense transference and countertransference processes emerged as I found myself becoming a container for D.'s internal experiences.

The quality of the relationship, in the intensity and the clarity with which one can feel the emotional experiences of the other, characterize psychotic transference phenomena. At that early stage, it was not yet possible to turn them into an object for contemplation and processing within the therapeutic encounter.

D. asked me in a straightforward manner what I thought about the events that he described to me, and I made sure to acknowledge the emotional experience that could be identified in his narrative, without expressing a position that could be considered judgmental. I emphasized the transition to parenthood as a charged and sensitive period. The loneliness that he experienced at that time, the lack of significant sources of support and the distress he encountered and felt trapped in, like a whirlpool. During those weeks, my conduct outside of the therapy room began to occupy D.'s attention, and he said that he noticed that I spoke to the ward head after one of our sessions. He was convinced that the conversation was about him and asked what messages about him were being relayed by me to other staff members. D. tried to figure out my position in relation to him and his world as if I were a foreign body that penetrated his complex system and whose activities and intentions needed to be mapped. What course was I taking? What forces influenced me? To whom was I loyal?

I will take a short break in the description of D.'s treatment in order to describe parallel processes that occurred with the staff, parallel to the psychotherapeutic treatment processes.

Opportunities to meet with patients in the ward vary and each staff member of the multi-disciplinary team has a different and significant perspective from which s/he can examine the patient's mental state and behavior, and contribute to the integrated assessment and treatment of the patient. The clinical psychologist's unique contribution lies in the ability to be in the transitional space formed between his role as a staff member involved in the ward's systemic processes of ongoing evaluation of the patient, and his role as psychotherapist, who allows his patient a personal space for emotional development based on constancy and continuity, together with containment and acceptance (Hinshelwood, 1986).

I find that as I begin individual therapy with a patient, I can bring his voice in a rich and unique way to the multi-disciplinary discussions. That voice enables the staff to further process their understanding and containment of the patient, a process that takes place in an informal manner and without necessarily being publicized as such. At times my role on the ward is to assist in managing a crisis, or aid with development and change; mostly, to assist the team in assessing processes as being transient and passing or rather stable and with continuity. It is quite conceivable that split off aspects of a patient's self-experience, a patient that I feel that I know well, are held by other staff members while I remain blind to them. Conversely, it can be difficult for staff to encounter aspects of the patient that are not revealed outside of the intimate therapeutic relationship.

Returning to D., to a great extent, his observations were accurate. I discussed his therapeutic process with ward staff members many times. However, I did so with utmost sensitivity to the content revealed, and for the importance of the patient continuing to feel that the therapeutic space remained safe and secure. For example, I would not reveal personal experiences and life events described by patients in sessions unnecessarily. However, I have on occasion informed staff members of a patient that held a dangerous grudge toward one of them, or of a dangerous conflict that was developing between patients. The therapeutic contract is clear to the patients from the start of our relationship, and I see such disclosures when made by the patient as a request for protection from further harm. In such cases, I am strict about transparency and find a way to accompany the patient to a position where he can be given more space for his words in facing the staff with his disclosure. In D.'s case, I began presenting the staff with specific aspects of D.'s experience of the loss and guilt with which he was coping, which was the basis for his seeking treatment. And I also gave voice to his ongoing distress in the ward, for over a decade after the murder. I helped the staff understand his experience, including his feeling as though he was not actually a patient on the ward and that he did not consider the various staff members as professional authority figures. That understanding gave rise to a great deal of empathy.

Six months after the beginning of therapy, the staff began reporting updates regarding the softening of D.'s relationship to other patients as well as staff. D. began to show interest and to participate in the ward group meetings, and his compliance with ward routine improved. It was difficult to pinpoint clear objective signs; however, the softened facial expression, eye contact, choice of words, his new way of physically positioning himself in the ward space, sufficed to indicate that a process of change was developing. I was left with questions: does he sense that there is hope that someone will understand? Is the staff undergoing a process that allows for new observations of D. and his needs? Apparently, all of the possibilities were embodied in the new developing space.

Unlike with my other patients, where communication with the staff was a clear and comfortable task for me, here with D. it was most complicated. His inquisitive questions preoccupied me, and I often felt that he was watching me intently. I noticed that I was making an effort not to have discussions with staff members within range of his vision, and my awareness of his whereabouts increased. I found myself carefully choosing my words, making sure not to reveal details or traces of issues that arose in our meetings, concerned that other staff members might then inadvertently mention in their communications with him.

Through my own supervision, I was able to understand my strong countertransference reaction to D.'s emotional experiences in his therapeutic relationship with me. I felt a tense suspension, if not a truly paranoid experience. Contrary to D., who found himself trapped in that experience for many years, for me there was great relief as I became able to observe and process my emotional experiences and to dissolve the anxiety that I had in facing him. The question of trust became a central and fragile issue. On realizing this, I was able to more correctly identify how to maintain a balance between my position as D.'s psychotherapist and my position vis-a-vis the ward staff, in my attempt to promote various systemic processes relevant for his progress.

I often found myself speechless, facing challenges that D. posed to me in our sessions, as he presented to me indisputable "facts," describing how random sentences that he collected from staff members in the past and present connected to form additional support for his tragic delusional story.

My answers remained vague, addressing only his subjective experience: "I see how important it is for you ...," "a lot of details that you connect create order ..." D. found it difficult to accept my struggles to preserve an emotionally empathic dialog in the therapy room and made great effort to control the direction of the reality in which his absolute truth validated and upheld his own perceptions (Searles, 1967).

At the end of a year of therapeutic work, D. informed me that the therapy was not progressing, that the sessions were repetitive and that he had nothing more to share. He asked to end our work together at that same meeting. His statement from our first session, in which he asked to limit the sessions between us echoed in me, and I tried to think of the meaning of his attempt to interrupt the process of creating a relationship between us that had progressed slowly but positively and meaningfully. Despite my attempts to create a space where it would be possible to bring up issues of separation and distancing, D. was decisive and asked me to sum up: "can you summarize for me in a few words what we talked about in our sessions?" I felt confused, shocked and even under attack. I found myself making an effort to organize my thoughts, a familiar experience during therapeutic sessions with this patient, forever creating a disturbing and disorienting experience in our relationship.

I described to him three layers of our work together: first, the processing of the distance from his son; second, the murder and the internal strengths that lead him to continue fighting for his inner truth; and third, the subject of trust built between us.

An unexpected separation, murder of soft and dependent parts that began to germinate ... A sudden ending that reflected the world of D. and of others in the forensic ward, a world full of disruptions, traumas, disappointments and pain without anyone to contain and process (Gallwey, 1996).

In the tension between voluntary and compulsory treatment, there is a moment in which the ward staff discusses the implications of the patient's request to end the treatment and the different possible modes of response. A space is created in which to discuss the patient's needs. A response is formulated by the team and provided to the patient concerning his choice to terminate and its implications. Sometimes there is understanding and empathy for the patient's request; other times a statement is provided to help the patient understand his stage in therapy in an attempt to return him to the therapeutic process. In this case, and after a multi-disciplinary team discussion, we responded to D. with an integrative message that commended his original request for therapy and his ability to be helped and make a change as experienced in the ward, alongside encouragement that in due course he would find a way to return to therapy.

The therapeutic work on the ward does not end with the cessation of individual therapy, and my relationship with D. continued from a slight distance. I noticed various changes in his behavior; responsiveness to the staff, his relationships with new patients on the unit, and even through my other patients' depictions of him, as a part of their life in the ward. On D.'s side as well, one could feel that he was eager to maintain contact; he greeted me happily when I came into the ward, and referred to me when he made comments about new patients in the ward. I was left with the feeling, perhaps hope, that eventually we would return to our work together.

About six months later, D. reached out to me for therapy, and after consulting with the multi-disciplinary staff, we resumed our sessions.

D. opened our first session with a request to help him deal with the psychiatric committee, which he appears before once every six months. The psychiatric committee is what stands between the patients and long-awaited leave. The committee's decision whether to continue a patient's involuntary hospitalization or allow a discharge process gives rise to many hopes for the patients, as well as much tension and suspicion. For D., over the years, the committee has come to represent that same system with which he has been struggling for years.

D. asked me to go over all of the summaries of the committees that examined him throughout the years so that I could try to help him understand the reasons for his failures to get leave thus far. This was a very concrete request and made me think that I was being exploited and used as an object to fulfill realistic wishes. Was this part of a plan that D. devised, in which I was an actor? In response to my moment of silence, D. asked: "what do you say?" I imagined myself coming to our session carrying his thick personal file, reading together the protocols of the various Committees, and I was appalled. What was he asking? That I should join him in a manipulative attempt to formulate sentences more "correctly"? A more sophisticated appearance before the persecutory system? How dangerous is this to the therapeutic alliance developed here, as I walk along a very narrow path?

"I am trying to understand what you are asking; indeed, all of the protocols are open to you." Here, suddenly, other needs arose, and D. began to painfully describe the high price he was paying for his long stay in the ward. "I want to meet someone and live with her; my family ... everyone is busy with his own issues, I have no place to return to, and soon there won't even be a chance." These words helped me look more empathically at D.'s request, and I saw before me a middle-aged man, stuck in the ward and in his inner world, asking to be in other places, building a life, a life that was totally destroyed. I made a place for this human experience within me and again by that felt that I regained my ability to sustain our threatened therapeutic transitional space (Winnicott, 1971). I suggested that I take time until our next session to think about how to respond to his request.

This is the place to stress how important support and supervision for the therapist are at these moments. In supervision, I could make a place for the many thoughts that flooded me during the meeting with D. I found that consultation with the ward staff helped me find the correct way to concretely bring in such external material into the session with D., without creating splits. The shared thinking with the staff helped me find in such a joint review with D. of the committee summaries, an opportunity for integration, for completing the picture and not for splitting it. Together with the ward head, we decided that the committee's experience, as it emerges from these written summaries, would be brought up and discussed with D.

I reviewed the various protocols. Committees in which D. appeared agitated and enraged. Throwing accusations at the committee members, seeing them as "part of the system," that they had "no mandate to judge him and the day will come when they will pay the heavy price together with many others." In other committees, he appeared reserved and organized, described the process he went through during hospitalization to understand his mental disorder and revealed insight into the deadly act he committed and expressed grief and remorse. D. swayed from extreme to extreme, and held on to a series of details that in a delusional manner became facts, that bound together and changed his life, refusing to let go and move on. The various committees saw him as manipulative and dangerous with no substantive change in his inner world.

I returned to the session with D.:

> I read the various protocols. I think that in general, it can be seen that there is a struggle for truth, your inner truth, and within the clashes with the committee you find yourself frustrated, again and again continuing long-term hospitalization with no progress. The committee experiences you as dangerous and often manipulative.

D. smiled:

> What do you think, that I would give them what they want? They'll give me two hours leave, and six months later increase it to four hours, I won't give them that pleasure, do you know how old I will be when I get out at that rate?

I continue: "it is indeed very long and not simple for you. However I see that there were also times that you tried to convey a different message, and to progress according to their rules." D. remained silent, and I added:

> It is not simple, on the one hand, you ask to return to be part of the life that goes on outside, on the other hand is your desire to maintain your truth, even to "show them" and to take revenge.

In response, D. began to describe a complex story full of intricate connections between various role figures in the public service. He told of letters that he wrote over the years, for which he never received satisfactory answers. Over the years, he accumulated a heavy burden and a strong will to reach the long-awaited moment when the truth would finally be revealed, the moment when he would triumphantly leave the ward. Being discharged and free was not enough; he had to leave a significant public mark.

Three months after the beginning of our second round of therapy, as his trust in our relationship grew stronger, he was able to share with me that he was continuing to devise various plans: plans to activate various agencies so that they would intervene and tip the scales in his favor.

While in our first round of therapy we dealt with D.'s relationship with his son and getting to know his history and the story of the murder, in this second period in his therapy, as his experience of trust deepened, we dealt with his missed life together with strong feelings of insult and humiliation, as well as with his desire to overcome the system and take revenge.

In our work together, in addition to bringing emotionally distressful content, familiar and part of human experience such as loss and a missed life, D. also brought a complex delusional system of beliefs. This polarization weighed heavily on the therapeutic relationship and on my emotional position as therapist.

At that stage, I tried to examine with D. ways to extend his emotional experience and allow an intermediate area, beyond swinging between feelings of either victory or defeat, either illness or health. I realized that in order for D. to develop empathy toward himself, he should be able to experience himself and his needs in a more complex manner. He needed to become empathic to the one who murdered, and be able to have moments of rest and quiet in his life; perhaps even rehabilitate what remained of his life. D. responded to that and shared: "you know, lately I began thinking about the family of the nurse that I killed … If there is something that I regret it is what happened to her." D. re-examined the dense and difficult event. The core of his beliefs did not change, but there were new additional feelings of authentic guilt, pain and remorse. Non-psychotic areas emerged during therapeutic encounters that allowed for emotional connections and growth.

In our therapy sessions, issues of the Committee and ways to progress in them receded, and more content appeared that related to the previous life that he had, to the person he once was, to achievements in his past life and to who he has become now, and has been for many years. A session that took place at that time became the epitome of our work in that period and the peak that heralded the end of that chapter. D. entered the session and commented that the patient who was in the session before him looked weak and poor: "it is hard to come in here after a person like that." A passing comment that signified for me an additional layer of D.'s ability to observe himself and the environment in which he lives, as well as recognition of me and my role in the ward.

> Lately you share with me the pain you feel and the difficulty of seeing the gap between who you were in the past, and your life today. To be part of this place is not an easy experience. Who are the people around me? Why are they here? Why me? A lot of questions.

D. remained confused and grasped the explanation that this was the most difficult place in the country, a place "that they knew that nobody would be able to find me." It suddenly occurred to me that carefully hiding his face in his hands during ward community groups was his way to avoid seeing his reflection mirrored back to him from his fellow patients. Being part of the community of patients was associated with pain and feelings that were hard for him to accept and contain.

In the next sessions, D was once again somewhat remote and reserved. He returned to talk about "treading water" and the repetition in the sessions and asked to terminate them. I again found myself holding the therapeutic process, describing to him the process of developing the relationship. However, for him, closeness and trust exposed pain and many losses, more than he could bear. This time I asked to allow for farewell sessions, three such sessions in which we could reflect on our work of the past eight months. The meanings reached, the trust that was built and how such developments were significant and not to be taken for granted. This time, D was able to touch on his experience of our sessions together:

> You know, Hilik, it does not really matter to me now whether you are from the Ministry of Health or from the police; your questions were those of a psychologist that is for sure. It was interesting talking to you. I am sure we will meet again.

This time as well, facing the second interruption in therapy, I remained with various thoughts regarding the achievements accomplished during the process. I am comforted by the fact that I am here, available for him; and if not me, then other therapists can find their way to meet D. in a transitional space. A space that will allow him to continue the process of building trust in another, in steps carefully taken, saturated with pain and sometimes with dread, but that will allow him change, development and creation of new connections, as he did during his therapy with me.

I also draw comfort from knowing that I will continue to support and help the ward staff see him in a fuller and more rounded way, and by that continue to be there for him as a benign therapeutic figure.

Summary

In writing this chapter, I tried to provide the reader with an as-near-as possible experience of the complexity felt when working as a clinical psychologist in a forensic maximum security ward. Behind the fences and the security precautions, there is a world rich with turbulent and volatile emotions, a world I sought to describe as found on the continuum of human experience. This "city of refuge" is a place of shelter for people with mental disorders that other inpatient units nationwide cannot contain, either owing to high risk or because of violent crimes committed by those that reside there. Here, these patients are protected from complex incarceration in prisons and are under the care of multi-disciplinary staff who seek to provide care and aid.

This safe space assumes different meanings when viewed through the patients' eyes. Often, they experience this space as being limiting and restricting. They find it difficult to build trust in clinical staff and find it hard to commit themselves to therapeutic processes whose aims are development and change. Most of the patients describe life histories riddled with trauma and distress, alongside serious difficulties in their judgment and with their insight into the complex relations present in the realities of their lives.

Throughout the therapeutic work in the forensic unit, we come across tensions that should not be settled, but rather recognized and acknowledged as such: whether the space is a safe and secure refuge or a closed and restrictive place; between seeing the team as supportive, containing and enabling development, or as rigid, reductive and employing coercive force; between a therapeutic position of empathy and sensitivity, to that of examining and assessing dangerous behaviors. All these create splits that correspond well with the mental complexities of the patients on the forensic ward. These polarities challenge our attempts to build a transitional space for the development of significant therapeutic processes, at times making it feel impossible.

I emphasized throughout the chapter, the importance of supervision processes and professional support that takes place within and without the ward. These supports help those of us who work in complex systems of pressure, to identify difficult feelings that reverberate within them: anxiety, persecution, aggression, anger and helplessness. Identification, holding, and containment of these feelings are crucial in order to enable teamwork in the ward and attain the best possible therapeutic work.

Entering the forensic ward, that isolated complex space I have tried to describe throughout this chapter, is accompanied by a sense of disconnectedness. Writing this chapter has enabled me to further emotionally process and share experiences that are oftentimes difficult to imagine as able to be shared.

Acknowledgment

I would like to thank Ms. Naomi Schwartz, the retired Head Psychologist of Sha'ar Menashe Mental Health Center, who accepted me for the position and guided me through important years of professional growth and development. Thank you for your understanding, acceptance, wisdom, and warmth.

Note

1 Translated from Hebrew by Mrs. Rena Kurs

References

Bion, W. R. (1962). A theory of thinking. *International Journal of Psycho-Analysis, 43*, 306–310.

Gallwey, P. (1996). Psychotic and borderline processes. In C. Cordess & M. Cox (Eds.). *Forensic psychotherapy: Crime, psychodynamic and the offender patient* (pp. 153–174). London: Jessica Kingsley.

Hinshelwood, R. D. (1986). The psychotherapist's role in a large institution. *Psychoanalytic Psychotherapy, 2* (3), 207–215.

Kahr, B. (2003). Series foreword. In R. Doctor (Ed.). *Forensic psychotherapy monograph series. Dangerous patients: A psychodynamic approach to risk assessment and management* (pp. vii–x). London: Karnac.

Kernberg, O. F. (1986). Identification and its vicissitudes as observed in psychosis. *International Journal of Psychoanalysis, 67*, 147–158.

Klein, M. (1946). Notes on some schizoid mechanisms. In M. Klein (Ed.). *Envy and gratitude and other works 1946–1963* (pp. 1–24). London: Hogarth.

Maruna, S., Matravers, A. & King, A. (2004). Disowning our shadow: A psychoanalytic approach to understanding punitive public attitudes. *Deviant Behavior, 25*, 277–299.

Minne, C. (2009). The dreaded and dreading patient and therapist. In J. Gordon & G. Kirtchuk (Eds.). *Psychic assault and frightened clinicians* (pp. 27–40). London: Karnac.

Ogden, T. (1980). On the nature of the schizophrenic conflict. *International Journal of Psychoanalysis, 61*, 513–533.

Searles, H. F. (1967). The schizophrenic individual's experience of his world. *Psychiatry, 30*, 119–130.

Winnicott, D. W. (1971). *Playing and reality*. London: Routledge.

Yakeley, J. (2009). Individual psychoanalytic psychotherapy for violent patients. In J. Yakeley (Ed.). *Working with violence. Basic texts in counselling and psychotherapy* (pp. 127–149, Chapter 9). New York, NY: Palgrave MacMillan.

Part 3

Assessment and Psychodiagnosis in Mental Health Inpatient Settings

Introduction to Part 3

Michael Siglag and Meidan Turel

Psychological assessment and psychodiagnostic investigation are central to psychologists' work, particularly in mental health inpatient settings. This has been the case for decades and is likely to continue to be true for the foreseeable future. During the early and mid-twentieth century, international pioneers in psychology and various medical specialties initiated development of numerous measures of cognitive and psychological functioning. Numerous assessment tools were developed in order to evaluate, quantify, and better understand the workings and complexities of the human mind. These tests were initially used for a variety of purposes in a range of settings, including measurement and screening in educational, military, and immigration settings. Over time, versions of many of these measures have become important tools, which are commonly utilized in inpatient and other mental health settings.

Many psychologists, along with close associates from medical and other fields, created measures that have become important for assessment in inpatient mental health treatment settings. Among those whose early work led to the development of measures that are used in assessment work today are: Romanian-American psychologist David Wechsler (developer of the Wechsler intelligence tests) (Wechsler, 1939), Swiss psychiatrist and psychoanalyst Hermann Rorschach (developer of the Rorschach Inkblot Test) (Rorschach, 1924), American psychiatrist Henry Murray (along with Christiana Morgan, developer of the Thematic Apperception Test or TAT) (Morgan & Murray, 1935) and American clinical psychologist Starke R. Hathaway and neuropsychiatrist J. Charnley McKinley (developers of the original Minnesota Multiphasic Personality Inventory or MMPI) (Hathaway & McKinley, 1940). American ego-psychologists Rapaport, Gill, and Schafer (1946) introduced a classic battery of tests that has been the model for personality and cognitive assessment for many psychologists working in mental health inpatient settings. These and other assessment pioneers have played significant roles in shaping modern psychodiagnostic, cognitive, intellectual, and personality assessment. Current versions of the assessment tools noted here are utilized by the psychologists whose work is described in the chapters of this part of the current volume.

Psychological assessment approaches initiated by these assessment pioneers continue to evolve and remain relevant and applicable today in mental health inpatient settings. Efforts to establish and refine measures of cognitive and psychological functioning have continued through the present, but psychologists have shown the greatest sustained interest in this process; i.e., it is primarily psychologists who have continued to carry out formal psychological and psychodiagnostic testing in various settings, particularly in mental health inpatient settings.

Modern psychologists often seek to understand cognitive and personality issues of those they test, just as their predecessors did. However, assessment questions asked now are often more targeted than those previously asked. In addition, today, psychologists have access to a wider array of assessment tools than their predecessors. Psychologists are trained to use more evolved methodology and better normed and researched measures than the tests developed by the pioneers of psychological measurement. In addition to broad measures of intellectual functioning such as the original and revised versions of the WAIS (Wechsler Adult Intelligence Scale), and measures of personality functioning such as the MMPI, Personality Assessment Inventory (PAI), and Rorschach Inkblot Test, numerous specific tests have been developed to assess more targeted questions about issues such as depression, posttraumatic stress, anxiety, dissociation, and many other dimensions of individuals' personality and psychological functioning.

Psychologists have contributed to the development and application of increasing numbers of measures designed to answer questions relevant to high-risk behaviors such as self-harm and suicide. Some aspects of testing have become particularly specialized, requiring training in particular measures and bodies of knowledge. For example, neuropsychological testing, a specialty with its own pioneers and unique measures, has increasingly evolved to access and evaluate interactions between the workings of the human brain, and cognitive and psychological manifestations of neurological functioning and disturbance.

Psychological assessment is a multistage and multidimensional process. The first stage of the assessment process typically involves consideration of referral questions, followed by test selection. Psychologists frequently consider an array of available measures that pertain to the particular questions about the patient they seek to understand. They have opportunities to choose relevant and specific measures most applicable to their questions. While many psychologists also perform thorough and comprehensive test batteries in order to carry out in-depth personality assessments, it has become common for psychologists to perform more focused assessments in response to specific referral questions, and to provide screening evaluations using targeted assessment tools that are designed to provide information about specific aspects of functioning. Important components of many psychologists' assessments include collateral information provided through observations and assessments undertaken by other professionals, relevant historical information about the patient, and comparisons with past testing when available, in addition to test results specific to the psychological evaluation.

In modern psychological work, certain types of questions beyond the scope of personality and cognitive functioning have become common. For example, as a result of the increasing interface between the legal and mental health systems, many psychologists address questions with psychological and behavioral dimensions such as violence and legal culpability. These type of questions are increasingly posed in both civil and forensic mental health treatment settings and frequently relate specifically to legal competency, violence risk, sexual violence risk, and malingering.

In psychological and psychodiagnostic reports, psychologists typically include a description of the results of assessment measures that were administered, the psychologist's interpretations of these results, conclusions pertaining to referral questions, and recommendations relevant to those conclusions. Psychologists base their conclusions upon a number of factors, in addition to their direct interactions with the individual being evaluated, and results of assessment measures performed. Recommendations may relate to safety issues, treatment, or other specific questions, such as sources of anxiety, degrees of depression, and internal strengths and resiliencies. While feedback is not built into the assessment process in all settings, to the extent possible, the sharing of assessment results, implications, and recommendations with the individual who participated in the evaluation is an important dimension of the assessment process. Such a step is incorporated into psychologists' ethical codes in many countries, including the American Psychological Association's ethical guidelines (American Psychological Association, 2017). The chapters in this part of the book provide a window into this process. The authors of each chapter describe the increasing recognition of the importance of psychologists' efforts to engage the individual being evaluated in the feedback and discussion process, in some instances indicating how feedback may impact treatment in profound ways.

This part of the current volume includes three chapters highlighting psychological assessment and psychodiagnostic work in mental health inpatient settings. The psychologists authoring these chapters describe efforts they made, through psychological testing, to increase their own and their treatment teams' understanding of hospitalized individuals.

Their explicit aims centered around the goal to help guide therapists' and teams' treatment.

The assessments described in the chapters here all fall within the long-standing tradition carrying out extensive test batteries in order to develop a comprehensive understanding of the individual being assessed. However, other dimensions of testing are also evident in these chapters. These include incorporation of measures to evaluate specific aspects of functioning, sensitivity to self-understanding and motivation of the patients being assessed, and utilization of psychological testing to influence and strengthen therapeutic interactions. The degree to which the three chapters incorporate these dimensions of assessment and the specific perspectives and approaches of their authors differ, in ways that will be described below. Despite the apparent differences in approaches and settings, though, the chapters are all representative of psychological assessment grounded in traditional psychodiagnostic models that can be used by the psychologist in current contexts and in support of varying treatment paradigms.

In the first of these chapters (Chapter 16), Biedermann, Ridenour, and Biel describe psychological assessment as carried out in a well-established private mental health inpatient treatment center in the United States, the Austen Riggs Center (ARC) in Stockbridge, Massachusetts. Psychologists at the ARC apply an assessment model developed under the leadership of some of the most highly regarded clinicians of the twentieth century, a model that continues to be practiced and valued through the present time. The work described here by the authors provides a window into a tradition in which psychoanalytic thinking shapes the primary model for both treatment and assessment in the inpatient setting. Thorough psychodiagnostic batteries are routinely carried out at the ARC as a central component of the clinical assessment and treatment process. Through the use of case examples, the authors provide compelling support for the value such assessment brings to the treatment endeavor.

In the next chapter (Chapter 17), psychologist Paul Saks describes testing and treatment in a very different inpatient setting, a state psychiatric hospital. Paul provides an account of his work in this setting, in which he engages a female patient in an extensive psychological assessment. He describes the important and significant influences the assessment process had on her treatment. Paul describes his use of psychodiagnostic tools to clarify and distinguish between psychosis and other severe mental states. He highlights the crucial function and treatment implications psychological testing can have when making nuanced diagnostic decisions while engaging in efforts to understand subtle and complex mental states. The reader is provoked by this chapter to consider the impact of the assessment process on a hospitalized individual in the midst of severe emotional and psychological distress and illuminates the potential for psychological assessment to assist in the process of healing and integration.

In the third chapter in this part of the book (Chapter 18), authors Shweta Sharma and Patricia Daza detail their approach to assessment at the Menninger Clinic, a private mental health inpatient facility based in Houston, Texas, with a long-standing tradition dating to the 1940s, which the authors describe as 'dynamic, collaborative, multidisciplinary, and person-centered.' The authors view a multifaceted approach to psychological testing as contributing to understanding the 'complexity of the whole person,' and see an important aspect of the assessment process as enhancing the patient's self-knowledge and mentalization. The approach highlighted in this chapter emphasizes efforts through assessment to also deepen the engagement of the patient as an active participant in the process of self-understanding. Through case examples, the authors portray how this patient-centered approach, along with increased understanding conveyed to therapists and other treatment team members, can help enhance therapeutic alliances and contribute to a more individualized, focused, and effective treatment process.

The three chapters in this part of the book examine the basic core of psychological assessment. In each of the chapters, authors describe their efforts to better understand patients' internal worlds and their behaviors and interpersonal interactions. Each psychologist considers a variety of factors including the patients' cognitive functioning, motivations, and psychological patterns, as well as the psychologists' diagnostic impressions or understanding. Psychological assessment measures, honed over years of use and refined by generations of psychologists, are used toward this end. To varying degrees, these authors, as is currently common for psychologists in general, take the process further. Specifically, engagement of the individual being assessed in the process of enhancing self-knowledge is understood by each of the authors here as an important, and perhaps a primary component of assessment. The current approach to assessment, articulated in psychologists' professional guidelines, supports psychologists shift from an approach to assessment as a passive process, with the assessor obtaining knowledge that may or may not be shared with the patient or individual participating in the assessment. The importance of engagement of the patient in the process and the patient's relationship with the assessor are increasingly being recognized as important to the assessment process. Utilization of assessment to enhance self-knowledge, educate team members and other therapeutic staff participating in treatment, and using assessment results to actively improve the focus and relevance of treatment efforts are described in these chapters as central goals of psychological assessment.

References

American Psychological Association. (2017). *Ethical Principles of Psychologists and Code of Conduct*. Adopted August 21, 2002. Effective June 1, 2003 (with the 2010 amendments to Introduction and Applicability and Standards 1.02 and 1.03 effective June 1, 2010). With the 2016 Amendment to Standard 3.04 adopted August 3, 2016. Effective January 1, 2017. Retrieved from: www.apa.org/ethics/code/ethics-code-2017.pdf

Hathaway, S. R., & McKinley, J. C. (1940). A multiphasic personality schedule (Minnesota): Construction of the schedule. *Journal of Psychology, 10*, 249–254.

Morgan, C. D., & Murray, H. A. (1935). A method for investigating fantasies: The thematic apperception test. *Archives of Neurology & Psychiatry, 34*, 289.

Rapaport, D., Gill, M., & Schafer, R. (1946). *Diagnostic psychological testing: The theory, statistical evaluation, and diagnostic application of a battery of tests: Vol. 2*. Chicago, IL: The Year Book Publishers.

Rorschach, H. (1924). *Manual for Rorschach Ink-blot Test*. Chicago, IL: Stoelting.

Wechsler, D. (1939). *The measurement of adult intelligence*. Baltimore, MD: Williams & Wilkins.

16 Psychodynamic Psychological Testing in the Mental Health Inpatient Setting

A Way of Listening, Learning, and Holding Patients and Psychotherapists

Christina Biedermann, Jeremy Ridenour, and Spencer E. Biel

In this chapter, we will illustrate the model of psychodynamic psychological testing at the Austen Riggs Center (ARC), a small, private, nonprofit psychiatric hospital in Stockbridge, Massachusetts, USA. The ARC specializes in the care of people with complex psychiatric problems who are often labeled treatment resistant in the broader psychiatric literature. Patients are referred from all over the world – from outpatient psychotherapists, college counseling centers, residential treatment centers, and other psychiatric hospitals. From a diagnostic perspective, most patients are struggling with complex, comorbid psychiatric diagnoses that have proven treatment refractory, often including personality pathology and sometimes psychosis. Approximately two-thirds of patients have histories of early deprivation, loss, and abuse, and approximately half struggle with substance abuse. Most have been hospitalized at least once and have had multiple episodes of self-destructive behavior; approximately half have made serious suicide attempts over the course of their lifetimes (Plakun, 2003).

The ARC encompasses a continuum of care organized to address different developmental learning needs. Whereas patients are initially admitted to the most intensive, hospital level of care, they can step down to programs focused on developing independent living skills, returning to school or work, or establishing more fulfilling interpersonal relationships. However, a core value runs through these levels of care, the commitment to an open setting. While there are many features comparable to other inpatient units (e.g., 24-hour nursing support, an integrated treatment team, an intensive program of therapeutic interventions), patients have full authority to come and go and live in relatively unrestricted environments. They are engaged in their choices and, thus, learn about the meanings, motivations for, and impact of their behaviors.

We will begin by introducing the testing model and its origins. Next, we will describe what we assess, how we assess and write about it, and how we teach the method. Finally, we will present the ways we integrate testing findings into the overall treatment effort, including treatment planning and facilitation, and the assessment of change. Throughout, we will reference testing material in order to illustrate the approach.

The Testing Model

At the Austen Riggs Center (ARC), patients are admitted for a comprehensive six-week evaluation and treatment. This includes intensive individual psychodynamic psychotherapy with a doctoral level psychologist or psychiatrist, psychopharmacological evaluation and medication management, the gathering of a thorough life history and three-generation family history, substance abuse and medical evaluations, immersion in a therapeutic community program, and psychological testing. At the end of the evaluation, the clinical staff gathers for a two-hour case conference; the patient briefly attends the meeting to help focus the conference according to what she identifies as most salient. Afterward, the psychotherapist synthesizes the discussion and offers the patient and, often, her family, a formulation of her difficulties, efforts to manage, vulnerabilities, and resources. This is an attempt to make sense of presenting problems, articulate their meanings and functions, and illuminate their contexts. In this endeavor, psychological testing plays an important role. It offers a unique perspective on the intrapsychic world of the patient, detailing, for example, her relational schemas, conflicts, defenses, thought quality and processes, as well as her abilities to name, manage, and use affects. At the ARC, we also use testing to assess therapeutic change. After patients have been in treatment for a year, they are eligible for another case conference, at which time the focus is on change since admission. For patients who are in treatment for multiple years, reassessment is available annually.

The Testing Model: Its Historical Roots

While the practicalities of the model and its applications at the Austen Riggs Center (ARC) are unique, the testing model itself is the result of the import and evolution of testing practices beginning with Robert Knight. In 1947, the ARC Board of Directors recruited Knight, an esteemed psychiatrist from the Menninger Clinic in Topeka, Kansas, to continue the transformation of the ARC into a psychoanalytic hospital. Originally, the ARC had been a treatment center for individuals suffering from neurotic and substance use disorders, using both occupational and psychological therapies. This approach was based on Austen Fox Riggs's idiosyncratic synthesis of pragmatism and psychoanalysis (Kubie, 1960).

In 1947, Knight became the Medical Director and brought with him a group of gifted clinicians and researchers from Menninger, including David Rapaport, Roy Schafer, Merton Gill, and Margaret Brenman (Friedman, 1990). Rapaport, a masterful theoretician of ego psychology and a pioneer of psychological testing, became the Director of Research at the ARC. Just prior to his arrival, he, with Rapaport, Gill, and Schafer (1945), had written the landmark texts, *Diagnostic Psychological Testing, Volumes I & II*. During this era, psychological testing was conceptualized as a preventive screening that would allow clinicians to detect premorbid pathology before flagrant decompensation (Menninger, Rapaport, & Schafer, 1947). In 1951, Erik Erikson arrived at the ARC. Erikson, whose work situated ego psychology in the context of lifelong psychosocial development, would exert a prominent influence on psychologists at the ARC and across the United States.

Roy Schafer served as the primary testing psychologist for over 5 years until 1952 when he left to become the Chief Psychologist at Yale Medical School (Piers & Shapiro, 2011). Schafer's reports were highly condensed psychoanalytic formulations, sometimes only 1–2 paragraphs that included a diagnosis and description of the patient's personality structure and symptoms. In 1953, David Shapiro assumed leadership of the testing service and the ARC began accepting postdoctoral psychology fellows who would go on to write reports under Shapiro's supervision. At that point the fellowship was 2 years; currently, it is a 4-year Accreditation Council for Psychoanalytic Education (ACPEinc) accredited psychoanalytic training program. While Shapiro's reports resembled Schafer's, Shapiro focused more on the patient's characteristic thought patterns and adaptive functioning. Shapiro (2012) had been highly influenced by Wilhelm Reich's (1949) novel ideas about character, especially the view that individuals actively act upon and construct their world rather than being passive agents governed by unconscious forces. Shapiro's experience of testing patients at the ARC eventually culminated in the publication of *Neurotic Styles* (Shapiro, 1965), a classic study in psychoanalytic personality theory.

At the same time, in the world of psychological testing, Ernest Schachtel published *Experiential Foundations of Rorschach's Test* (Schachtel, 1966), a phenomenological approach attending to the affective and perceptual aspects of the Rorschach that was distinct from Rapaport's more explicit cognitive focus on thought organization (Lerner, 2007). Schachtel, influenced by the interpersonal analyst and social critic Erich Fromm (Smith, 2009), emphasized the value of an experience-near approach in which the examiner immersed herself in the subjective world of the patient. Both Schachtel (1966) and Schafer (1954) stressed the interpersonal context of the testing situation and the potential transference/countertransference factors that might influence the patient's responses (Lerner, 2007). Schachtel's influence was evident on Riggs psychologists' testing reports, particularly in the 1970s, as examiners increasingly commented upon their subjective reactions to patients rather than relying solely upon diagnostic labels.

In 1978, then Medical Director Otto Will commissioned Sidney Blatt to begin a research project using the psychological testing files to assess patient outcome (Blatt, 2006). Blatt collaborated on the project with Riggs psychologist Richard Q. Ford (who later became Director of Psychological Testing at the ARC), which led to the publication *Therapeutic Change: An Object Relations Perspective* in 1994 (Blatt & Ford, 1994). In the 1990s, under Ford's supervision, testing reports at the ARC began to increasingly emphasize the developmental contexts in which the patient's self-representations, relational schemas, and affects were linked in a psychodynamic formulation. More discrete psychodynamic diagnoses fell away. In 2004, J. Christopher Fowler and colleagues conducted a similar research project with updated measures and a new sample of ARC patients, again finding that patients showed improvements in behavioral and personality functioning along trajectories dictated by their personality styles, and that changes in projective testing correlated with meaningful behavioral change (Fowler et al., 2004).

The Testing Model: Current Practice

Currently, psychological testing at the ARC culminates in a concise 1–2 page report. The report is based on data from the Human Figure Drawings, Thematic Apperception Test (Murray, 1943), Rorschach Test (Rorschach, 1951), and Wechsler Adult Intelligence Scale – fourth Edition (WAIS-IV) (Wechsler, Coalson, & Raiford, 2008). There is also an optional neuropsychological screening that can be administered at any time during a patient's treatment to evaluate the need for a more comprehensive neuropsychological evaluation. The testing battery, largely unchanged since being assembled by Rapaport, Gill, and Schafer (1945, 1946), presents patients with a range of tasks organized along a continuum of structure and interpersonal demands. The cognitive component of the assessment, the WAIS-IV, has the most structure and provides the patient with the most interaction with the examiner. It calls upon patients to exercise their intellectual capacities in the domains of verbal comprehension, perceptual reasoning, working memory, and processing speed, providing them with problems to solve, words to define, and puzzles to arrange. The TAT offers the second highest degree of structure. It is comprised of relatively clear pictures of people in various states and modes of interaction, though much is left to interpretation. The patient is asked to create narratives including characters' thoughts, feelings, and behaviors, and is left largely alone to do so. The Human Figure Drawings and the

Rorschach are the final two tests, with the latter affording the least amount of structure. For the Human Figure Drawings, the patient is asked to draw herself and others, whereas on the Rorschach the patient is asked to state what an ambiguous visual stimulus might look like. As the level of structure provided by the tests diminishes, patients are increasingly called upon to bring forward their internal models and means of organizing experience.

No objective or self-report assessment measures are included in the battery as priority is given to measures most able to assess the patient's intrapsychic world, rather than her symptoms or behaviors. Furthermore, all of the psychological testing at the ARC is administered and interpreted without knowledge of the patient's history. This approach allows those interpreting the data to work exclusively from how the patient responds to the testing stimuli. It is an examination of the ways the patient thinks, sees, and reacts to the world, rather than an effort to make sense of her history. While both of these decisions, i.e., to forego the use of objective or self-report measures and to work without reference to the patient's history, prioritize inquiry into patients' intrapsychic worlds, they also limit what we can say about patients' behavioral functioning and descriptive diagnoses.

The tests administered are evaluated using both quantitative and qualitative approaches; the Rorschach Test is currently scored using the Comprehensive System (Exner, 2002). Qualitative approaches are psychodynamically informed and include the study of narrative, sequential, and content elements. We are also interested in how the patient uses structural elements of the stimuli, including its form and features. Inferences about the patient's capacities and vulnerabilities are derived from converging data points, while divergent data points are tracked in order to continually test and develop alternative hypotheses. This approach is phenomenological in its effort to describe the patient's experience, and structural in its attempt to outline the patient's levels of functioning across a variety of domains. While it sometimes informs the psychotherapist's diagnostic efforts, unlike psychological testing in other settings this inquiry is not designed to yield diagnosis or categorization. Instead, we try to provide a more nuanced, personalized description of each patient. The testing, for example, might yield information about how and when a patient's reality testing falters, rather than just classify a patient as psychotic. This approach yields particularly important data when working with patients with severe psychopathology who are often oscillating between borderline and psychotic levels of functioning.

For example, Ms. A. was admitted to the ARC following a major decline in functioning. After her divorce, Ms. A. became agoraphobic and barricaded herself in her room. She developed a shopping addiction, spending thousands of dollars on Disney paraphernalia (e.g., stuffed animals) that reminded her of her favorite childhood movies.

When her friends came to visit, they found her apartment in severe disarray. She was intensely anxious and suspicious that her neighbors had been stealing her beloved Disney movies.

On psychological testing, Ms. A. exhibited a wide range of functioning, at some points appearing to be in the borderline range while at other times appearing more psychotic. For instance, on Rorschach Card IX, Ms. A. saw an "awesome lava lamp with mixing colors," before then declaring it was an "ugly and hideous color mix." She frantically continued to offer five more responses as she chopped up the stimulus into more manageable parts. Consistent with a borderline level of functioning, Ms. A. struggled to register and contain the affectively arousing stimulus and used primitive defenses (i.e., splitting and devaluation) in an effort to organize it. Instead, on Rorschach Card X, Ms. A. tried to integrate discrete parts of the blot, ultimately seeing "whales mixed with baby chicks." This contamination response on the Rorschach is evidence of severe thought disorder. She merged two distinct animal species in a completely implausible manner. In addition, on Rorschach Card II, Ms. A. saw "two Christmas elves wearing Santa hats hi-fiving, like twins reflecting each other," before later adding, "the bodies aren't touching." In this response, her thought processes were clear, though the content was somewhat regressive (i.e., Christmas elves). She insisted the figures reflect each other and their bodies not touch, suggesting Ms. A. was trying to limit the intensity of contact between them. Then, on Card III, Ms. A. saw "two deer wearing bowties" whose heads became "chicken heads with beaks." Later, she commented that they resembled her pet cats who have "human heads." It was evident that she was registering the humanoid bodies on the card (hence the cats with human heads); however, her perceptions became highly fluid and categories blended together. She turned to trying to personalize the response, though this did not stabilize her. Whereas Ms. A. provided a more conventional response to Card II when she could limit the arousal of interpersonal connection, she became significantly more thought disordered when presented with the more sexualized bodies on Card III. Across both the TAT and Rorschach, Ms. A. fluctuated between these different levels of functioning. Studying the contexts in which her thinking became more disordered (e.g., when she produced more complex, integrated percepts, or when overstimulated) illuminated what motivated the variability.

Alongside evaluating the patient's cognitive capacities and screening for cognitive deficits, the cognitive assessment is considered in light of the patient's psychology. Further, in looking at the test battery as a whole, we have the opportunity to track cognitive functioning across tests. For example, we might gain information about perceptual processes from the Rorschach or temporal sequencing and narrative coherence from the TAT. As cognition is intimately intertwined with character, we strive to understand how psychological conflicts and resources shape and are shaped by cognitive styles, strengths, and weaknesses. The optional neuropsychological screening allows for further inquiry into cognitive functioning should there be concerns as to whether there are additional components contributing to the patient's presentation that might require a more comprehensive neuropsychological evaluation.

Assessment of risk for self-destructive or suicidal behavior is also frequently of interest to referring clinicians. While testing is limited in its ability to predict suicidal behavior, we integrate two approaches to identify risk. The first is a sign approach, as offered by both the Suicide Constellation (S-CON) in the Comprehensive System (Exner, 2002) and the Implicit Risk for Suicide Index (IRSI) developed and researched at the ARC by J. Christopher Fowler (Fowler, Hilsenroth, & Piers, 2001). The development of the IRSI was an effort to derive an index of theoretically grounded factors that might contribute to a patient's risk for self-destructive behavior. It includes, for example, scores associated with the presence of unbearably painful affect, boundary confusion, and a sense of oneself as damaged. However, in the spirit of acknowledging each patient's unique psychological makeup and recognizing the limitations of sign-based approaches, we primarily use these indices as markers suggesting we should look at the patient's risk particularly carefully. Ultimately, however, we rely more on our understanding of the patient's particular vulnerabilities, including, for example, how she understands and uses death in narratives, her capacities to manage affects, impulsivity, use of the body, and vulnerabilities to boundary disturbance.

This testing approach assumes the patient is offering her most adaptive solutions to her troubles. To understand them as such, it is often helpful to use a developmental perspective. This perspective helps organize and integrate data by linking information about various aspects of functioning. We might, for example, check our hypotheses about a patient's ability to establish boundaries between herself and others with the defenses she most often uses. For example, are boundaries stable enough to enable the processes involved in projective identification? Using a developmental lens not only establishes a framework in which to understand the data but also a reference point against which to consider outstanding or discrepant data points. Contradictory data points might suggest a range of functioning, for example, or multiple lines of development. The developmental frameworks of Anna Freud (1963), Margaret Mahler (1968), D. W. Winnicott (1965), and, more recently, Peter Fonagy (1991), Otto Kernberg (1995), Sidney Blatt (1991), Drew Westen (1991), and Martin Leichtman (2013) have proven particularly helpful in these endeavors.

Looking at Ms. A.'s testing, she was working at the developmental task of establishing a stable position from which to perceive and engage the world. She sorted and structured stimuli in an effort to achieve a stable subjectivity, particularly with regard to integrating bodily arousal into her self-concept. This capacity is normally developed, to a significant measure, through empathic holding, containment, and responsiveness in relationships. However, there are myriad ways in which these processes can be derailed, contributing to the sense of unsuccessful integration and identity diffusion Ms. A. suffered. The ways in which she was attempting, and struggling, to create a stable self-concept were clear on the testing. For example, on TAT Card 14, Ms. A. depicted a man in an "enclosed brick space" who was opening a window to let in light and air. She then insisted that there were no other signs of life – no grass, no trees, and no people. Holding this story in mind, on Rorschach Card V, Ms. A. saw a "bat or butterfly" in "an identity crisis." She then reversed aspects of the animal, unable to settle on the positions of the head and tail, and chopped off its wings. Abruptly, she personalized the response by bemoaning the fact that she had forgotten to wear her butterfly necklace, before concluding, "This is just having an identity crisis." One way of linking these data points that is consistent with the whole of Ms. A.'s testing is to consider them reflective of her attempt to build a self-structure at minimal risk for arousal, so as to attain a modicum of self-coherence. The brick space she referred to represents such a foundation, as she was careful to limit the character's exchange with the environment to protect against it crumbling. The butterfly on the Rorschach too was an effort at establishing a stable percept, but it was shaky as she initially struggled to define it as either a bat or a butterfly, and ultimately, she dissembled it into parts. Further, her attribution of an identity crisis to the percept showed how easily her thinking could become animistic and unbounded. She lost distance between herself and the card, seeing outside of herself what she struggled with inside. In animating the card, she attributed agency and causality to it, suggesting difficulties with logic and reality testing. Ultimately, she groped for her necklace as a concrete identity marker, something fixed, familiar, and tangible around which to orient.

Practicalities and Training

The patient completes the battery with three postdoctoral psychology fellows: one administers both the Human Figure Drawings and TAT, one the WAIS-IV, and one the Rorschach. The fellow administering the Rorschach writes the report. The data are then scored by each examiner and brought to a two-hour seminar. In the seminar, the three fellows gather together with the supervising staff psychologist and other fellows who help analyze the data. The patient's psychotherapist and other team members (e.g., social worker or psychopharmacologist) are also invited, though they are asked to observe silently to allow the psychologists to work exclusively from the data. Three times a year, the testing schedule is adjusted so that the seminar time is devoted to the study of a 4-year curriculum covering fundamental theoretical, research, and practical aspects of psychodynamic psychological testing. These include various means of assessing movement responses on the Rorschach, affect regulation, thought disorder, body representations, suicide potential, defenses, object relations, development, cognition, and ego functioning, as well as the assessment of therapeutic change.

In the testing seminar, the data are reviewed in exceptional detail, with close attention paid to each word. Line by line and percept by percept, the seminar participants delve into this bracketed field of study to examine what otherwise might get lost in the faster pace and interpersonal noise of patient–clinician interactions. When we are assessing change with patients who have been in treatment over a year, we compare each response to the one given the year before. At this slower pace, we are able to methodically study the patient's use of language (e.g., repeated signifiers), perceptual processes, and the interplay of character and cognition. We also engage thoughtfully in our own associative play, open to the unconscious as we make, question, and refine links between data points across layers of perception and experience. Throughout, we are checking, challenging, and elaborating each other's perspectives. From this, we build a model of the patient's mind and, when re-assessing, track her processes of change. Fellows often say the ways they learn to listen to testing data profoundly influence the way they listen to themselves and their patients across clinical contexts.

After the seminar, the fellow writing the report meets with the testing supervisor for an additional hour to review outstanding data, make and check inferences, and begin conceptualizing and outlining the report. The supervision model is one of apprenticeship. Anchored in its own developmental frame, it is based on the supervisor and supervisee collaborating to establish, revisit, and amend learning goals over the 4 years of the supervisee's postdoctoral fellowship. Initially, for example, fellows may need help scoring tests and understanding basic conceptual material discussed in the seminar, as well as developing the creativity and finesse necessary to successfully manage and describe patients' behaviors and their reactions to them. As they grow more confident with the tasks of synthesizing the data and writing reports, advanced fellows may be assigned full testing batteries outside the seminar, first under the direction of a supervisor and then independently.

Regardless of the supervisee's skill level, the testing supervisor reviews the report for accuracy and conceptual and stylistic clarity. The supervisor gives dialogic feedback, inviting the supervisee to respond to her thinking, whether it be about grammatical edits or more substantive, conceptual issues. This process is a collaborative and sensitive one, particularly as it involves the intimate task of reviewing the supervisee's writing. Further, fellows are often learning an entirely new form of clinical writing distinct from the clinical documentation, research, and data-focused psychological testing reports that are more familiar. In contrast, these evocative, highly condensed narratives are a sort of art, intended not only to communicate findings clearly but also to bring the reader closer to the patient's experience.

Whether it be the development of writing skills or case conceptualization, or about one's functioning as a learner in a group, this model of supervision attends to and assumes that direct feedback will be a reciprocal process between the supervisor and the supervisee. Each supervisor and supervisee brings her own dynamics and edges of growth to the endeavor and relies on the other for feedback in order to continue developing. These conversations happen in scheduled annual reviews, as well as in less formal, ongoing ways. As the supervisory relationship develops, all aspects of growth take place: confusion and clarity, frustration and achievement, regression and forward movement. The testing supervisors also meet periodically to discuss and reflect on their functioning as supervisors and assess fellows' learning needs. As needed, they also attend each other's seminars to generate more effective means of supervising.

Lastly, in this model, the data analysis and learning occur in a group context. Much as Schachtel (1966) and Schafer (1954) suggest using data from the patient-examiner relationship, the group process in the seminar often provides useful data. While leading the seminar, the testing supervisor monitors the group's countertransference, which may be either concordant or complementary to the patient's experience. A seminar for a patient who works to dull states of arousal with obsessive, isolative speech, for example, might take on a lifeless tone, or, in sharp contrast, a hysterical, giddy tone as if to compensate. At other times, the group process is less linked to the patient and more to the expectable group dynamics of a group working together over several years. Fellows adopt various roles, and dynamics of pairing, competition, and envy inevitably surface. If these dynamics impede either individual learning or group functioning, the supervisor addresses them directly.[1]

Informed by all of these processes and guided by the supervisor, the fellow designated to write the report ultimately writes a short report that aims to be evocative of the patient's experience and free of jargon. The report is given to the psychotherapist and included in the Case Conference Abstract, the document compiled at the culmination of the patient's six-week evaluation. At the case conference, staff who have contributed to the Abstract present brief summaries of their reports. This affords the fellow practice communicating the complex ideas in the testing report in a manner accessible to professionals of other disciplines.

As the psychotherapist synthesizes and presents the formulation generated at the case conference to the patient, she might consult with the fellow who wrote the report if assistance is needed in finding a way to integrate and communicate the testing findings. This again is an opportunity for the fellow to speak about the clinical applications of testing in an accessible and useful manner. If the psychotherapist requests it, the fellow is available to meet with the patient, or the patient and psychotherapist together, to provide testing feedback. These requests are always considered in light of the current state of the transference and countertransference, and the potential implications of bringing a third person outside of the therapy dyad into the treatment situation. A psychotherapist caught in an increasingly intense transference may hope to bring in a third party for an outside perspective, for example, or she might be colluding with a transference in which she has been cast as inept.

The Integration of Testing into the Treatment Effort

In addition to informing the psychotherapist's assessment of the patient and training fellows to listen in a particular way, this approach to psychological testing enhances the quality of care we provide in several invaluable ways. Psychodynamic psychological testing is a unique tool in treatment planning, facilitation, and reassessment. When we assess a patient, we are gleaning information about how she perceives, makes sense of, and responds to the world around her. Going beyond symptom checklists, isolated IQ scores, descriptive diagnoses, or descriptions of discrete personality traits without account for their meanings and contexts, we learn about the conditions under which the patient is most able to achieve and sustain or, conversely, to lose, stability. Thus, we can use testing findings to provide a scaffolding on which to anticipate, understand, facilitate, and reassess treatment as it unfolds.

At the Austen Riggs Center, we do not go so far as to make treatment recommendations given the limitations of our data set. We have no knowledge of past treatments and, more importantly, believe the intricacies of any particular psychotherapy relationship are far more complex than we can speak to with authority. Rather, psychotherapists independently integrate the testing findings into their work. For example, they might use them to achieve optimal distance with a patient or to be more sensitive to the needs of a disorganized patient. Most often, psychotherapists say they value the reports for their consistently clear illumination of aspects of the patient they recognize but would not otherwise have been able to articulate as if to say, "Ah, that's what I've been feeling."

One particularly useful contribution of testing to these ends is its ability to detect discrete forms of thought disorder that, when present, often play a central role in patients' struggles. Unrecognized differences between how a psychotherapist and patient perceive, make sense of, and respond to the treatment situation are often at play in the kinds of impasse that lead to treatments devolving and patients ultimately being deemed "treatment resistant." These troubles are often difficult to detect without testing, especially for patients who are verbally gifted and able to hide their confusion beneath sophisticated verbiage. By thought disorder, we mean the processes underlying illogical thinking and reasoning (e.g., loose associations), perceptual confusion and impaired reality testing, linguistic disturbances and neologisms, and boundary disturbances. As noted earlier, we attend to the contexts in which these troubles occur, as well as to the conditions that help the patient recover. Perhaps more interpersonal structure, a less ambiguous environment, more interpersonal distance, or less affective stimulation might be helpful. Further, rather than conceptualizing disordered thinking as absolute or strictly indicative of deficit, we consider how apparent breakdowns in thinking might be breakthroughs, how lapses in organization might be on the way to reorganization that is more complex and adaptive, and how disorganization and disintegration might be serving protective functions (Leonhardt et al., 2016).

Psychotherapists also use testing to anticipate transferences and better understand situations in which confusing or split-off transferences emerge. This can be useful not only to the therapist but also to the treatment team. When treatment team members are agitated, confused, anxious, or exhausted, it often signals the presence of uncontained or disorganized transferences and countertransferences. In such instances, psychotherapists routinely feel pressed to manage their patients and control their behavior. The impulse is to act. In the throes of such pressures, reviewing the testing can function as a sort of ballast around which to reorient and restabilize. This is also true in moments of frustrating or deadening impasse. Even the report's abiding assumption that the patient's behaviors, however stultifying or enraging, are her best efforts to manage can often help a beleaguered psychotherapist rediscover empathy and curiosity. It is a document just beyond the fray that holds clinicians both in its provision of valuable information and in its reminder of this essential stance.

On Ms. A.'s psychological testing report, there were two prominent object relations paradigms: 1) an admired, sexualized other with whom Ms. A. maintained a dedifferentiated relationship, and 2) a formless empty other that was difficult to locate. During the early phases of Ms. A.'s treatment, these relational schemas were evident in Ms. A.'s highly chaotic relationship with her team members. Ms. A. largely ignored the nursing staff, treating them as useless and insignificant because they were not doctors. This resulted in the nurses feeling both useless and defeated, not knowing how they could assist Ms. A. In contrast, Ms. A. idealized her therapist. She began dressing like her and often acted in sessions as if she could finish her therapist's every sentence. She also spoke in an overly familiar manner, referencing episodes in her life without actually explaining what had happened. She appeared to harbor the fantasy she and her therapist shared the same mind. However, over time Ms. A. became increasingly anxious in her psychotherapy and hypervigilant to her therapist's sexuality. When her therapist inquired about Ms. A.'s sexual history, Ms. A. immediately asked, "Are you asking because you're a lesbian?" This culminated in a deeply paranoid transference in which Ms. A. interpreted her therapist's curiosity as a perverse interest in her sexuality. Ms. A. had difficulty thinking about her ideas about her therapist, regarding her impressions as absolute reality. She seemed to be suffering the confusion and lapses in reality testing the testing had identified, particularly as her affective arousal became more intense and the psychotherapy focused on issues of intimacy and Ms. A.'s body. Ms. A.'s means of managing, and her object world more generally, became increasingly dominated by primitive defensive splitting. She was desperately trying to maintain her fragile self-structure. Staff members discussed their vexing relationships with Ms. A. during treatment team meetings in an effort to use their experiences to better understand Ms. A.'s relational schemas. The psychotherapist integrated the psychological testing into the discussions, using its description of Ms. A.'s internal world to provide language and context for these conversations. Ultimately, the team recommended a psychotherapy consultation in hopes it would provide space for reflection on the impasse and the transferences/countertransferences fueling it.

Finally, psychological testing facilitates treatment by assessing change. In longer-term treatments, it is important both to allow room for processes to unfold and to periodically gauge the overall efficacy of the interventions. By using the same testing protocol at annual intervals, we are able to track both major and minor shifts. Sometimes responses on the Rorschach and stories on the TAT initially look quite similar, but close attention to detail reveals subtle changes. We might see changes in affect tolerance and regulation, reflectiveness, maturity, the range and flexibility of defenses, or the patient's sense of agency and self-direction. We might also track the coherence and complexity of the patient's self and object representations, and the capacities therein to secure containment and proceed developmentally. We sometimes see significant shifts on one type of task and not on another, outlining the edge of the patient's growth or the conditions needed to sustain it.

Assessing the complexities of change using psychological testing is a complicated task, as, often, patients seek treatment because they are barely managing using brittle coping strategies. During treatment, they gradually come to sacrifice these maladaptive efforts, which then threatens to expose the core trouble. At this point in treatment, patients may be more agitated and disorganized, but on their way to developing more stable, adaptive ways of being. Differentiating disorganization in the service of growth versus as a signal of a malignant reaction to treatment is difficult, and, sometimes, only time can tell. This is another context in which developmental frameworks are helpful, as they suggest a trajectory against which to compare the patient's presentation.

Ms. A. underwent repeated testing after a year of treatment. On the initial testing, Ms. A. evidenced disorganized thinking and poor reality testing. She produced the severely thought disordered response mentioned earlier on Rorschach Card III, "two deer wearing bowties" whose heads became "chicken heads with beaks." On the second testing, she saw "two deer with a bowtie in the middle and a skull at the bottom." Though she said she considered casting the bowtie as the deer's heart removed from the body, she decided against it. Further, she commented that she was not trying to integrate all the percepts into a single response, but, rather, to offer multiple, discrete responses. In fact, on the initial testing, she gave a single response to Card III; whereas on the follow up testing, she produced three. Her newfound abilities to decelerate, deliberate, and decide upon her responses suggested greater control of her perceptual field. With this, she was able to selectively ignore stimuli that might otherwise have disturbed her thinking. Additionally, her responses on the second testing were significantly less thought disordered as her perceptions were more stable and realistic. It is as if she had begun to experience herself as being more in charge of her ideas rather than swept away by a chaotic stream of thoughts and feelings.

Conclusion: A Way of Listening, Learning, and Holding

In this chapter, we have laid out the model of psychodynamic psychological testing done at the Austen Riggs Center. We have addressed its origins and practicalities, as well as the ways it serves multiple training and treatment functions. This model is costly in terms of the clinical staff time and, thus, the financial resources it requires. Multiple examiners are involved in administering and analyzing each data set, and the psychology fellow and supervisor collaborating on the report spend much time writing, reviewing, and discussing it. That said, the value, in our estimation, far exceeds the costs if the testing is considered a combined clinical service and educational provision, and the range of its clinical applications are recognized. This way of testing tailors, contains, and assesses treatments, and it offers unparalleled insight into the workings of the human mind and its means of change that are applicable far beyond the testing situation.

Note

1 See Chapter 20 by Valerie Sims (this volume) on supervision regarding these issues.

References

Blatt, S. J. (1991). A cognitive morphology of psychopathology. *The Journal of Nervous and Mental Disease*, *179*(8), 449–458.

Blatt, S. J. (2006). A personal odyssey. *Journal of Personality Assessment*, *87*(1), 1–14.

Blatt, S. J., & Ford, R. Q. (1994). *Therapeutic change: An object relations perspective*. New York, NY: Springer Science & Business Media.

Exner, J. (2002). *The Rorschach: A comprehensive system. Volume I: Basic foundations* (4th ed.). New York, NY: Wiley.

Fonagy, P. (1991). Thinking about thinking: Some clinical and theoretical considerations in the treatment of a borderline patient. *The International Journal of Psycho-analysis*, *72*(4), 639.

Fowler, J. C., Ackerman, S. J., Speanburg, S., Bailey, A., Blagys, M., & Conklin, A. C. (2004). Personality and symptom change in treatment-refractory inpatients: Evaluation of the phase model of change using Rorschach, TAT, and DSM-IV Axis V. *Journal of Personality Assessment*, *83*(3), 306–322.

Fowler, J. C., Hilsenroth, M. C., & Piers, C. (2001). An empirical study of seriously disturbed patients. *Journal of the American Psychoanalytic Association*, *49*(1), 161–186.

Freud, A. (1963). The concept of developmental lines. *The Psychoanalytic Study of the Child*, *18*(1), 245–265.

Friedman, L. J. (1990). *Menninger: The family and the clinic*. New York, NY: Alfred A. Knopf.

Kernberg, O. F. (1995). *Object relations theory and clinical psychoanalysis*. Lanham, MD: Jason Aronson.

Kubie, L. S. (1960). *The Riggs story: The development of the Austen Riggs Center for the study and treatment of the neuroses*. New York, NY: P. B. Hoeber.

Leichtman, M. (2013). *The Rorschach: A developmental perspective*. London: Routledge.

Leonhardt, B. L., Kukla, M., Belanger, E., Chaudoin-Patzoldt, K. A., Buck, K. D., Minor, K. S., Hamm, J A., & Lysaker, P. H. (2016). Emergence of psychotic content in psychotherapy: An exploratory qualitative analysis of content, process, and therapist variables in a single case study. *Psychotherapy Research*, *28*(2), 264–280.

Lerner, P. M. (2007). On preserving a legacy: Psychoanalysis and psychological testing. *Psychoanalytic Psychology*, *24*(2), 208.

Mahler, M. S. (1968). *On human symbiosis and the vicissitudes of individuation: Infantile psychosis*. Vol. 1. New York, NY: International Universities Press.

Menninger, K., Rapaport, D., & Schafer, R. (1947). The new role of psychological testing in psychiatry. *American Journal of Psychiatry*, *103*(4), 473–476.

Murray, H. A. (1943). *Thematic Apperception Test: Manual*. Cambridge, MA: Harvard University Press.

Piers, C., & Shapiro, D. (2011). *Personality and psychopathology*. New York, NY: Springer.

Plakun, E. M. (2003). Treatment refractory mood disorders: A psychodynamic perspective. *Journal of Psychiatric Practice*, *9*, 209–218.

Rapaport, D., Gill, M., & Schafer, R. (1945). *Diagnostic psychological testing: The theory, statistical evaluation, and diagnostic application of a battery of tests* (Vol. 1). Chicago, IL: Year Book Publishers, Inc.

Rapaport, D., Schafer, R., & Gill, M. (1946). *Diagnostic psychological testing: The theory, statistical evaluation, and diagnostic application of a battery of tests* (Vol. 2). Chicago, IL: Year Book Publishers, Inc.

Reich, W. (1949). *Character analysis*. New York, NY: Orgone Institute Press.

Rorschach, H. (1951). *Psychodiagnostics: A diagnostic test based on perception* (5th ed. rev.). Oxford: Grune & Stratton. (Originally published 1921).

Schachtel, E. (1966). *Experiential foundations of Rorschach's test*. New York, NY: Basic Books.

Schafer, R. (1954). *Psychoanalytic interpretation in Rorschach testing*. New York, NY: Gruner Stratton.

Shapiro, D. (1965). *Neurotic styles*. New York, NY: Basic Books.

Shapiro, D. (2012). Theoretical value of psychological testing. *Journal of Personality Assessment*, *94*(6), 558–562.

Smith, B. L. (2009). A Boston Yankee: Paul M. Lerner and the heart of assessment. *Journal of Personality Assessment*, *91*(1), 9–14.

Wechsler, D., Coalson, D. L., & Raiford, S. E. (2008). *WAIS-IV: Wechsler adult intelligence scale*. San Antonio, TX: Pearson.

Westen, D. (1991). Clinical assessment of object relations using the TAT. *Journal of Personality Assessment*, *56*(1), 56–74.

Winnicott, D. W. (1965). *The maturational processes and the facilitating environment: Studies in the theory of emotional development*. London: The Hogarth Press and the Institute of Psycho-Analysis.

17 "Listening to the Music of the Mind"

The Uses of Psychological Assessment in the Diagnosis of Psychotic Disorders in a State Psychiatric Center

Paul Saks

Psychological assessment can play a vital role in diagnosis and treatment planning within the confines of psychiatric inpatient units. The title of this chapter references a response on the Thematic Apperception Test (TAT) that speaks to the potential power of a psychological assessment to aid clinicians in the process of experiencing and better understanding "the music of a patient's mind." A full battery of tests including cognitive instruments, objective personality measures, and projective tests can help provide more accurate diagnoses, inform strength based treatment plans and potentially allow patients better outcomes in both the hospital and in the community.

Accurately diagnosing individuals upon admission to an inpatient unit should be an extremely nuanced and complex process (McWilliams, 2011). For an example of data representative of the commonality of inpatient diagnoses indicating psychosis, the Pennsylvania State Psychiatric System reported that in 2010, 1171 out of 1609 inpatients were diagnosed with schizophrenia or another psychotic disorder (Zimmerman, 2011). In the initial intake, admitting clinicians must provide a diagnosis shortly after meeting a patient, often depending upon records from transferring facilities, emergency rooms, jails, and prisons that can be inaccurate. Aside from the fact that crucial elements such as personality disorders, traumatic brain injuries, and developmental disorders can be missed or misdiagnosed, the often idiosyncratic way in which psychotic disorders manifest can be lost beneath diagnostic labels. Inaccurate or incomplete diagnoses can affect the course of treatment, limit potential outcomes, and bind patients to inappropriate labels that stay with them across multiple admissions. This is not to fault the admitting clinicians in inpatient facilities. Decisions must be made rapidly. There can be unspoken pressures to assign a psychotic disorder diagnosis for insurance purposes, and treatment must begin for patients who are obviously acutely symptomatic and potentially dangerous to themselves or others.

The nature and missions of state facilities have changed rather dramatically during the past 20 years (Webster & Harmon, 2006). The process of deinstitutionalization that dominated inpatient mental health care since the advent of anti-psychotic medication over half a century ago is currently referred to by names such as "community focused care." The process has heralded a dramatic downsizing both in the number of beds available and in the average length of stay of those who are admitted to such facilities (Torrey et al., n.d.). A premium is placed upon the rapid assessment, stabilization, and discharge of patients, with many resources being dedicated to the creation of realistic community based after-care services (Fisher, Geller, & Pandiani, 2009). Patients who require longer-term treatment are usually those who present with complicated profiles, symptoms that do not respond to a multiplicity of standard treatments, co-morbid disorders, criminal or forensic histories, and patterns of failed attempts to live in the communities (Fisher, Geller, & Pandiani, 2009).

In an environment with decreasing inpatient resources, psychological assessments utilize empirically validated instruments that can aid clinicians in the assigning of more meaningful diagnoses and targeted treatment plans that are individually designed to work with both the strengths and weaknesses of patients. Furthermore, they lead to the creation of nuanced and complex profiles of the human beings who are being treated. In the experience of this writer, clinicians' focus on strengths and unique talents is often lost in the process of assessing pathology; by losing that focus, clinicians can lose the opportunity to reach the oft-times remarkable and creative individuals who have had their lives shattered by severe mental illness. This strength-based approach is an important element of the Consumer Recovery Model (Bellack, 2006), which is linked to positive outcomes in longitudinal studies of success in the community. A comprehensive assessment can be a way to explore that which makes individuals in state hospitals remarkable, resilient and vibrant individuals beyond that which makes them sick. Clinicians informed by testing can thereby better understand the dynamic issues that manifest as symptoms. While medications can be highly effective in reducing acuity, they often do little to treat the emotional, relational, and traumatic precursors that trigger these symptoms.

This writer contends that there is a language to psychosis, and if clinician and patient can co-create meaning a degree of integration and healing can begin. Testing can start the process of finding meaning in the idiosyncratic worlds of psychotic individuals. It is through this shared sense of meaning that treatment providers can better understand patients and can help them develop the coping mechanisms needed to face the harsh realities, histories, and circumstances of their lives.

The Case of "Elaine"

Elaine was a young woman who found herself in a state hospital after spending several months in a city hospital; she had been brought there by Emergency Medical Services after she was found wandering in the streets. She was unclear about her age and reported that she had been raped, kidnapped, and imprisoned by drug dealers. She was observed to be disorganized and circumstantial and once admitted the description of her rape became increasingly disorganized and illogical. Collateral information indicated that she had a pattern of presenting at hospitals with accounts of sexual assaults. She refused to provide contact information fearing that her mother would be raped; she further stated that her parents, who were vacationing in an exotic place, would come to take her home to their mansion. At the city hospital, she attacked and injured a physician. Collateral information further indicated that she had a history of violence directed at her family.

When she was first admitted to the state hospital, Elaine had assumed a name that ultimately proved to be false. She also denied any psychiatric symptoms, and presented a history that was riddled with grandiose and bizarre details. She insisted that "Elaine" (her actual name) was a different and "bad" person who was in jail; though she always preferred to be called by her assumed name, she was eventually willing to respond to her legal name as well. At different points during her stay, Elaine reported that she been born and raised on a ship cruising in the Bermuda triangle, that she was a famous "DJ," and that she had been married in a ceremony attended by a donkey, a tiger, and a little pig (a scene from Winnie the Pooh). She spoke often of being a "pageant queen," and, claimed that, since infancy, she was the winner of several crowns. Her speech would shift from logical and insightful to language verging on word salad. Interestingly, Elaine was a brilliant poet and artist (she attended a poetry therapy group and was able to prolifically and seemingly without effort, create sophisticated poems). While her spoken communication was often disorganized, her written work was well crafted and eloquent.

Elaine's treatment team posed numerous questions concerning her diagnosis; were her observed symptoms the delusions and thought disordered patterns of schizophrenia? One colleague suggested that she was possibly malingering in order to escape from pending legal charges in other states; another suggested Dissociative Identity Disorder as a possible diagnosis. Once Elaine's identity was confirmed, records and collateral information indicated that she had an extensive psychiatric history beginning at age 16, when she was initially diagnosed with schizophrenia. Elaine had a significant substance abuse history that included heroin, marijuana, and cocaine. She reported several instances of early trauma, including being raped by a school employee.

Elaine's presentation raised complicated and engaging questions. Because of her complex symptom profile she was referred for testing. Elaine was given a battery with the following tests; Wechsler Test of Adult Reading (WTAR, Wechsler, 2001), Wechsler Adult Intelligence Scale – fourth edition (WAIS-IV, Wechsler, 2003), Delis–Kaplan Executive Functioning System (D-KEFS; Trail Making Test, Delis, Kaplan, & Kramer, 2001), Minnesota Multiphasic Personality Inventory – second edition (MMPI-2, Ben-Porath & Tellegen, 2008/2011), Millon Clinical Multiaxial Inventory – third edition (MCMI-III, Millon, Millon, & Davis, 1997), Projective Drawings (House, Tree, Person, Kinetic Family), Thematic Apperception Test (TAT; Murray, 1943), Rorschach Inkblot Test, Comprehensive System Scoring (Exner, 2007). The focus of discussion in this chapter will highlight cognitive measures and projective tests; while important information from the MMPI-2 and the MCMI-III will also be referenced, in terms of personality assessment, the chapter will highlight the use of projective tests.[1]

Cognitive Assessment

To Kraepelin, cognitive deficits, "a characteristic state of feebleness," truly differentiated *dementia praecox* from other forms of madness (Kraeplin, 2014); for most patients, it represented a gradual, degenerative process for which there was little hope of recovery. For many clinicians and researchers, schizophrenia is characterized by significant cognitive deficits and limitations in the areas of memory, processing speed, and executive functioning (Forbes, Carrick, McIntosh, & Lawrie, 2009; Johnson-Selfridge & Zalewsky, 2001; Lee & Park, 2005; Reichenberg & Harvey, 2007). Cognitive impairments in schizophrenia are believed to reflect underlying neurological vulnerabilities to the illness since they precede illness onset, are stable over time, persist when symptoms begin to remit, and are associated with frontal and medial temporal lobe dysfunction (Michel et al., 2013).

Identifying cognitive impairment across a variety of domains is an element in the current diagnosis of schizophrenia (Michel et al., 2013). Those who receive the diagnosis are assessed as performing an average of 2.0 standard deviations below healthy controls on many tests of cognitive functioning (Keefe & Fenton, 2007), with deficits in working memory being particularly prominent. However, meta-analyses (Grot, Potvin, & Luck, 2014; Hedman, Van Haren, van Baal, Khan, & Hulshoff Pol, 2013) suggest that evidence of specific declines are not robust and confounding factors such as the side effects of medication must be taken into consideration. There is not always a clear etiology for neuropsychological impairments when co-morbid disorders exist. There are, for example significant overlaps in memory tasks between schizophrenia and major depression. It has been estimated that only about 25% of those diagnosed with schizophrenia would have scores outside of the average range if data were normally distributed (Williamson, 2006).

Tests of Intelligence: The Wechsler Adult Intelligence Scale, Fourth Edition (WAIS-IV)

Elaine's battery began with an administration of The Wechsler Adult Intelligence Scale, fourth edition (WAIS-IV; Wechsler, 2003), a test of general intellectual ability (Appendix 1). The standard administration of the WAIS is comprised of 12 subtests spanning four index domains of cognitive functioning; verbal comprehension (VCI), perceptual reasoning (PRI), working memory (WMI) and processing speed (PSI) (Wechsler, 2003). In a variety of settings, the WAIS-IV is used extensively to assess cognitive ability, with persons diagnosed as schizophrenic showing impairment relative to comparison subjects on most tasks. Though much of the research to date relies on data acquired using the WAIS-III, Michel et al. (2013) suggest that those diagnosed with schizophrenia and control group performance were comparable on tasks measuring crystallized verbal knowledge. In contrast, the schizophrenia group performed below controls on measures of perceptual reasoning, working memory, and processing speed, with significantly greater impairments on the latter than those observed on all other index measures. A 2016 meta-analysis by Hedman et al., cautiously suggested that patients diagnosed with schizophrenia experience cognitive decline over time.

When using tests such as the WAIS for psychodiagnosis, it is often helpful to look first at overall, broad assessments and then move to performance in specific domains (Cohen, 2007). Considering Elaine's diagnosis, and her early onset of symptoms and shortened formal education, a Full Scale (FSIQ) score of 83, placing her in the 14th percentile, was higher than what one would predict. However, there was considerable scatter between her Index Scores, suggesting that her FSIQ was not a unitary measure of her overall functioning and thus should be approached with a degree of caution. Elaine's General Ability Index (GAI), another estimate of general intellectual functioning which pertains to only verbal and visual reasoning and is believed to better capture disparate levels functioning (Wechsler, 2003), fell within the Borderline range (GAI = 93, 32nd percentile). Elaine was administered the Wechsler Test of Adult Reading (WTAR), an assessment that has demonstrated validity for examination of premorbid function (Wechsler, 2001). The WTAR uses a reading-recognition paradigm requiring the reading of and pronunciation of words, in the absence of comprehension of word meaning. This test maximizes the subjects' previous learning of a word, for word recognition provides a relatively stable measurement of ability in the face of cognitive decline (Putnam, Ricker, Ross & Kurtz, 1999). Elaine's WTAR scaled score of 86 was in the 18th percentile and was slightly lower but still within the interval of her predicted WTAR score (93, 73–113, 90%; Wechsler, 2001) based upon her level of education. Furthermore, the WTAR can be used to generate a predicted, premorbid FSIQ, which in the case of Elaine was 90 (Wechsler, 2001). Thus, Elaine was performing at a level that suggested some impairment and decline, but was not significantly below her predicted levels based upon her education. Furthermore, her performance was not the two standard deviations below healthy test groups (Borderline–Extremely Low ranges) suggested by her diagnosis of schizophrenia.

Research suggests that crystalized verbal intelligence is the domain that remains most stable in the face of schizophrenia (Williamson, 2006). Elaine's Verbal Index (VCI) was a relative strength, as she performed within the Average range. It was interesting to note that Elaine's best performance was in the domain of perceptual reasoning, which traditionally is seen as more susceptible to impairment and decline due to schizophrenia, in contrast to verbal measures which tend to be the most resistant to impairments related to schizophrenia (Michel et al., 2013). It is important to note that there was also a degree of scatter within this index, and that to understand the causative factors, one must look beyond the numbers to the quality of Elaine's responses. In the Vocabulary subtest, Elaine achieved her lowest score. She consistently lost points because she became disorganized by what appeared to be powerful affective reactions to some of the questions. One of the responses involved her saying, "Blood ... there is blood everywhere ...." On more than one occasion, Elaine's tangential style of speaking and rapid, loose associations prohibited her from articulating her knowledge in a linear and coherent manner. Such reactions, coupled with verbal and perceptual reasoning scores that fell well within the Average range, suggested the presence of either positive psychotic symptoms or mood symptoms that were interfering with her cognition, as opposed to the presence of the more cognitively based symptoms of schizophrenia, dementia or some other organically based disorder.

Elaine's relative performance was impaired in the domains of processing speed (Low Average) and working memory (Borderline). Her perceptual reasoning index was also likely affected by slow processing speed, as she scored lowest on the one timed task, Block Design. While studies suggest that memory and processing speed represent areas of particular impairment for persons diagnosed with schizophrenia, slow processing speed, issues with attention and concentration, and impairments in working memory are also suggestive of Mood Disorders and in particular depression (Cohen, 2007). Cognitive testing may be useful in identifying general areas of impairment, but personality testing creates understanding of these potential deficits. With Elaine, it was therefore important to further explore the specific contributing factors to her cognitive weaknesses through the use of personality tests.

The importance of using information gained from cognitive testing to highlight Elaine's strengths cannot be overstated. Despite years of psychotic symptoms, homelessness, incarceration, substance use, psychotropic medications, and institutionalization, Elaine was functioning at nearly an average level in many domains, and at a place that is relatively close to her premorbid predictions. While she experienced a degree of disorganization and intrusion when attempting to communicate ideas, she could think abstractly, was able to draw facts from her base of knowledge and could creatively solve problems and puzzles. Such strengths could be crafted into her discharge plan, while giving her hope of success in the future (Bellack, 2006).

Tests of Executive Function: Delis-Kaplan Executive Functioning System (D-KEFS)

Neuropsychological measures of executive functioning have long demonstrated that the performance of patients with organic brain dysfunction differs from that of normal control subjects (Johnson-Selfridge & Zalewsky, 2001). Theories that try to link schizophrenia to dysfunctional brain regions stem at least in part from the generalization of hypotheses based on observed corollaries from brain injury, dementia, and other organic pathologies. Behavioral changes associated with frontal lobe damage include impairments in foresight, spontaneity, and judgment, as well as difficulty with abstract reasoning, problem-solving, concrete thinking, and the planning and sequencing of complex behaviors (Johnson-Selfridge & Zalewsky, 2001); similar deficits are associated with those diagnosed with schizophrenia (Gold & Harvey, 1993; Williamson, 2006).

Several instruments have been developed to assess executive functioning; these include the Delis–Kaplan Executive Functioning System (D-KEFS), Wisconsin Card Sorting Test (WCST), and the Halstead Category Test (HCT). While the research is not as robust as that concerning brain injury, most studies consistently document impaired performance of participants diagnosed with schizophrenia as compared to normal control participants on measures of executive functioning (e.g., Beatty, Jocic, Monson, & Staton, 1993; Blanchard & Neale, 1994; Braff et al., 1991; Butler et al., 1992; Goldberg et al., 1990; Heaton et al., 1979; Kinney, Yurgelun-Todd, Watemaux, & Matthysse, 1994). For example, those diagnosed with schizophrenia are noted to have difficulty with the WCST, completing fewer categories and demonstrating a tendency to perseverate on the same category (Van der Does & Van den Bosch, 1992).

The D-KEFS is a battery of nine tests that were developed to measure various abilities typically subsumed under the domain of executive functions, such as abstraction, problem-solving, response inhibition, set-switching, and planning. Elaine was administered the Trail Making Test (Appendix 2), which consists of five subtests that assess visual-motor coordination, cognitive flexibility, and speed. The Visual Scanning subtest required Elaine to quickly scan and mark a target number among a field of other numbers. The Number Sequencing subtest required Elaine to visually scan a field of numbers and draw a line connecting numbers of ascending order. The Letter Sequencing subtest required Elaine to scan a field of letters and draw a line connecting them in ascending order. The Number-Letter Switching subtest required Elaine to visually scan a field of letters and numbers and connect them in alternating and ascending order, which is an assessment of cognitive flexibility. The Motor Speed subtest required Elaine to quickly draw a line over a dotted-line, which assesses her ability to quickly execute motor behaviors. The significant discrepancy between Elaine's Average performance in the Motor Speed and Visual Scanning subtests and Impaired and Borderline performance in the other subtests suggested that while her motor skills appeared relatively intact, her impairment of performance in the other subtests is likely a result of a deficit in visual attention and/or her ability to quickly process information.

These findings suggest that Elaine struggles to make meaning out of visual information when it is presented to her in a rapid and/or complex manner. This deficit in processing speed is consistent with some of the possible executive functioning impairments associated with schizophrenia (Johnson-Selfridge & Zalewsky, 2001). That being said, while there were areas of impairment, there were also areas of relative strength, as Elaine displayed average functioning in visual scanning and motor skills.

Personality Assessment: Objective Measures of Personality

Objective personality inventories have many uses and advantages in the environment of state hospitals. They also have notable disadvantages including their reliance upon patient self-report and requirements for literacy, as well as the high degree of concentration and patience needed to complete a measure with hundreds of items.

Elaine's full battery included the Minnesota Multiphasic Personality Inventory – second edition (MMPI-2), Millon Clinical Multiaxial Inventory – third edition (MCMI-III, Millon, Millon, & Davis, 1997), two widely used measures (Aiken & Groth-Marnet, 2005). Though not discussed in detail in this chapter, they will be briefly mentioned here. Both Elaine's MMPI-2 and MCMI-III were notable for patterns of random responding and were thus considered invalid. While not formally interpreted in her report, these instruments do indicate that Elaine was in a state that can be described as acute psychological turmoil, characterized by extreme states of depression, agitation and paranoid ideation.

Personality Assessment: Projective Tests

Projective tests can provide an invaluable lens through which the personality functioning and dynamics of a patient are interpreted. Projective testing can provide information to supplement and clarify data gathered using objective measures. If the ultimate goal of a battery of tests is to create a portrait of an individual, the process of using projective tests can be akin to deconstructing a tapestry; each individual thread, of limited value on its own, serves a purpose in bringing forth a complicated work of art. Understanding how each thread contributes to the larger piece is crucial in understanding how an individual functions in the world and how psychopathologies may impact how he or she navigates life.

Before discussing specific tests and their interpretive value, the following general guidelines are suggested as a strategy when employing a full battery of projective tests. First, it is critical to look for patterns and themes across tests. The essence of a projective test involves presenting subjects with varying levels of ambiguous stimuli, and providing them with space within the testing process to allow for their inner experience to become manifest in their perceptions and comprehensions of that stimuli. At any particular moment of a person's life, certain narratives will dominate the ways in which they perceive themselves and how they relate to others and the world. In the experience of this writer, these crucial narratives will appear as recurring themes that appear repeatedly in projective responses.

As will be noted throughout this case study, Elaine expressed themes of the sexualizing and brutalizing of women, desires to reunite with lost loved ones, and most predominantly a fragile and amorphous sense of self that was defended by idealized fairytales and fantasies. There was also a persistent thread of projected paranoid beliefs, wherein people were envious of her exceptional qualities and consequently were always ready to sabotage her successes. The closer that Elaine was forced to confront the realities of her life and the feelings that they invoked, the more outlandish, bizarre and disorganized her defending fantasies became. Thus, for all of their problematic elements, Elaine's psychotic symptoms seemed to be serving a protective though maladaptive function, implying that treating clinicians may have been met with resistance as they attempted to encourage her contact with reality. Lest testing become solely an exercise of pathologizing and finding weaknesses, Elaine demonstrated strengths as well; her fantasy world was remarkably creative, poetic, informed by literature and popular culture and filled with a powerful and at times ironic sense of humor.

Finally, throughout the process, she demonstrated a true capacity for empathy and a powerful desire to be connected to others. These strengths would be crucial elements in developing an effective treatment and discharge plan.

The Thematic Apperception Test

The Thematic Apperception Test is a projective test developed by Henry Murray in 1938 consisting of 20 picture cards usually depicting one or more people in ambiguous situations; the recipient is asked to tell a story about what is happening in the picture and what the characters are thinking and feeling. In an inpatient setting, the administrator may need to query more than with other subjects; though it is important to allow for patient projection, a skilled administrator will prompt for thoughts about what happened before or after the depicted scene or elaboration upon the thoughts and feelings of the characters.

Several scoring systems have been used with the TAT (Cramer, 1996). The system derived from Murray (1943) is rarely used today due to insufficient reliability and validity. The Social Cognition and Object Relations Scale-Global Rating Method (SCORS-G; Stein, Hilsenroth, Slavin-Mulford, & Pinsker-Aspen, 2011) is a system for coding narrative data that has been applied to the TAT. Content analysis of the TAT has been used in risk assessment for sexual violence (Pam & Rivera, 1995), perception of self as it relates to gender (Pollack & Gillian, 1982), aggression and risk for future violence (Murstein, 1965), and antisocial behavior (Purcell, 1956).

Elaine provided detailed and at times affect-laden responses to the 13 cards that were selected for her assessment. Content analysis was performed, focusing on thematic content, reality testing, and logic, defense mechanisms, internal structure and coherence, basic interpersonal themes, attitudes toward gender and sexuality, themes of violence and aggression, and the possible presence of depression, hopelessness or suicidality.

Using the TAT in this way allows for the creation and exploration of narrative. In the case of an inpatient evaluation like Elaine's, the administration of the TAT provides a semi-structured environment in which a clinician can begin to explore the possible narrative themes that serve as the foundation for psychotic symptoms. If psychosis is an attempt to "not know" that which is too painful to be experienced, the act of creating a narrative through a measure like the TAT may serve as an access point for clinicians to begin the process of translating psychotic process into a shared language. Elaine's responses on three cards will be presented and discussed, as they provide striking examples of how such data can be used in a larger battery of tests.

Card 1

Response: He's listening to the music in his mind to get the feel and vibe for this song. It's a prayer of worship to the violin, and he needs to strum it just right to get the right music. He reads the music and gets into the vibe and emotions of what he's playing, and he becomes an award-winning violinist because his parents let him do what he wanted.

Commentary: Card 1 depicts a boy sitting before a violin and has been associated with pressure to achieve, reactions to authority, mediating self-discipline, and discovering agency. Elaine's response immediately declares that she turns to her inner world over the conventions of objective reality. To get the "feel and vibe" of the song, and indeed life, it would seem that Elaine listens to the "music in her mind," her constructions of how life should be rather than the facts that she must face. Even the boy's style of play is rebellious, for violins are traditionally not strummed. There are few rules or restrictions, for parents (who are absent and passive with the exception of a mention at the very end) let their son "do what he wanted." In choosing to live in such a way, Elaine soon slips into the world of grandiose fantasy, as the boy in her story becomes famous due to the environment created by these distant yet idealized parents. As a response, it speaks to Elaine's psychotic defensive structures, namely withdrawal, introjection, and dissociation. When faced with difficult circumstances, Elaine will turn inwards upon the path of fantasy.

Card 2

It's a funeral. Looks like they have a younger sister wise in the Bible, and she's ready to find someone to do … "what men do." The man is getting ready to plow a field while his pregnant wife waits for him. At the end, he plows a great field and she gives birth to babies and her sister goes off to find love. (Examiner: Before?) She's waiting on the side of the road. (Examiner: Funeral?) What? Are you writing what I said? Not funeral. The man is thinking, "if I treat this horse right, I'll be able to take care of this family." Proud. The woman is thinking, love … that he chose her and she's very proud. The other woman … is nervous … what if he doesn't like me?

Commentary: Here, Elaine begins to give some clue as to the dynamics of her inner world that invoke psychotic defenses. Overall, Elaine required more prompting than she did in her first story, and told a story that was more disorganized and seemingly less intended for presentation to others. She immediately declared the scene a "funeral," an idea which likely evoked unbearable feelings that she eventually retracted and denied; it is possible that she became upset with the idea that her distressing feelings were being written down and were thus made more real and less susceptible to her psychotic defenses. It is a card that suggests themes of fertility and budding sexuality, which in the world of the victim of sexual abuse may have been perceived as the death of innocence and childhood; it may have been an indication that being exposed to adult sexuality led to the death of the person that she might have been. Elaine indicated ambivalence about men. Initially, her response is laden with sexual innuendo (the plowing of fields), where women are treated as sexual property and exist to satisfy the inevitable desires of "what men do." Worth and value for a woman is dependent upon the validation of others, and there is anxiety about not being chosen; this is an important theme that will appear across tests. It is further possible that both women in the card represent societal ideals (good mother and pure, innocent girl) in which Elaine feels she has fallen short. While she tries to be positive and organize herself in the end, the card ultimately suggests a subject that deals with trauma and psychotic level defenses.

Card 14

It's a silhouette of a man staring up at the stars. He's astrologically advanced, and he's into the stars. You want a Starburst? (Examiner, "No thank you.") The window was shut, and it was a very dark room. Saw the stars in the sky and wanted to count them. What candle should I light? Like the universal candle … is there one he should light to watch the stars and write about it? He is feeling anxious … what are the stars going to say next? After, he goes back to the army … planet Mercury is going into the sun. I know this because of my birthday, it's like 666, and I was in the room and everyone was staring at me so I worked for Hustler and they send me $2000 every month. I have a new home. But yeah, back into the army. It's going to help things; he's going to Romania; I have a house there … actually it's a castle. I talked to my daughter about it.

Commentary: Elaine's response is tangential, rife with idiosyncratic references, and fused episodes from her personal history with elements from the card and seemingly random momentary thoughts. The card itself is among the most ambiguous; the shadowy figure of a man in a darkened room near what could be seen as a light-filled, open window. In other protocols, it can evoke stories involving suicide or seeking hope for the future in the midst of dark circumstances. In the midst of overpowering, dark stimuli, Elaine responds with manic defenses and grandiose psychotic fantasy. This is her most incoherent response, with a narrative that respects only the rules of her internal logic. An important illustrative moment occurred when she offered the examiner a piece of candy. From some theoretical perspectives (Eigen, 1993; Matte-Blanco, 1988; Searles, 1961) psychotic thought process is exemplified by idiosyncratic associations and symmetrical condensations of seemingly unrelated objects. The darkness of the drawing inspired thoughts of the night sky, night sky to astrology and stars, and this to a Starburst candy. While perhaps feeling overwhelmed by darkness, Elaine was seeking the comfort of a sweet and reaching out for some form of interpersonal connection with the examiner. The invocation of astrology may represent a desire to assert some form of control, to make some sort of sense of the unknowable, but ultimately she is rendered helpless and waits for "what the stars will say next." By the end of the narrative, she refers to her ex-husband (going into the army), her ongoing themes of sexualization and degradation and ultimately attempts to create a happily-ever-after ending in a castle with her daughter, which is a creation of fantasy. Such a response provides crucial information in working with Elaine, for it provides a snapshot of the defensive quality of her psychotic symptoms, giving insight into what conditions trigger her (depressive affect and references to her traumatic past) to subsequently retreat. It also suggests that in the midst of such a "breakdown" there exists the desire for interpersonal connection, opening a door for her to reach out to others and ultimately learn to better tolerate reality.

Projective Drawings: The House-Tree-Person Protocol

Drawings, which have been used as projective measures since the 1920s, can provide invaluable insight into the developmental, cognitive and emotional status of patients (Oster & Crone, 2004). While there remains controversy as to the reliability and validity of projective drawings (Swenson, 1968), their use, especially with children and families, continues to be extensive. There are a variety of ways in which projective drawings can be used with children, adolescents, and adults to aid in the diagnostic process. One advantage of using drawings is that while most instruments rely almost solely on verbal responses, techniques such as the House-Tree-Person protocol allows patients struggling with unprocessed trauma or cognitive impairment to access an alternate means of expression (Hammer, 1997). In a sense, the examinee is allowing the examiner to be part of a co-created transitional space (Winnicott, 2005) that transcends words. This can allow for the expression of things that may otherwise go unsaid.

Numerous protocols for test administration and interpretation have been developed for the use of drawings in assessment (Bolander, 1977; Burns, 1987; Hammer, 1997; Leibowitz, 1999). These include the Goodenough–Harris Drawing Test (Harris & Goodenough, 1963) and the Machover Draw-A-Person Test (Machover, 1949). Today, the most commonly used technique is the House-Tree-Person (H-T-P) drawings; the three objects represent a common familiarity to people across ages while presenting powerful opportunities for free association

(Oster & Crone, 2004). The author of this chapter uses a modified version of this technique that employs five drawings; a house, a tree, two people (of different genders), and a kinetic family. The instructions for the test are purposefully simple and ambiguous; the examinee is given separate sheets of paper and is asked to draw the figures without comment as to type, size, or condition (Oster & Crone, 2004). The order represents a sequence of gradually increasing complexity, thus making personal responses more likely as the test progresses (Hammer, 1997). Following the completion of all five drawings, the examiner asks a series of questions to encourage further associations and reflection upon the drawings. By framing the questions in terms of the drawn externalized objects, in the experience of this writer, examinees are more likely to freely and more safely discuss their own thoughts and feelings through projected narratives.

As a strategy for interpretation, it is helpful to look at each drawing in terms of thematic elements both specific to each figure and in the context of the entire H-T-P, as well as clinical history, behavioral observations and information gathered from other measures (Oster & Crone, 2004). One can consider developmental quality and age appropriateness of the drawings, attention to detail and possible inclusion of extraneous objects. A brief discussion of the various figures in the H-T-P and two of Elaine's drawings (Figures 17.1 and 17.2) and verbal responses will be presented here.

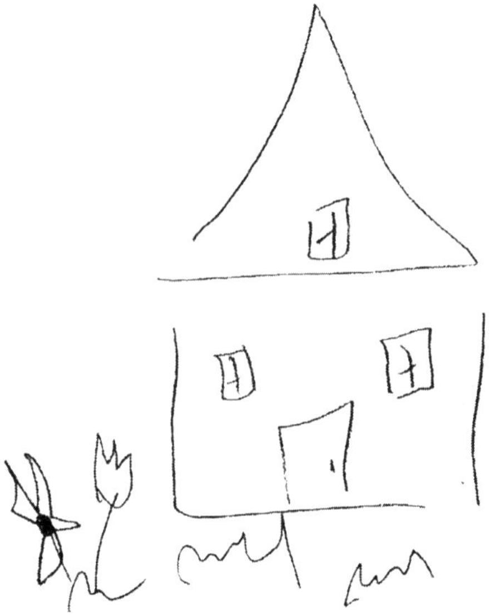

Figure 17.1 'Elaines's house drawing'

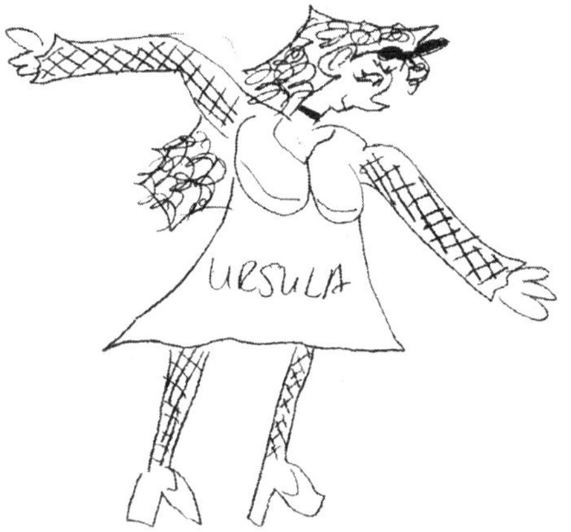

Figure 17.2 'Elaine's human figure drawing'

The house drawing has been associated with self-concept particularly regarding interpersonal dynamics experienced in a familial setting, including events and relationships that may have taken place within the various households in which the examinee has lived. (Malchiodi, 1998). Elaine's house, as portrayed in Figure 17.1, was notable for thin, disconnected walls which can be indicative of a weak, fragmented, and vulnerable sense of self, connected to a roof that is disproportionately large and prominent, suggesting her tendency to retreat into fantasy. Her comment that "a wolf can blow it down" is further evidence of how she may feel vulnerable in a world filled with predatory dangers. The presence in the foreground of extraneous details (flowers and shrubs) suggests that Elaine feels insecure in the world, and looks for a sense of control through idealized interpersonal relationships; her statement that the house most needs "flowers and love" supports this. That these crucial elements in her self-conception are barely recognizable further suggests that while she may have fantasies of what she needs to feel happy, these relationships are unrealistic and she is ill-equipped to actualize them. The multiple barred windows suggest that while Elaine desires relationships with others, she has difficulty actually establishing contact. Finally, in naming her house the residence of Smurfs when questioned, Elaine returns to the fairytale and fantasied themes that recur throughout her testing; for one who so strongly desires relationships, the ones she describes are with the idealized and unobtainable dreams of her childhood.

Human figure drawings are most clearly and directly associated with the examinees' perceptions of who they are and how they wish to be seen in the world (Oster & Crone, 2004). Human figures tend to elicit portrayals of body image, sexuality, trauma, perceptions of personality characteristics, and self-concept. The second of Elaine's two figures (she chose to create a little boy in a baseball cap as her first) is portrayed in Figure 17.2, a sexualized caricature of Ursula the sea witch from the Little Mermaid. This is a pattern that repeatedly appears in her projective test responses, in which Elaine draws from fairytale or fantasy archetypes to portray people. Dressed in fishnets, high heels and a black choker, Ursula's high hemmed dress extenuates her large breasts. Elaine describes her as "short-tempered" and liking "dancing" and "cheerleading." It is possible that her swirling, long hair characterizes a dependence on fantasy life to escape from the sexualized and degrading role that women are forced to play; the choker serves as a clear demarcation between mind and body in the drawing.

The Rorschach Inkblot Test

The Rorschach Inkblot Test can provide various forms of data to aid the clinician in diagnosing a severe mental disorder. It can be particularly useful in helping to detect severe mood disturbance and subtle psychotic thought processes (Weiner, 1966, 1998) that may be missed in an initial interview (Cohen, 2007). Though the 10 inkblots have remained unchanged since Hermann Rorschach picked them from a larger collection based partly upon his work with both non-clinical and schizophrenic adults, many methods for scoring have been used; these include Rapaport, Gill, and Schafer (1946), Schafer (1954), and Klopfer (1946). The use of the Exner Comprehensive System (2002) and the Rorschach Performance Assessment System (Meyer et al., 2011) currently provide extensive psychometric data and a large body of empirical literature to support the validity and reliability of the assessment.

Two of Elaine's responses will be presented in Tables 17.1 and 17.2 for a discussion of content before an overall discussion of the findings related to her scored Rorschach protocol (Appendix 3).

Table 17.1 'Sample of Elaine's Rorschach Card 1 Responses'

Card I.1. A bat flying through the night to his beloved Vampyra.	There's a pin right there, so when she pins him against the wall she pins him right here. That's his chompers, and here's his wings. The vampire is his master. He's the color of midnight, so you can't see when he flies. [flying through the night?] Wings are open. [Open?] Spread that way. [Beloved Vampyra?] Because she's his master, she's not in the picture. [The night?] Because bats only come out at night. He's bigger than most bats, so it has to be a vampire's.

Table 17.2 'Sample of Elaine's Rorschach Card 10 Responses'

Card X.2. The Queen of Hearts.	The Queen of Hearts, here's the two footmen, and she's painting the roses red. Have you seen Alice in Wonderland? People tell me I need to get out of Lala Land, but I have children and we like to watch it. Where's my little monkey boys? He'd wear glasses. I have four boys and one ... he was voted most popular in Pre-K[indergarten]. [Queen of Hearts?] The queen of hearts wears red. [Two footmen?] Because they're both blue, and here's their eyes and mouth. You know, I got the mother of the year award. It was so nice ... I love my kids.

While a full analysis of all of Elaine's responses or the data provided and scored using the Exner Comprehensive System is beyond the scope of this chapter, a brief summation of the most cogent points help to understand the ways in which severe mental disorder can manifest in a Rorschach protocol. In terms of content, as seen in Tables 17.1 and 17.2, samples of Elaine's responses evidence themes that are consistent with the other projective measures. Immediately upon seeing the first card, Elaine associated to an internal fantasy world and experienced a breakdown in logic as the ambiguity of the card led to idiosyncratic responses riddled with Special Scores and images from the world of horror and science fiction movies. One can extrapolate that this is her basic defensive style when faced with ambiguous or stressful situations (Weiner, 1966). As seen in these two examples in Tables 17.1 and 17.2, when human figures were perceived, they were inevitably interpreted as fictional or fantasy characters (The Queen of Hearts, Vampyra, (H) responses). This speaks to her distorted perception of people and relationships based upon her inner experience. This powerful nonexistence of "Pure H" (human) responses was also a factor that elevated her Suicide Constellation to near-clinical value (seven out of the required eight factors). The protocol culminated in her response from "Alice in Wonderland" on Card X, which represented a significant distortion of reality by internally mediated coping mechanisms. Though she attempted to end the protocol in a positive light by discussing the love she has for her children, it was divorced from the task at hand. There were themes of powerful depressive affect (three Morbid responses, elevated Vista responses (3r + (2)/R [0.07] < 0.33), and low self-esteem (High Morbid, FQ-FM responses), suggesting that her flight into fantasy was a means of obliterating these intolerable feelings.

Elaine's protocol was notable for the high number of Special Scores, and in particular the presence of two Contaminations, two "ALOGS" and five Deviant responses, Lvl 2; these strongly suggest a highly idiosyncratic and at times bizarre way of perceiving the world. Specifically, Elaine struggled with coming to reasonable conclusions about events transpiring around her, while maintaining any form of logical flow or connection between her thoughts and associations. Thus, Elaine's ability to function in the world was likely compromised by arbitrary, circumstantial reasoning and moments in which loose and scattered ideation confused both Elaine and the people with whom she was attempting to interact. As suggested by the two responses provided, her thinking operated from its own logic and was likely to become bizarre when contemplating the nature of people and their actions.

Consistent with her performance in other instruments, Elaine's pattern of responses was strongly suggestive of the diagnosis of a schizophrenia-spectrum disorder. Additionally, her perceptual distortions appear to be provoked by emotionally arousing situations that generate and intensify her dysphoric affect; that relationship between impaired cognition and powerful affective states was an indication that a diagnosis of schizoaffective disorder was appropriate to consider. The Rorschach thus further supported a large body of evidence that Elaine's psychotic thought processes were inextricably related to feelings of depression, which fueled her other symptoms.

Using Testing in Treatment Planning

A reoccurring challenge of conducting psychological testing involves transforming often massive amounts of data into a coherent narrative that can be useful both to the treating professionals and the patient. What may be important for the former, may actually prove distressing or harmful for the latter. This writer encourages interns and externs to abandon overly technical language and communicate in a style that is accessible to a multidisciplinary team of mental professionals as well as their patients. A report should include strengths, a sense of hope for the future, and recommendations that are concise, targeted to deficits, and can be put into action. Furthermore, psychological assessments should always be accompanied by verbal feedback for both the treatment team and the patient; reports can be misinterpreted and overwhelming, and it is crucial to sit down and discuss the meanings and implications of the testing.

Taken in totality, Elaine's battery suggested that although she presented in a grandiose manner, her idealized identity was created to cope with a poor self-image, several early traumas, and interpersonal losses. Her fragile, psychotic defenses functioned to manage intense and unbearable affect states. Elaine's severe depressive states and traumatic past impelled her to seek safety and comfort from emotional pain through short-term, maladaptive means such as substance use, and retreating into a world of pure fantasy and ultimately psychotic disorganization. She struggled to form logical and reality-based impressions of the people and events around her. The resulting paranoid, and at times bizarre, distortions served mainly to make Elaine feel more depressed, anxious, and disconnected from reality. While she retained cognitive strengths, facilities such as processing speed and attention were severely compromised by emotional distress and internal preoccupation. Deficits were not likely to be the result of organic dysfunction. As Elaine retreated into psychotic defenses, she confounded and pushed away interpersonal attachment with others, leading her to become more isolated and perpetually divorced from the real relationships she desperately desired.

Feedback to Elaine conveyed that she was an extremely creative person who exhibited many strengths. However, it was also conveyed to her that she had clearly been through many terrible things in her life and that these traumas had left her prone to feelings of great sadness and loss. As a result, she had used drugs and acted out in ways that had caused many problems for her. Furthermore, when she started to experience really bad feelings, her creative mind would start to create stories in which she would escape, and that it was possible that she would get confused between what was happening in her mind and what other people considered to be reality. She was able to hear this, discuss the fact that it was indeed frustrating when other people did not understand her and dismissed the things that she truly felt were true. Slowly, she was beginning to question certain delusional beliefs.

As a result of testing, Elaine's treatment plan was adjusted to accommodate the gathered information. Regarding her diagnosis, it was clear across measures that she exhibited psychotic symptoms and patterns consistent with a diagnosis of schizophrenia; however, a powerful mood component was also evidenced, suggesting the strong possibility of schizoaffective disorder. Furthermore, there was strong evidence of a traumatogenic etiology underlying and exacerbating both psychosis and mood; her history of substance use and reckless behavior were likely attempts to self-medicate sequalae of trauma, that ultimately fueled further psychotic disorganization and mania. Her medication was adjusted to factor in this mood-related component to her experience and led to a reduction of symptoms, which allowed her to engage more thoughtfully in psychosocial and dynamic modes of treatment.

Elaine engaged in almost six months of weekly psychotherapy, through several stages of treatment. When confronted by painful realities in the context of a safe and supportive relationship, Elaine gradually became more able to stay in the room with her therapist, while in the past, she would have fled to tropical islands and enchanted gardens.

Elaine's schedule of therapy groups was also modified. Her use of psychotic and dissociative defenses coupled with acting out behaviors led to a referral to a modified DBT (Linehan, 1993) group, in which she focused upon using mindfulness to better tolerate the realities of the moment. Her experiences of trauma led to placement in a trauma-informed treatment group (Herman, 2007), in which Elaine learned to verbalize her experiences and ask for support from others who had also suffered from unspeakable losses; this set Elaine on the path of forming real relationships over the self-imposed isolation of psychotic defenses. She was in a substance recovery group, and this part of her treatment was better informed by insight into the nature of the feelings and experiences she was attempting to self-medicate through substance use (Khantzian, 1995). Finally, and perhaps most importantly, the obvious brilliant creativity of her inner world led to a referral to a poetry therapy group led by this writer. Elaine was nothing short of brilliant in this group and demonstrated an ability to quickly and seemingly spontaneously write affectively powerful, technically sophisticated, and poignant poems. The group provided her with a creative outlet to express experiences of trauma in an artistic form, perhaps allowing her to process and make sense of unbearable feelings in an organized and interpersonal manner (Saks, 2006). Elaine was discharged to a community residential program several months after her battery was completed, having demonstrated significant progress during her hospitalization.

Conclusion

Psychological testing is an essential tool to better understand the experience of patients contending with psychotic disorders. By using an analysis of both cognitive and personality measures to "listen to the music of their minds," clinicians can not only provide some clarity to the diagnostic procedure but provide idiographic meaning to syndrome labels that could otherwise obscure the uniqueness and humanity of the people that we serve.

The chapter will conclude with a poem written by Elaine. It lays bare in an eloquent and devastating written form the feelings that once she had managed though psychotic withdrawal; the creation of this work was perhaps made possible by a course of treatment that began with a comprehensive assessment. It is reprinted with her permission.

Am I Really Loved?
Help me lord for I have sinned
Please grant my innocence back again
Do you love me?
Do you care?
All this hatred I can't bare
I hate myself
I hate my life
Should I cut it with this knife?
Cut through veins, through flesh so deep
If I die, who will weep?

Exner, J.E. Jr. (2007). *A Rorschach workbook for the comprehensive system* (5th ed.). Asheville, NC: Rorschach Workshops.

Fisher, W.H., Geller, J.L., & Pandiani, J. (2009). The changing role of the state psychiatric hospital. *Health Affairs, 28*, 676–684.

Forbes, N.F., Carrick, L.A., McIntosh, A.M., & Lawrie, S.M. (2009). Working memory in schizophrenia: A meta-analysis. *Psychological Medicine, 39*(6), 889–905.

Gold, J.M., & Harvey, P.D. (1993). Cognitive deficits in schizophrenia. *Psychiatric Clinics of North America, 16*, 295–312.

Goldberg, T.E., Ragland, J.D., Torrey, E.G., Gold, J.M., Bigelow, L.B., & Weinberger, D.R. (1990). Neuropsychological assessment of monozygotic twins discordant for schizophrenia. *Archives of General Psychiatry, 47*, 1066–1072.

Grot, S., Potvin, S., & Luck, D. (2014). Is there a binding deficit in working memory with patients with schizophrenia? A meta-analysis. *Schizophrenia Research, 158*, 142–145.

Hammer, E.F. (1997). Advances in projective drawing interpretation. Springfield, IL: Charles C. Thomas Publisher, LTD.

Harris, D.B., & Goodenough, F. (1963). *The Goodenough-Harris Drawing Test*. New York, NY: Pearson.

Heaton, R.K., Vogt, A.T., Hoehn, M.M., Lewis, J.A., Crowley, T.J., & Stallings, M. (1979). Neuropsychological impairment with schizophrenia vs. acute and chronic cerebral lesions, *Journal of Clinical Psychology, 35*(l), 46–53.

Hedman, A.M., Van Haren, N.E., van Baal, C.G., Khan, R.S., & Hulshoff Pol, H. E. (2013). IQ changes over time in schizophrenia and healthy individuals: A meta analysis. *Schizophrenia Research, 146*, 201–208.

Herman, J. (2007). *Trauma and recovery: The aftermath of violence–from domestic abuse to political terror*. New York, NY: Basic Books.

Johnson-Selfridge, M., & Zalewsky, C. (2001). Moderator variables of executive functioning in schizophrenia: Meta analytic findings. *Schizophrenia Bulletin, 27* (2), 305–316.

Keefe, R., & Fenton, W. (2007). How should *DSM-V* criteria for schizophrenia include cognitive impairment? *Schizophrenia Bulletin, 33*, 912–920.

Khantzian, E.J. (1995). Self-regulation vulnerabilities in substance abusers: Treatment implications. In Dowling, S. (Ed.), *The psychology and treatment of addictive behavior* (pp. 17–41). Madison, WI: International Universities Press.

Kinney, D.K., Yurgelun-Todd, D.A., Watemaux, C.M., & Matthysse, S. (1994). Obstetrical complications and trail making deficits discriminate schizophrenics from unaffected siblings and controls. *Schizophrenia Research*, 12, 63–73.

Klopfer, B. (1946). *The Rorschach Technique: A Manual for a projective method of personality diagnosis*. New York, NY: World Book Co.

Kraeplin, E. (2014). *Lectures on clinical psychiatry*. Charleston, SC: Nabu Press.

Lee, J., & Park, S. (2005). Working memory impairments in schizophrenia: A meta-analysis. *Journal of Abnormal Psychology, 114*(4), 599–611.

Leibowitz, M. (1999). *Interpreting projective drawings: A self psychological approach*. Ann Arbor, MI: Edwards Brothers.

Linehan, M. (1993). Cognitive-behavioral treatment of borderline personality disorder. New York, NY: Guilford.

Machover, K. (1949). *Personality projection in the drawing of the human figure*. Springfield, IL: Thomas.

Acknowledgment

The author would like to thank Dr. Nikaya Becker-Matero ongoing assistance and support made the writing of this chapter p

Note

1 The administration of tests was performed by Charles Burton, ps intern; interpretation and analysis were performed under the super this writer.

References

Aiken, L.R., & Groth-Marnet, G. (2005). *Psychological testing and assessm* ed.). New York, NY: Pearson.

Beatty, W.W., Jocic, Z., Monson, N., & Staton, R.D. (1993). Memory ar lobe dysfunction in schizophrenia and schizoaffective disorder. *J Nervous and Mental Disease*, *181*, 448–453.

Bellack, A. (2006). Scientific and consumer models of recovery in schiz Concordance, contrasts, and implications. *Schizophrenia Bulleti* 432–442.

Ben-Porath, Y.S., & Tellegen, A. (2008/2011). *MMPI-2-RF (Minnesota M Personality Inventory-2-Restructured form): Manual for administration, sc interpretation*. Minneapolis, MN: University of Minnesota Press.

Blanchard, J.J., & Neale, J.M. (1994). The neuropsychological signature phrenia: Generalized or differential deficit? *American Journal of Psychi* 40–48.

Bolander, K. (1977). *Assessing personality through tree drawings*. New Y Basic Books.

Braff, D.L., Heaton, R., Kuck, J., Cullum, M., Moranville, J., Gra Zisook, S. (1991). The generalized pattern of neuropsychological d outpatients with chronic schizophrenia with heterogeneous Wiscon Sorting Test results. *Archives of General Psychiatry*, 48, 891–898.

Burns, R.C. (1987). *Kinetic house-tree-person drawings: K-H-T-P: An inte manual*. New York, NY: Routledge.

Butler, R.W., Jenkins, M.A., Sprock, J., & Braff, D.L. (1992). Wiscon Sorting Test deficits in chronic paranoid schizophrenia: Evid a relatively discrete subgroup? *Schizophrenia Research*, *7*, 169–176.

Cohen, L.J. (2007). Psychological testing in inpatient psychiatry. In Bc (Ed.), *New psychological tests and testing research* (pp. 1–33). New Y Nova Science Publishers, Inc.

Cramer, P. (1996). *Storytelling, narrative, and the thematic appercep* New York, NY: The Guilford Press.

Delis, D.C., Kaplan, E., & Kramer, J.H. (2001). Delis-Kaplan Executive System (D-KEFS). Retrieved from: www.pearsonclinical.ca/en/proc duct-master/item-105.html

Eigen, M. (1993). *The psychotic core*. Lanham, MD: Jason Aronson, Inc.

Exner, J.E. Jr. (2002). *The Rorschach: A comprehensive system* (4th ed.). H NJ: John Wiley and Sons.

Malchiodi, C. (1998). *Understanding children's drawings*. New York, NY: The Guilford Press.

Matte-Blanco, I. (1988). *Thinking, feeling and being*. New York, NY: Routledge.

McWilliams, N. (2011). *Psychoanalytic diagnosis: Understanding personality structure in the clinical process* (2nd ed). New York, NY: Guilford Press.

Meyer, G.J., Viglione, D.J., Mihura, J.L., Erard, R.E. & Erdberg, P. (2011). *Rorschach performance assessment system*. New York: Rorschach Performance Assessment System, LLC.

Michel N.M., Goldberg J.O., Heinrichs R.W., Miles A.A., Ammari N., & McDermid Vaz S. (2013). WAIS-IV profile of cognition in schizophrenia. *Assessment, 20*(4), 462–473.

Millon, T., Millon, C., & Davis, R.T. (1997). *Millon Clinical Multiaxial Inventory-III (3rd ed.) – Manual*. Minneapolis, MN: National Computer Systems.

Murray, H.A. (1943). *The thematic apperception test*. Cambridge, MA: Harvard University Press.

Murstein, B. (1965). *Handbook of projective techniques*. New York, NY: Basic Books.

Oster, G.D., & Crone, P.G. (2004). *Using drawings in assessment and therapy: A guide for mental health professionals* (2nd ed.). New York, NY: Routledge.

Pam, A., & Rivera, J. (1995). Sexual pathology and dangerousness from a thematic apperception test protocol. *Professional Psychology: Research and Practice, 26*(1), 72–77.

Pollack, S., & Gillian, C. (1982). Images of violence in thematic apperception test stories. *Journal of Personality and Social Psychology, 42*, 159–167.

Purcell, K. (1956). The TAT and antisocial behavior. *Journal of Consulting Psychology, 20*(6), 449–456.

Putnam, S.H., Ricker, J.H., Ross, S.R., & Kurtz, J.E. (1999). Considering premorbid functioning: Beyond cognition to a conceptualization of personality in postinjury functioning. In Sweet, J.J. (Ed.), *Studies on neuropsychology, development, and cognition. Forensic neuropsychology: Fundamentals and practice* (pp. 39–81). Lisse, The Netherlands: Swets & Zeitlinger Publishers.

Rapaport, D., Gill, M., & Schafer, R. (1946). *Diagnostic psychological testing, Volume II*. Chicago, IL: The Year Book Publishers.

Reichenberg, A., & Harvey, P.D. (2007). Neuropsychological impairments in schizophrenia: Integration of performance-based and brain imaging findings. *Psychological Bulletin, 133*(5), 833–858.

Saks, P. (2006). Reflections of no man's land; symbolization, symmetry, experience and memory through poetry of the first world war. (Panel Member) Narrative Matters Conference on Psychology and Literature, Halifax, British Columbia, Canada.

Schafer, R. (1954). *Psychoanalytic interpretation in Rorschach testing*. Oxford: Grune & Stratton.

Searles, H.F. (1961). Schizophrenic communication, *Psychoanalytic Review, 48A* (1), 3–50.

Stein, M.S., Hilsenroth, M.J., Slavin-Mulford, J. & Pinsker-Aspen, J.H. (2011). *Social Cognition and Object Relations Scale: Global Rating Method (SCORS-G; 4th ed.)*. Boston, MA: Unpublished manuscript, Massachusetts General Hospital and Harvard Medical School.

Swenson, C. (1968). Empirical evaluations of human figure drawings: 1957–1966. *Psychological Bulletin*, *70*, 20–44.

Torrey, E.F., Entsminger, K., Geller, J., Stanley, J., & Jaffe D.J. (n.d.). *The shortage of public hospital beds for mentally ill persons*. Retrieved from www.treatmentadvocacycenter.org/storage/documents/the_shortage_of_publichospital_beds.pdf

Van der Does, A.J.M., & Van den Bosch, R.J. (1992). What determines Wisconsin Card Sorting performance in schizophrenia? *Clinical Psychological Reviews*, *12*, 563–583.

Webster, S.L., & Harmon, S.H. (2006). Turning the tables: Inpatients as decision makers in the treatment mall program at a state hospital. *Psychiatric Rehabilitation Journal*, *29*, 23–225.

Wechsler, D. (2001). *Wechsler test of adult reading* (WRAT). [Assessment instrument]. San Antonio, TX: Harcourt Assessment.

Wechsler, D. (2003). *Wechsler intelligence scale for Adults* (4th ed.). [Assessment instrument]. San Antonio, TX: Pearson.

Weiner, I.B. (1966). *Psychodiagnosis in schizophrenia*. New York, NY: John Wiley & Sons, Inc.

Weiner, I.B. (1998). *Principles of Rorschach interpretation*. Mahwah, NJ: Lawrence Erlbaum.

Williamson, P. (2006). *Mind, brain and schizophrenia*. New York, NY: Oxford.

Winnicott, D. (2005). *Playing and reality*. New York, NY: Routledge.

Zimmerman, B. (2011). *Pennsylvania State Hospital System Length-of-Stay, Demographics & Diagnoses Report For 2010*. Retrieved from www.dhs.pa.gov/cs/groups/webcontent/documents/report/p_010895.pdf

Appendix 1

WAIS-IV Scores

WAIS-IV Index	*IQ Score*	*Qualitative Description*	*Percentile*
Verbal Comprehension	93	Average	32nd
Perceptual Reasoning	94	Average	34th
Processing Speed	81	Low Average	10th
Working Memory	71	Borderline	3rd
Full Scale	83	Low Average	13th
General Ability	93	Average	32nd

WAIS-IV VCI Subtest	*Standard Score*	*Qualitative Description*	*Percentile*
Similarities	9	Average	37th
Vocabulary	7	Low Average	16th
Information	10	Average	50th
Comprehension	8	Average	43rd

WAIS-IV PRI Subtest	*Standard Score*	*Qualitative Description*	*Percentile*
Block Design	6	Low Average	9th
Matrix Reasoning	10	Average	50th
Visual Puzzles	11	Average	63rd
Picture Completion	8	Average	25th

WAIS-IV WMI Subtest	*Standard Score*	*Qualitative Description*	*Percentile*
Digit Span	4	Borderline	2nd
Arithmetic	6	Low Average	9th

WAIS-IV PSI Subtest	*Standard Score*	*Qualitative Description*	*Percentile*
Symbol Search	6	Low Average	9th
Coding	7	Low Average	16th

Appendix 2

D-KEFS Trail Making Scores

D-KEFS Trail Making	*Scaled Score*	*Qualitative Description*	*Percentile*
Visual Scanning	9	Average	37th
Number Sequencing	2	Impaired	<1st
Letter Sequencing	2	Impaired	<1st
Number-Letter Switching	4	Borderline	2nd
Motor Speed	10	Average	50th

Appendix 3

Rorschach Protocol Score

Card	Resp. No	Location and DQ	Loc. No.	Determinant(s) and Form Quality	(2)	Content(s)	Pop	Z Score	Special Scores
I	1	Wo	1	FMa.FC'o		(A),Ls, Hh	P	1.0	ALOG, DR2, DV, AG, PHR
II	2	W+	1	FMp.CF-		(Hd),Hx, (A)		4.5	CP, CONTAM, MOR, PHR
III	3	W+	1	mp.CF-		Cg		5.5	
IV	4	Wo	1	FMa.FVu		(A),Hx, Ls		2.0	AG, PER, PHR
V	5	Wo	1	FMa-		(A)		1.0	PER, DR2, ALOG
VI	6	W+	1	ma.FTu		Sc,Ex,Fi		2.5	AG, MOR
	7	W+	1	Ma.TF-		(H),Sc,Fi, Ay		2.5	AG, PSV, DR2, PHR
VII	8	Wo	1	Fu		Sc		2.5	PER, DV
	9	W+	1	ma.VF.YFo		Ay,Fi,Ls		2.5	DR2, DV2, MOR
VIII	10	Wv	1	C		Ls,Sc			
	11	W+	1	Fo		An,Ad		4.5	
IX	12	W+	1	FMa.CF-		A,Sx,Fi, Hx		5.5	FAB2, COP, PHR
	13	W+	1	FMa.FC-		A,Sx,Na		5.5	COP, PSV, FAB2, PHR
X	14	Wv	1	Ma.Co		Bt,Hx			DR2, PHR
	15	W+	1	Ma.CF-	2	(H),Art, Cg,Bt		5.5	COP, PSV, CONTAM, PER, PHR

18 The Role of Psychological Testing in an Inpatient Psychiatric Setting

A Mentalizing Approach

Shweta Sharma[1] *and Patricia Daza*

Meaningful psychiatric psychodiagnostic work demands an understanding of the whole person. The psychologist using psychological tests can play a crucial role in helping treatment providers appreciate the complexity of the whole person. This chapter discusses psychodiagnostic work in the treatment of hospitalized psychiatric patients. The authors detail an approach to diagnosing and treating that is dynamic, collaborative, multidisciplinary, and person-centered, reflecting a longstanding testing tradition that began evolving at the Menninger Clinic in the 1940s. The chapter highlights the role of clinical psychologists on multidisciplinary teams and in the diagnostic process. The psychologist uses a battery of psychological tests to systematically investigate the nature and meaning of the patient's psychological problems. Patients are enlisted as partners in the testing process, and their active engagement is sought to reach an understanding of their difficulties and how treatment can be of help.

The Indian parable of six blind men and the elephant beautifully captures the nature of the multidisciplinary psychodiagnostic work in psychiatric inpatient settings. As the story goes, the six learned blind men gather together to learn about the elephant. To make sense of the unknown in front of him, each man goes on to inspect it. As it happens, each man inspects a different aspect of the elephant. One probes a very round, smooth, and sharp object and warns the others that they are dealing with a spear. Another grapples with a tall, wide-girthed, thick pillar-like thing and announces that it is very much like a tree, and so on. The conclusion of each man is specific to the aspect of the elephant he examines and how he interacts with that part. Only by synthesizing their observations into the whole are they able to arrive at some accurate description of what is in front of them. Of course, being able to describe is not the same as understanding the elephant. To determine how to proceed requires the next step of getting to know the elephant.

In psychodiagnostic work, the task is to understand the individuals, who have their own observations and understanding of their troubles.

We clinicians are, in fact, blind to the perspective and understanding of the person that we are trying to help, notwithstanding our professional knowledge of the human mind and behavior. Furthermore, our disciplinary training can result in our developing a narrow focus that may overly simplify the complexity of the person. No doubt, we are more likely to arrive at an accurate description and understanding of the person by listening to their own understanding and by including diverse perspectives. We may even go a step further and suggest that all psychodiagnostic work must be geared toward using diverse perspectives to explore, elaborate, and expand the personal understanding of the patient. We will employ the technical term *mentalizing* (Fonagy, 1989) for this focus on understanding and holding the patient's mind in mind. Put simply, mentalizing refers to attending to and understanding the basis of mental states such as thoughts and feelings in oneself and others. Promoting mentalizing facilitates mutual emotional attunement; promotes understanding of self, others, and relationships; and fosters trust in others as resources for social learning, which is the basis for effective psychotherapeutic treatment (Allen, 2013; Allen & Fonagy, 2014; Fonagy & Allison, 2014). Most crucial is the effort to engage the patient in a *mentalizing stance* that promotes non-judgmental curiosity about mental states in oneself and others (Bateman & Fonagy, 2016).

This chapter is written from the perspective of clinical psychologists who engage in psychodiagnostic work using psychological testing with patients presenting complex psychiatric problems in an intensive inpatient multimodal intermediate-term treatment setting. We, the authors, are part of a multidisciplinary treatment team, but in this chapter, we will highlight the role of the clinical psychologist. In the chapter's opening section, we outline our thinking about the diagnostic work with patients in general, as well as the issues particular to our unique treatment setting. We describe the treatment setting, the composition of the treatment team, and our historical roots as well as current models of assessment that exemplify some of the principles that guide our work. To credit the pioneers of our longstanding testing tradition and provide even a brief summary of the developments that have occurred over more than a half-century is beyond the scope of this chapter; however, we help the reader situate our kind of diagnostic work in its specific historical and treatment context. The case examples[2] are organized around the diagnostic topics that we illustrate, and focus on the contribution of the psychological testing. In the spirit of being transparent, as well as attempting to be instructive in our approach, we interweave explanations about test interpretation in general with specific case material. The chapter concludes with a summary of our experience and conclusions from the diagnostic work as it pertains to all treatment settings.

Our Diagnostic Philosophy

The diagnostic work we aspire to practice is based on a way of thinking and engaging with the patient and the data that aims not to identify the problem in the person but to understand the person with the problem (Shectman, 1979). As Menninger, Mayman, and Pruyser (1963) posited,

> It is diagnosis in the sense of understanding just how the patient is ill and how ill the patient is, how he became ill and how his illness serves him. From this knowledge one may draw logical conclusions regarding how changes might be brought about in or around the patient which would affect his illness.
>
> (Menninger, Mayman, & Pruyser, 1963, p. 7)

In this sense, the enterprise of diagnosis is about understanding how and why patients struggle the way they do, which is less a matter of identifying and putting them into a category but, instead, understanding the ways in which they are trying to suffer less and are both taken and served by their illness and suffering. The most challenging and perhaps the most important aspect of the diagnostic work is enlisting active collaboration from the patient and engaging the patient and their families as active members of the diagnostic team. As such, the diagnostic work focuses on engaging the patient and the family in establishing and maintaining a mentalizing stance.

In this respect, the aim of the psychological testing, which is the focus of this chapter, is not to arrive at a *Diagnostic and Statistical Manual of Mental Disorders* (DSM) or *International Classification of Diseases* (ICD) diagnosis. Rather, it is to understand the patient's experience in order to provide meaningful information to the patient about his/her struggles and to assist the clinicians puzzling about how to help the patient. This model of assessment includes inquiry into the patient's cognitive, affective, and behavioral functioning, and is also broadened to include the goal of orienting and preparing the patient for treatment. This aspiration may include using test findings for delineation of the patient's vulnerabilities, increasing understanding of the obstacles or challenges to developing the therapeutic alliance and the conditions that facilitate the building of, or cause disruption to the alliance; making explicit the patient's implicit assumptions or expectations around help and help-seeking; and identifying areas of vulnerability to emotional dysregulation. The task is to develop a shared formulation of the patient's experience and the focus and goals of treatment. Developing a shared understanding is the basis of empathy for and establishing connection with the patient, and sets the foundation for the psychotherapeutic work and the treatment process. Ideally, the testing process gives the patient an experience of mentalizing, a corrective experience of understanding oneself and being understood by the other that then acts as a therapeutic intervention and furthers the treatment.

Our Roots

To briefly provide the relevant historical context, the use of psychological testing as a diagnostic tool began evolving at the Menninger Clinic during the 1940s under the leadership of the psychologist David Rappaport. Through his extensive data collection and detailed research, he demonstrated the psychodiagnostic value of a battery of psychological tests. He developed a systematic approach to the interpretation of test responses and an understanding of the response process based on conceptualization derived from ego psychology and psychoanalysis. The following fundamental assumption forms the basis of Rappaport's philosophy of diagnostic testing:

> Every behavior segment bears the imprint of the organization of the behaving personality, and permits – if felicitously chosen – of reconstructions of the specific organizing principle of that personality ... It is assumed that these behavior segments bear the imprint of the organization of the subject's personality, and therefore it is expected that the test performance will be revealing of that personality.
>
> (Rappaport, 1967, pp. 339–340)

Rapaport's systematic approach to test responses, which has been extensively documented and discussed by him and others (see Rapaport, Gill, & Schafer, 1968), helped clinicians understand the cognitive, affective, and behavioral factors underlying the patient's functioning. These clinically and conceptually driven methods of data analysis, synthesis, and hypothesis formulation help bring to light the uniqueness of the person and significantly add to the empirical sources of knowledge available to the treatment team. The case examples discussed in this chapter share this approach to inference making and synthesizing test data that is part of this longstanding tradition which remains highly relevant to this day. The psychologist uses a battery of tests to sample the patient's behavior across a range of situational demands that vary in terms of external structure, ambiguity, relational demands, and medium of self-presentation (Bram & Peebles, 2014), and uses the cross-sectional data to understand the person being assessed. The focus is on understanding the patients' experience, stimulating the patient's curiosity, and engaging the treatment team in exploration and clarification of their interpersonal experiences with the patient. Engaging the patient in a reflective process, employing test materials and responses, exemplifies in a microcosm the kind of psychotherapeutic work we endeavor to conduct throughout the hospital treatment (Allen et al., 2017).

Therapeutic Assessment

The attitudinal stance of interest in and respect for the person along with the collaborative nature of inquiry and engagement with the patient are increasingly being incorporated in current advancements in conceptualizing and conducting the assessment process. Steve Finn's model of Therapeutic Assessment (TA) champions the spirit of collaborative inquiry (Finn, 1996). TA is a semi-structured form of collaborative assessment (Finn, 1996, 1998; Finn & Tonsager, 1997) that enlists the patient as an active collaborator in everything from specifying the goals of the assessment, to collecting collateral information and interpreting test findings. In TA the psychologist uses a flexible battery and begins standardized testing with tests that seem most transparently related to the patient's main concerns. Following every standardized administration, patients are engaged in collaborative and targeted discussion of their response to the test and their test responses, in order to collaboratively explore various working hypothesis and to arrive at new understandings. Psychological tests are employed as "empathy magnifiers" (Finn & Tonsager, 1997, p. 375) with the goal of providing patients with a new experience and new information about themselves that might then stimulate curiosity and thereby broaden their understanding of self, others, and relationships. This new experience opens the door for and allows the patient to develop new insights that promote change in relationships. TA is often used as a consultation to a patient–therapist dyad who are feeling stuck in therapy and to revise or define new goals. We believe that TA is an improvement upon many of the principles of diagnostic testing; it is a practice we hold close to our hearts.

Treatment Setting

The Menninger Clinic is a psychiatric hospital that provides intensive multimodal intermediate-term treatment. Patients struggling with severe, chronic, and multiple psychiatric problems immerse themselves in a psychotherapeutic milieu of peers and staff members for a period of six to eight weeks. Many of the patients have had several partially effective or failed trials of outpatient treatment and/or multiple hospitalizations (Fowler et al., 2015). Among the patients admitted between July 1, 2012, and June 30, 2016 (N=2216), more than half endorsed suicidal ideation within the month prior to the admission, one-third reported at least one suicide attempt during their lifetime, and among those reporting at least one suicide attempt (N=679), an average of 2.25 attempts were reported per person (A. Madan, personal communication, February, 2017). The treatment at the Clinic is organized around the immersion in the therapeutic community of the staff and the peers. The development of intensive therapeutic relationships provides multiple and rich opportunities for emotional experiencing and expression that fosters understanding of self, others, and relationships. The treatment is heavily weighted toward group interactions and interventions, and much of the treatment occurs in patients' informal interactions. Peer relationships, as well as the interactions with members of the nursing staff, provide a rich environment for interpersonal engagement, feedback, and regulation, and greatly enhance the understanding that depends on the expertise of the treatment team. This emotional, relational engagement in combination with psychoeducational and skill-building groups (Allen, O'Malley, Freeman, & Bateman, 2012) provide impetus for the challenging task of building trust in others as a resource for social learning, and fosters the development of agency and hope to move forward. The therapeutic community is organized into different demographic groups including young adults, adolescents, and professionals, among others. The aspects of the social milieu, time (average length of stay of 45 days), and the treatment team make the treatment setting atypical and provide the condition for the diagnostic work outlined in this chapter.

To the extent that a mentalizing stance can be maintained, the social milieu and the extended time provide the team and the patient the opportunity to engage in a rich interpersonal process in the service of understanding the patient. Patients are invited to reflect on their interpersonal functioning with staff and peers in real time. This emotional engagement, practicing, experiencing, and expressing emotions, entails developing understanding of self, others, and relationships and comprises interpersonal regulation of distress. For the psychologist, the immersion with the patient in the social milieu adds to the rich data source of the patient-examiner relationship and enhances the use of the test data for promoting a reflective stance and providing a mentalizing experience. Such an immersion provides rich opportunities for empathic understanding of the patient's narrative of suffering, the implicit relational assumptions, and the patterns of destabilization and recovery, all of which fundamentally influence the unfolding of the treatment process. As the treatment unfolds, the psychologist, by being part of the process, has the advantage of using the test data to both understand and influence the unfolding of the treatment. The psychologist in this treatment setting is both the treatment provider for the patient and the diagnostic consultant to the treating professionals on the treatment team (Allen, 1981). Furthermore, as the patient becomes immersed in the therapeutic community, the psychologist also has the advantage of returning to the test data to develop meaningful working hypotheses about the transference-countertransference enactments, the struggles or ruptures in the alliance with the treatment team, and the treatment impasses, when and as they arise.

Treatment Team

The treatment team is a multidisciplinary composite, and members bring their expertise to the study of the biological, intrapsychic, and interpersonal functioning of the patient. The social worker, psychologist, nurse, psychiatrist, rehabilitation specialist, chemical dependence counselor, eating disorder specialist, dietician, chaplain, mental health associate, and the *patient* and the patient's family – all engage in a partnership in the conviction that only in this way can patients develop a thorough and comprehensive understanding of their suffering, cultivate hope for help and alleviation of suffering, and develop a pathway to effective and healthy coping and problem-solving. An assumption behind the multidisciplinary diagnostic is that the psychiatric problems are complex and associated with the problems in living; thus, warranting the need for diverse perspectives in the understanding of the problems. Each member of the team studies the problem from their disciplinary vantage point and contributes to the diagnostic work-up. The team seeks to reach a diagnostic understanding that synthesizes the contributions from all participating members, including the patient and his/her family.

The next section will demonstrate aspects of the diagnostic work as we aspire to practice it by using case examples. We focus primarily on the role of the clinical psychologist, on the diagnostic team and on the diagnostic process.

When Discrepancy Arises

In this example, we illustrate a not so uncommon diagnostic scenario of discrepancy between the diagnostic impression from the test data and the clinical impression accepted by most of the treatment team. The presence of discrepancy poses a diagnostic challenge for the treatment team, and the team is obliged to wrestle with the contradictory impressions of the patient until they arrive at a more coherent and a complex understanding of the patient. This is not an easy task. The team members are vulnerable to being pulled into the mindset of the ancient learned "blind men" and can find themselves amassing data to support their impression of the patient, and may inadvertently lose sight of the patient. The team must resist the strong pull to deem one impression more accurate than another. The secret to working with discrepant impressions of the patient is to think "both-and" rather than "either-or." In one type of this discrepancy between the test and non-test (clinical) data, the treatment team perceives the patient as higher functioning than the test data suggests or vice versa. This may occur because psychological tests and assessment procedures are often able to clarify and illuminate that which is not so easily accessible clinically, especially in a short time period, that is, the structural organization of the patient's personality. The psychologist on the team can play a crucial role during the diagnostic challenge of discrepant clinical and testing impressions of the patient by studying the test data and looking for when, and under what conditions, one or the other aspect of the patient's functioning emerges as prominent.

Clinical Presentation

Danielle, a woman in her late 20s, sought treatment at the Clinic because she had been feeling stuck in depression for a long time despite receiving pharmacological and psychotherapeutic treatment on an outpatient basis, a course of electroconvulsive therapy, and two acute hospitalizations. She had been diagnosed with bipolar disorder, was prescribed antipsychotic medications, and had finally felt stabilized on a medication prescribed for mood stabilization. However, she had started struggling after her roommate, with whom she was in an open sexual relationship, broke-up with her.

Despite her complex clinical presentation, Danielle quickly settled into the therapeutic community. She responded to the structure of the hospital unit and the support of the peers and the staff, with improvement in her mood. She worked with her psychiatrist to slowly and gradually taper off several medications, which included anti-depressants, psycho-stimulants, and mood stabilizers. In individual therapy, she identified several issues to focus on, including lack of self-compassion and over-reliance on others for a sense of self and worthiness. In family therapy, she focused on broaching the subject of her sexuality with her parents, addressing her mother's tendency to fix her problems, and her mother's need for her own therapy. On the eating disorder track, she admitted to difficulties with body image and over-eating. She revealed fears that she was different because she was heavy and would never find a man. Danielle related well with the staff and peers. She carried herself in a mature manner, presented as focused and motivated, and was very well liked. In her informal interactions, she showed minimal self-doubt, over-reliance on others, confusion, or volatility, tendencies that had been characteristic of her attachment relationships in her life outside the hospital. In contrast with her history of significant struggles with emotional dysregulation, in treatment she presented as emotionally well contained. She also stood out in the community for her accomplishments. Unlike most of her peers on the unit, she had completed a college degree and had been able to hold a steady job.

Psychodiagnostic Work

The test data from a battery of self-report and performance-based measures showed that Danielle suffered from significant precariousness in her ostensible maturation. The data suggested that underneath her confident outer presentation, she felt weak, inadequate, and helpless. She displayed a tendency to deny her painful subjective reality by behaving as if she were untroubled – not guilty, needy, angry, or demanding – and functioning well. This contradiction between her outer presentation and inner experience was reflected in the evaluation by way of the discrepancy in her test data. For example, on the Minnesota Multiphasic Personality Inventory – 2 (MMPI-2; Butcher, Dahlstrom, Graham, Tellegan, & Kaemmer, 1989) content scales, she showed no elevations that would have suggested low self-esteem. Inconsistent with this lack of concern related to self-esteem on this self-report measure, her Rorschach percepts (Rorschach Performance Assessment System, R-PAS; Meyer, Viglione, Mihura, Erard, & Erdberg, 2011) made several references to beauty, fancy jewelry, clothing, and exotic fruit or places. Responses with such content are known to reference the fragility, vulnerability, and precariousness of the sense of self (Schafer, 1954). It also was interesting that Danielle's Rorschach had multiple reflection responses. Reflection responses are empirically, clinically, and conceptually established as associated with grandiosity and self-absorption (Weiner, 1998; Mihura, Meyer, Dumitrascu, & Bombel, 2013). Furthermore, she showed a tendency to justify her responses on the Rorschach with "past experiences or prior knowledge." Such personal responses (PER) are known to be suggestive of anxiety about the adequacy of one's answers (Weiner, 1998). Her self-justifying style conveyed her sensitivity to being perceived as lacking or not credible.

Guided by the psychoanalytic conceptualizations of a hypervigilant or shy narcissistic character (Gabbard, 1989; Akhtar, 2000), the examiner developed a hypothesis that Danielle consciously denied or covered up (reflected in her MMPI-2 self-report) her unstable and fragile self-worth (her Rorschach percepts) that likely made her feel less valued, less important, and fearful of being exposed and judged as lacking and not credible. The data from the social milieu supported this working hypothesis. On the unit, she presented as an intelligent, confident, and articulate, even somewhat charismatic woman. She had quickly become the leader in the community of the peers, and the unit staff perceived her as mature, motivated, responsible, and all-in-all a model patient.

In addition to the hidden vulnerabilities, the test data suggested significant obstacles to Danielle's openness to learning in relationships. It showed that her relational expectations of criticism and judgment and (less conscious) anxieties about needing and depending on others made it extremely challenging for her to trust others. The data showed that Danielle related in a manner that excluded any relational input. Inside the interior of her interactions with people, she engaged with projected and imagined aspects of herself instead of engaging with and taking in the other. This again was discrepant with Danielle's report of a good working alliance with the treatment team, and the treatment team's experience of collaborating with her on treatment issues.

The examiner sought Danielle's help in understanding the discrepancies between the test findings and her presentation. Danielle responded by idealizing the examiner. She openly discussed her disappointment in people, seeing others as not intelligent or knowledgeable enough to appreciate her unique complexity. When the examiner encouraged her to take a risk to show her vulnerabilities she devalued staff and peers to support her self-protective style of keeping an emotional distance. Her response to the feedback provided further support for the challenge of developing an alliance with her. Although her style of keeping an emotional distance limited her opportunity to have a new relational experience and kept her lonely and trapped in her internal world, to her it seemed the only rational and intelligent response to uncaring, unresponsive, or controlling others. Her devaluation of others was an effective way of protecting herself against feared rejection and abandonment, which partly had its roots in her early experiences with a clinically depressed mother.

The opportunity to appreciate Danielle's fragility, while also holding in mind her high functioning self, arose in treatment when she felt criticized by a staff member. She became emotionally dysregulated when she requested to cancel a session and heard staff's response as a judgment of her commitment to treatment. Although the treatment team validated her distress, she could not be comforted and was enraged. The treatment team, based on their perception of her high functioning self and at that point of the alliance with her, expected her to be able to reflect on this hurtful interpersonal experience with them. Danielle, on the other hand, had felt severely injured and had retreated to a place of extreme mistrust and expectation of relational malevolence everywhere. In this instance, the discrepant impression was setting up a reciprocal interaction, characterized affectively by both the patient and the team feeling misunderstood and becoming frustrated. This interaction had the potential to create an impasse in treatment. The examiner returned to the test data and used it to understand and make the affects, of both the patient and the treatment team, explicit. Understanding the team's surprise and confusion as a function of Danielle's discrepant functioning allowed the team to move toward appreciating Danielle's internal struggle underlying the interpersonal struggle. Feeling validated, the treatment team was then able to be curious about the intensity of Danielle's hurt and asked her to help them understand her internal experience. Being approached by the team in this way allowed Danielle to overcome her shame and opened the door for a new relational experience of being interested in, "seen," and possibly understood.

Hidden Dynamics that Complicate Treatment

Some patients tend to live out their intrapsychic conflict in the interpersonal realm, leading to splits in the patient's internal experience and self-representation playing out externally in the team. The team members find themselves divided in their response to the patient. Or, some patients can unconsciously recreate their family dynamics by pulling various members of the team into specific roles, which can then be understood as an expression of the patient's inner struggle in action rather than words. A thorough diagnostic understanding requires ongoing alertness to these issues and communication among various team members, including the patient. The psychologist can contribute to the diagnostic understanding by being alert to these issues in the testing protocol and by describing internal splits in the personality organization of the patient and its implications for countertransference reactions (e.g., Fowler, 1999; Fowler, Hilsenroth, & Handler, 2000).

Clinical Presentation

Ava, a married woman in her mid-50s, the mother of three children, presented to the Clinic with a history of depression, anxiety, and significant physical health problems. She was admitted to the Clinic after she injured herself with the intent to end her life. She had previously struggled with suicidal thinking in the context of an argument with her daughter that concerned her son's heavy drug use. She had a previous history of abusing laxatives for a period of six months to lose weight. She described a difficult relationship with her husband and reported that he was emotionally and sexually abusive. Her trauma history was also significant for a sexual assault at age 15 and the traumatic experience of diagnosis and treatment of cancer. She had received some outpatient treatment but not consistently.

Ava was pleasant, friendly, and very well-liked by the staff and her peers. Among other things, the diagnostic team was puzzled by her report of feeling traumatized by her husband. Some members of the team believed her while others questioned the report. Notably, in the course of treatment, her husband had confirmed Ava's self-report about his abusive behaviors. Ava was referred for testing to better understand her personality style.

Psychodiagnostic Work

First and foremost, the examiner took note of Ava's overall demeanor, which was girlish, naïve, and even flirtatious – unlike what would be expected from a middle-aged woman. The examiner's subjective experience of Ava converged with the themes of adolescent rivalry, jealousy, and competitiveness that dominated her TAT (Thematic Apperception

Test; Murray, 1943) stories. It was interesting also to note that on the Rorschach, Ava had difficulty describing and explaining the basis of her percepts. Furthermore, on both the TAT and the Rorschach, Ava disparaged herself in a flippant and almost frivolous manner. The examiner felt pulled in to rescue, comfort, encourage, and support Ava.

The compilation of test data – the global, impressionistic, and affect-laden cognitive style (Shapiro, 1965); frivolous, immature, and dependent relating with the examiner; and themes of jealousy and competitiveness on the TAT stories, led the examiner to tentatively hypothesize the presence of a hysterical character style. To garner further support for her inference and to test her hypothesis, the examiner invited Ava to reflect upon her TAT stories. Ava responded with several "I don't know," "I am so uncreative," "I am terrible at this." Guided by psychoanalytic conceptualizations of hysterical character (McWilliams, 2011), the examiner developed the inference that Ava tended to repress negative affect. It was then interesting to note that Ava's test data were not infused with traumatic content or themes and did not show trauma-related disruption in reality testing or reasoning, despite her presenting concerns about trauma. This discontinuity in test data and self-report led the examiner to infer, based on both the psychoanalytic conceptualization of hysterical character and trauma model (Peebles-Kleiger, 2012), about a need for a dissociative and/or repressive barrier against trauma as a way to protect herself from the danger of getting overwhelmed. More importantly, it helped the examiner appreciate the diagnostic team's puzzlement around Ava's report of feeling traumatized, despite her husband's confirmation of her self-report.

The examiner used the test data to help team members understand each other's response to Ava. The early disbelief of her traumatic experiences among some team members could be clarified and explored as a reflection of Ava's internal struggle. The examiner used the test data to stimulate curiosity in the diagnostic team about their disagreement, in the service of developing a more complex understanding of Ava's intrapsychic and interpersonal dynamics. In this instance, the test data helped the treatment team members step back and move out of the dynamic of the split and move toward integration in the treatment team. It clarified the underlying dynamics impacting Ava's struggles as well as the treatment, alerted the diagnostic team to the transference and countertransference dynamics that were playing out in treatment, and brought into sharp focus the treatment goal of integration of the dissociative and/or repressed aspects.

Changing the Story: Embracing Colors

This is an example of collaborative inquiry that occurred during hypothesis testing, and the testing of limits phase, transforming the patient's treatment. Collaborative inquiry can help open the door for a new experience for patients and can help them rewrite the narratives of their suffering. The stories we tell ourselves shape us and the testing experience can help change problematic or incomplete stories by helping patients tune in and listen to themselves. That is, the testing can be used to stimulate empathic self-engagement and develop greater narrative coherence by promoting reflection and curiosity.

Clinical Presentation

George, a man in his early 20s, was admitted to the Clinic due to feelings of "disconnect" and chronic suicidality. He admitted to feelings of depersonalization, living as if he were in a dream, starting at age 15. One year prior to the admission, his symptoms had worsened with an increase in suicidal thoughts, intent, and planning, despite ongoing outpatient treatment. George did not enter treatment with hopes of getting better. Instead, he wanted to satisfy his parents by giving treatment one last chance. His own stance was that he was "just done" with his life and "it is time to move on." George denied feeling depressed but did endorse depressive symptoms of low energy, initial insomnia, social withdrawal, and diminished interest.

Psychodiagnostic Work

As part of his treatment, George was asked to participate in psychological testing. He agreed and was administered the TAT, the Rorschach, and the MMPI-2. George had a creative bent. He enjoyed creative writing. He used the test stimuli to show his creativity and generated a rich, although highly intellectualized protocol. Test data suggested that he was quite emotionally sensitive. He felt weak, unattractive, inadequate, and uncomfortable in social situations, and expected rejection by others. He was a hypervigilant individual who experienced the human world as dangerous and messy, and preferred keeping distance from others whom he characterized as "full of greed and lust." This also seemed to be his way to make others subhuman – perhaps a projection to preserve his own self-worth. His indifference and detached stance suggested a defense against discomfort with closeness, fear of betrayal, and self-protective denial and repression of emotional needs. One of George's TAT stories, on card 14 (i.e., a silhouette of a figure in a window against a dark backdrop) stood out. Unlike the rest of the test data, the character in this story revealed the hidden yearning for acceptance. On this card, he told the following story:

> This boy, you probably see him more than you actually realize. He is always there. He is kind of part of the backdrop. You might not notice him, but he is always just around the corner. He is always on

> the outside looking in. He follows around the real people, hoping to be like them. In a way, he despises everything they stand for, their greed and their lust and their meaningless little lives. But he wants nothing more than be accepted by them. Every night he sits at his window and looks outside. He watches the street. At first, the business people, then the drinkers, and then just the homeless wander the streets. And even those homeless, he wonders, "why can't I be like them?" And he looks to the sky every night, and he prays. He is not even sure anymore if anyone is really listening. That boy is always around but is never quite there. Even standing in the light somehow he is always shrouded in the shadows forever looking at the real world through his window.

The examiner developed the hypothesis that George's difficulty engaging with the diagnostic team might be due to his need to repudiate intense dependency needs because they stirred unbearable shame and disgust in him. After all the tests were administered, the examiner decided to read the TAT stories with George and asked him to reflect on any connection with his own life. The examiner wanted to test the hypothesis about repudiated dependency needs and assess how open George might be to noticing his self-protective intellectual stance and to speaking about what lies behind his distancing armor. The examiner also wanted to acquire treatment-relevant data about George's ability to self-reflect and engage with the examiner and stimulate curiosity, reflection, and self-discovery in him. The examiner set up a follow-up meeting with George and read out aloud the above-mentioned story, letting him know in advance that she was interested in his thoughts and feelings about the character in the story, and how he may relate with the character. Upon hearing the story, George became extremely emotional. He broke-down crying. He revealed that the story touched a nerve regarding his wish to be part of things like other people and his feelings of extreme loneliness. He felt so emotional that he could not continue talking with the examiner. He appropriately requested to end the session to have some time by himself. The following day he shared that he could not remember ever having such a strong emotional reaction. This display of extreme emotionality in the context of a safe and trusting relationship and supportive environment transformed his experience of a "breakdown" into a "breakthrough." Previously, he had experienced displays of emotionality as being potentially damaging to others, but his experience with the examiner suggested to him that sometimes emotions can help people feel closer. Connecting with his emotions made George feel alive and human, more emotionally engaged with others, and gave him hope. He began to appreciate himself as emotionally alive rather than dead. Notably, George always dressed in black and just as he began to recognize and experience his emotions, he began to wear more vibrant clothing.

Is There a Thought Disorder?

One unique contribution of psychological testing is its ability to assess patients' reality testing and reasoning with more efficiency and specificity that can be achieved through clinical interviewing alone. Reality testing refers to the patient's accuracy of perception and ability to differentiate between subjective internal experience and objective external characteristics of objects, people, and actions. Reasoning refers to the patient's "way of organizing observations or sensory information to reach conclusions, often about causality" (Kleiger, 1999, p. 122). Reasoning is associated with the assessment of a thought disorder or disordered thinking and includes the assessment of the logic of the patient's reasoning, style of making connections among ideas and feelings, ability to move within an appropriate level of conceptual abstraction (not too overly abstract or too overly concrete), and ability to screen irrelevant, socially inappropriate, and emotionally raw subjective experience in a constructively communicative fashion. Testing provides more refinement than simply providing yes-no answers to such referral questions as "Is there a thought disorder?" Test data can be used to assess

> the stylistic details of the patient's lapses in reality testing and reasoning, the severity of the lapses, the conditions under which the lapses occur, the patient's awareness of and attitude toward their lapses, their ability to recover from lapses, and the conditions that facilitate recovery.
>
> (Bram & Peebles, 2014)

Understanding and assessing for the presence of such indicators could help differentiate among various diagnostic conditions such as schizophrenia, bipolar disorder, and less severe conditions, and has crucial implications for treatment.

Clinical Presentation

John, a man in his mid-20s with a diagnosis of bipolar disorder was admitted to the Clinic for further assessment and treatment. At the age of 19, he had experienced a manic episode in the context of amphetamine and opiate use. He had felt stabilized on a medication prescribed for mood stabilization for years, but a year previously he began to struggle again. The month prior to his admission, he had been hospitalized for a couple of weeks owing to ideas of reference, including the belief that he was being watched through the computer, the radio was playing in tune with his emotions, and that the specific modes of technology were directed at him in a special way to control his life. John was referred for psychological testing to clarify contributors to his symptoms and for diagnostic clarity; the possibilities that the treatment team had raised included bipolar disorder or schizoaffective disorder.

Psychodiagnostic Work

John was hesitant to engage in testing but agreed to comply with the treatment team's request. Both in his response to the TAT and the Rorschach, he was noted to lose task focus. In his stories and percepts, he tended to move too far afield and slip off track, and the examiner had difficulty following his story or the percept. His associative elaborations indicated increased distance from reality such that the perceptual reality became less and less significant and the unusual content of the associative processes became abundantly evident. However, he seemed aware of this fanciful play and was noted to enjoy playing with highly affectively charged language and colorful references. Also, during the inquiry phase, when he elaborated on his responses, the justification for them was readily seen by the examiner. John also showed a tendency toward magical thinking, whereby he attributed to the entire inkblot content that was based on only a portion of it. But again, he was aware of his "reaching out," or "extrapolating," or "stretching" in these instances.

John's perceptual distortions, strained reasoning, and the tendency to pull ideas together in a way that made sense of the situation but sacrificed his attunement to the conventional reality were not diagnostically specific. These distortions and strained reasoning could arise in multiple, widely ranging clinical circumstances (e.g., schizophrenic spectrum illness, bipolar spectrum illness, immature ego development, and playful creativity). Notably, the content was playful, jocular, and excited. Furthermore, his attitude, delivery, and/or commentary were jocular. He clearly embellished his responses, but his perceptual accuracy remained intact, and his thinking retained coherence. Also, there was no evidence of penetration, distortion, or deterioration of body/ego boundaries. As such, the examiner viewed the data as consistent with a bipolar spectrum illness, versus schizophrenia.

In addition to providing information about John's reality testing and reasoning the test data elaborated on his self-experience. The test data offered repeated and converging evidence that John felt hungry for admiration and validation as special, unique, and/or gifted. The feelings of inferiority and inadequacy seemed to color his self-experience with unhappiness, hurt, and pain. He seemed to find relief in hypomanic denial of anxiety-arousing and depressing aspects of his life situation or self-limitations or depressed, needful, and hostile feelings. The examiner empathized with John's fear that his playful, whimsical mind could get infested by negative, dark thoughts, and invited him to use treatment to understand and accept his depressing thoughts and feelings instead of being afraid of them. The examiner then worked with the treatment team to understand that John was likely to enter treatment with underlying mistrust and lack of belief that relationships could be helpful or sustaining. Moreover, his relational expectations and anxieties about needing and depending on others were likely to interfere with trust and collaboration in the treatment of his bipolar disorder and treatment compliance. While medication might play a significant role in his treatment, John needed mindful and sensitive responsiveness to his brittle self-esteem and relational ruptures in treatment. With this understanding, the repairing of John's vulnerability to emotional dysregulation in the context of a lack of an internalized helpful, caring, and collaborative other became the focus in treatment.

Conclusion: Mentalizing the "Elephant"

We believe that every psychological testing experience has the potential to clarify diagnostic dilemmas and guide treatment planning in meaningful ways. Psychological test data is a rich source of valuable treatment-relevant information and can be used to inform treatment providers about factors that facilitate and hinder the work of therapy. It can illuminate the hidden psychological forces driving the patient's suffering so that an accurate treatment focus can be developed and tailored interventions can be recommended. Most important, however, is that the focus on non-judgmental understanding of the patient's mental processes and interactions undertaken by the psychologist and the patient during the testing can serve as a model for the whole treatment. Psychological testing can be used as a stimulus to orient the patient to the treatment in general. In the context of promoting reflection and curiosity, the experience of being understood in testing can provide new emotional experiences and foster the trust of others as resources for social learning. Meaningful psychodiagnostic work demands an understanding of the whole person. Through this work, the psychologist can turn the psychodiagnostic problem of understanding the "elephant" into an asset and use it to promote a mentalizing stance in patients and treatment teams.

Notes

1 The authors would like to thank Dr. Jon G. Allen and Dr. Hector Y. Adames for their comments on an earlier draft of this chapter.

2 Case examples are composites. Personal information about patients is changed or disguised in order to protect confidentiality.

References

Akhtar, S. (2000). The shy narcissist. In J. Sandler, R. Michels, & P. Fonagy (Eds.), *Changing ideas in a changing world: The revolution in psychoanalysis – Essays in honor of Arnold Cooper* (pp. 111–119). London: Karnac.

Allen, J. G. (1981). The clinical psychologist as a diagnostic consultant. *Bulletin of Menninger Clinic, 45*, 247–258.

Allen, J. G. (2013). *Mentalizing in the development and treatment of attachment trauma*. London: Karnac.

Allen, J. G., & Fonagy, P. (2014). Mentalizing in psychotherapy. In R. E. Hales, S. C. Yudofsky, & L. Roberts (Eds.), *American Psychiatric Publishing textbook of psychiatry* (6th ed., pp. 1095–1118). Washington, DC: American Psychiatric Publishing.

Allen, J. G., Fowler, J. C., Madan, A., Ellis, T. E, Oldham, J. M., & Freuh, B. C. (2017). Discovering the impact of psychotherapeutic hospital treatment for adults with serious mental illness. *Bulletin of the Menninger Clinic, 81*, 1–38.

Allen, J. G., O'Malley, F., Freeman, C., & Bateman, A. W. (2012). Brief treatment. In P. Fonagy & A. W. Bateman (Eds.), *Handbook of mentalizing in mental health practice* (pp. 159–196). Washington, DC: American Psychiatric Publishing.

Bateman, A., & Fonagy, P. (2016). *Mentalization based therapy for personality disorders*. Oxford, London: University Press.

Bram, A. D., & Peebles, M. J. (2014). *Psychological testing that matters: Creating road map for effective treatment*. Washington, DC: American Psychological Association.

Butcher, J. N., Dahlstorm, W. G., Graham, J. R., Tellegen, A., & Kaemmer, B. (1989). *Minnesota Multiphasic Personality Inventory – 2 (MMPI-2): Manual for administration and scoring*. Minneapolis, MN: University of Minnesota Press.

Finn, S. E. (1996). Assessment feedback integrating MMPI-2 and Rorschach findings. *Journal of Personality Assessment, 67*(3), 543–557.

Finn, S. E. (1998). Teaching therapeutic assessment in a required graduate course. In C. Handler & M. Hilsenroth (Eds.), *Teaching and learning personality assessment* (pp. 359–373). Mahwah, NJ: Lawrence Erlbaum Associates, Inc.

Finn, S. E., & Tonsager, M. E. (1997). Information-gathering and therapeutic models of assessment: Complementary paradigms. *Psychological Assessment*, 9(4), 374–385.

Fonagy, P. (1989). A child's understanding of others. *Bulletin of the Anna Freud Centre, 12*, 91–115.

Fonagy, P., & Allison, E. (2014). The role of mentalizing and epistemic trust in the therapeutic relationship. *Psychotherapy, 51*, 372–380.

Fowler, J. C. (1999). Transitional relating and healthy play in treatment. *Journal of Personality Assessment, 72*(2), 218–223.

Fowler, J. C., Hilsenroth, M. J., & Handler, L. (2000). Martin Mayman's early memories technique: Bridging the gap between personality assessment and psychotherapy. *Journal of Personality Assessment, 75*(1), 18–32.

Fowler, J. C., Madan, A., Allen, J. G., Ellis, T., Mahoney, J., Hardesty, S., & Oldham, J. M. (2015). Improvement in health-related quality of life among adults with serious mental illness receiving inpatient treatment: A prospective cohort study. *The Journal of Clinical Psychiatry, 76*(5), e632–e638.

Gabbard, G. O. (1989). Two subtypes of narcissistic personality disorder. *Bulletin of the Menninger Clinic, 53*, 527–532.

Kleiger, J. H. (1999). *Disordered thinking and the Rorschach: Theory, research, and differential diagnosis.* Hillsdale, NJ: Analytic Press.

McWilliams, N. (2011). *Psychoanalytic diagnosis* (2nd ed.). New York, NY: Guilford Press.

Menninger, K., Mayman, M., & Pruyser, P. (1963). *The vital balance.* New York, NY: Viking Press.

Meyer, G. J., Viglione, D. J., Mihura, J. L., Erard, R. E., & Erdberg, P. (2011). *Rorschach Performance Assessment System: Administration, coding, interpretation, and technical manual.* Toledo, OH: Rorschach Performance Assessment System.

Mihura, J. L., Meyer, G. J., Dumitrascu, N., & Bombel, G. (2013). The validity of individual Rorschach variables: Systematic reviews and meta-analysis of the comprehensive system. *Psychological Bulletin, 139*, 548–605.

Murray, H. (1943). *Thematic Apperception Test manual.* Cambridge, MA: Harvard University Press.

Peebles-Kleiger, M. J. (2012). *Beginnings: The art and science of planning psychotherapy.* New York, NY: Routledge Taylor & Francis Group.

Rapaport, D. (1967). The theoretical implication of diagnostic testing procedures. In M. M. Gill (Ed.), *The collected papers of David Rapaport* (pp. 339–340). New York, NY: Basic Books.

Rapaport, D., Gill, M., & Schafer, R. (1968). *Diagnostic psychological testing.* New York, NY: International Universities Press.

Schafer, R. (1954). *Psychoanalytic interpretation of Rorschach testing.* New York, NY: Gruen & Stratton.

Shapiro, D. (1965). *Neurotic styles.* New York, NY: Basic Books.

Shectman, F. (1979). Problems in communicating psychological understanding: Why won't they listen to me? *American Psychologist, 34*(9), 781–790.

Weiner, I. B. (1998). *Principles of Rorschach interpretation.* Mahwah, NJ: Erlbaum.

Part 4

Clinical Psychology Internship and Supervision in the Mental Health Inpatient Setting

Introduction to Part 4

Michael Siglag and Meidan Turel

Psychologists' formal education concludes with their clinical psychology internship experiences, the culmination of years of intensive study and training. Internships provide the final groundwork of supervised practical experience before students become full-fledged clinical psychologists.

Despite common international aims to provide this professional foundation, the way internship programs are structured and carried out in different countries varies. For example, graduate students in the United States typically start their internships after they have completed their academic classroom work and several practicum-training experiences. They spend 1 year, typically full-time (or less frequently 2 years, half-time) in internship training. Most students seek acceptance in American Psychological Association (APA) accredited programs. APA accredits programs in inpatient settings, outpatient or community-based settings, college or university counseling center settings, and other settings, in which people of all ages receive treatment. 'Psychology interns' in the United States may treat adults, adolescents, and children. They are not typically required to complete any of their internship training in an inpatient setting, though many do. Interns may still have additional requirements to complete, such as a doctoral dissertation or project, before they complete their graduate education. In the United Kingdom, the achievement of a doctorate in clinical psychology entails 3 years of supervised placements (three days per week) in various settings that may or may not include inpatient units, depending on placement availability at the time of training. While not termed 'internship' training, the supervised experience that is required before completion of the Clinical Psychology doctorate appears to fulfill the same function. In Israel, the internship program takes place over 4 years, with internship training consisting of part-time experiences during each of those 4 years, with a required inpatient setting placement for a minimum of 1 year. Other countries have their own unique processes.

Preparation for the internship experience begins early in graduate school through students' establishment of clinical interests and goals.

Deciding where to apply for internship training requires serious and difficult consideration of immediate and long term professional goals. The process of applying and being accepted to internship or training programs can be stressful, fraught with obstacles and uncertainties. As with any other significant life or job event or change, internship placements can require significant personal adjustments. And the professional impact on the intern of the internship training program itself can be profound, influencing one's career in both expected and unpredictable ways.

Despite their significance, internships do not mark the end of one's professional growth. After completing their internship program training requirements, psychologists will face numerous additional professional hurdles and continued requirements throughout their careers, some of which entail further formal training and credentialing. Requirements differ between countries, but may include obtaining extended supervision prior to obtaining psychology licensure, completing postdoctoral training, passing licensing exams, fulfilling continuing education requirements, acquiring licensure in order become a credentialed supervisor, completing specialized training and passing additional evaluations in order to establish a specialty, passing tests or completing additional requirements in order to obtain employment or establish one's own practice, and fulfilling specific professional stipulations in order to maintain licensure and additional credentials.

But the internship period is unique. It marks the transition between being a student and being a professional. The experiences one has during internship training can help provide a solid basis for a fulfilling and rewarding career. Internship experiences can help evolving professionals to define or alter career interests and goals, deepen and broaden experience that can be built upon after the internship period, and develop professional relationships with peers and senior colleagues that may have long term professional and personal impact. Interns can grow through the quality of supervision they experience, or miss such opportunities if supervision is less than adequate. For many, what is most significant about the internship undertaking is that it provides the clinical experience of working in a more independent way. During the internship, students are still provided significant support and supervision, but with a diminishing safety net and with greater autonomy as the internship progresses. This may be the most potentially transformative aspect of the internship program, providing challenges that require both professional and personal growth.

Perspectives of both supervisors and interns are provided in the four chapters that comprise this part of the book. Authors provide detailed descriptions of their experiences supervising or participating in internship programs in inpatient mental health settings. Internship programs share many commonalities. Perhaps foremost to all internships is the provision of supervision and training. Yet each internship site's way of meeting intern's needs, and each intern's experience, is necessarily unique. The chapters in this part provide examples of the spectrum of the internship experience.

Daria Mamon (Chapter 19), writing as a predoctoral intern, describes experiences in mental health inpatient facilities, initially as a practicum student and culminating during her year-long experience as a psychology intern in a state psychiatric hospital in the United States. In her chapter, she focuses on the professional growth the internship afforded her, presenting case examples of therapeutic work with patients who challenged her skills and preconceptions. These experiences increased her self-awareness and growth as a therapist. Her encounters highlight a sensitivity to aspects of both the inpatient setting and the patients she worked with. She conveys awareness of the impact of an institutional setting on those being treated there, including their mental distress and loss of autonomy. She also reveals the initial impact that the inpatient setting and the individuals residing and treated in such settings can have on an early career psychologist with little previous exposure to this type of setting. Finally, she articulates the pressures she felt that were particular to her role as an intern, and the importance of mentoring and supervision in helping her both navigate this environment and assist with her growth as a clinician and professional.

Valerie Sims (Chapter 20) provides the perspective of an administrator and supervisor of interns in a predoctoral psychology internship program based in an inpatient psychiatric facility administered by the state of Colorado. Her chapter focuses on programmatic efforts made to anticipate many of the personal and professional challenges interns face during their training. Valerie elucidates and provides examples that enable the reader to see how training programs and facilities attempt to address such challenges through supervision, formal training programs, selection of relevant clinical and training experiences, encouragement of peer support and input, and in other ways. She addresses many issues encountered by interns and internship training programs, including the diverse types of prior experience and skill sets of interns, the importance of tailoring supervision to account for such variation, and the challenge of striking a balance between support, education, and evaluation. To accomplish this, Valerie provides an overview and examples that illuminate a process that is intended to help interns to thrive. An overarching theme of this chapter is recognition and understanding of the clinical internship as a path psychologists take toward increased autonomy and professional independence.

Patricia Daza and Shweta Sharma (Chapter 21), through their supervisory role and perspective, describe the internship experience at the Menninger Clinic, a private inpatient facility in Houston, Texas. The work described in this chapter deals with challenges facing psychology interns when dealing with potential and actualized patient suicide. It takes place in an inpatient program where young adult patients, many of whom present with a high risk of suicidal behavior, receive treatment. The authors provide the reader with a sense of the precariousness and potential for loss that can characterize inpatient mental health work, particularly with individuals presenting a high suicide risk. They elucidate how patients' vulnerability interfaces with the relative inexperience of psychology interns. Despite comprehensive assessment, treatment team support, treatment planning in which the patient is engaged as an active participant, as well as expert supervision guiding treatment, the patients treated in such settings are vulnerable and at times end their lives despite all efforts. The authors of this chapter describe aspects of the personal and professional impact of losing a patient as a result of the patient's suicide. They present their perspective on why, despite the potential risks, they see it as important and valuable for psychology interns to train and work in settings treating individuals with a high potential for attempting suicide. Furthermore, they enumerate the supportive supervision and program tools provided in cases when psychology interns, as well as other staff, are challenged by a patient's suicidality.

The final chapter (Chapter 22) in this part is by Karin Reddie, a clinical psychology intern who describes her work and experience providing psychotherapy in an acute closed ward in a public psychiatric inpatient facility in Israel. Karin provides a window into inpatient treatment encounters that she experienced as more intense and challenging than those she faced during her outpatient training period, providing opportunities to learn and grow in ways that were not possible in those outpatient settings. At times impressionistic, at times direct, and at times turning to professional literature to assist in her descriptions, she captures in words her encounters and her personal reactions to the therapeutic work she performed on an inpatient ward, concentrating on her therapeutic connection with a man she worked with in psychodynamically oriented psychotherapy in this often extreme environment. The importance of self-awareness, supervision, and the evolution of a way of understanding her experiences and therapeutic work come to the forefront in this evocative chapter.

Internship training in mental health inpatient facilities provides unique challenges and opportunities for trainees to grow and develop as clinical psychologists. Patients encountered and treated by interns in such settings may be more vulnerable, may present a higher risk of engaging in behaviors that put themselves and others at risk, and are more likely to be suffering greater levels of psychological disturbance and disorganization than patients treated by interns in many other settings. The environmental and clinical challenges in mental health inpatient settings are unique and can be disturbing for the caregiver as well as for those treated in such settings. For those supervising and training psychologists in these settings, awareness of and sensitivity to both the challenges and the opportunities for growth adds a dimension to training not present in most other settings, but experienced by many as worthwhile, rewarding, and leading to a more well-rounded and better-trained psychologist. The experiences and encounters described in these chapters demonstrate some of the ways in which training in inpatient settings can be carried out in ways that benefit the trainees, supervisors, and others who work with psychology interns, the facilities, and most importantly, those patients whom interns engage with in their clinical work.

19 A Clinical Psychology Intern's Experience of Training in an Inpatient Unit

No Training Wheels

Daria Mamon

Reflecting on my training experiences over the past 6 years of graduate school, my inpatient work stands out as a crucial part of my development as a clinical psychologist. I always knew I wanted to work in an inpatient setting; it seemed to be the most interesting, "hard-core," and intense work I could do in professional psychology. This work forced me to confront uncomfortable parts of myself, question what I know, and notice my own reactions, all of which allowed me to understand my patients' experiences in a deeper way. I enjoy this (sometimes) painful process as I feel that I'm learning and growing both as a person and a clinician, which is rewarding and satisfying.

People who are admitted to an inpatient psychiatric unit are often in their most acute mental state; this is where I learned about severe psychopathology from close up. It may be that another part of my attraction to work in this "hard-core" setting is the feeling of being "special" by being able to tolerate acute distress, dysfunction, and personality disorganization. It is not for everyone. It is also a place where people are restricted; rights are temporarily or permanently taken away, doors are locked, basic human functioning is dependent upon *another*; going to the bathroom, eating snacks, wearing belts, shoelaces, and scarfs, and access to personal possessions are all mediated by a treatment team's judgment calls and a step-wise process of increased privileges. It is sometimes hard to find something patients *are* allowed to do.

Even beyond the logistical aspect, there is something very primal in the way that many patients are dependent on us, as staff, for basic emotional survival, which perhaps fulfills our narcissistic needs to be the strong, nurturing, and capable *other*. It is a one-sided, very intimate encounter in which the patient is much more exposed, both literally and figuratively. I have seen my patients naked, restrained, and incontinent. I suspect that often having myself and other staff witness them in these states was just as uncomfortable for them as it was for me. There are not many settings in which the therapist has such a close view of a patient's daily life and experience. Seeing patients in their most vulnerable and acute states, stripped of typical environmental and psychological guards, might often feel invasive to both parties. The sense of boundaries in an inpatient unit is so much different than in outpatient work, and that can often feel unsettling. The psychologist's role is much more encompassing than it is in outpatient settings where patients typically have a stronger capacity to care for themselves emotionally, physically and materially.

As a trainee, I've found that many of the patients I worked with have had a great impact on me and that these emotional and relational experiences have affected my professional and personal development. In attempting to convey how working in this environment has formed my understanding of my patients and myself as a psychologist, I have chosen to describe my work with several of my patients who to date have had the greatest influence on my development as a clinician. Grappling with this material throughout the years, and in writing this chapter, I was reminded of how challenging it is to put into words this experiential, raw, human encounter. I hope these cases will demonstrate some of my experiences.

Case Vignettes

Case Number 1: Suzanne

My first experience as a therapist was with a 52-year-old woman diagnosed with chronic schizophrenia. Although this was very early in my training, I believe that in many ways my relationship with her was instrumental in my choice to continue with inpatient work. Working with Suzanne was nothing like what I imagined it would be like to work with a person with schizophrenia. When I began meeting with her, most of her presenting issues were negative symptoms of schizophrenia. I recall how emotional our first meeting was for me. We went outside, off the ward, to sit in a grassy area. She wanted to sit in the cafeteria close to others. I tried explaining that I wanted a quiet area where we could talk, only us. She agreed, so we sat down, and I introduced myself. I spoke with her about the times I would be meeting with her and the purpose of our meetings. I told her I was there for her, and that we would talk about whatever she wanted. She appeared quite satisfied and immediately asked me: "So what do you want to talk about?" I was taken aback as I assumed (and had prepared myself) for her to flood me with raw, difficult, and perhaps shocking information about her life and experiences of psychosis. I said we could talk about whatever *she* would like. She appeared a little confused and again asked about what I wanted her to tell me. I suggested that she tell me about herself. She said that she wanted to be thin. I asked her why this was important for her, and she answered: "It's the best; if you are thin, everyone loves you." I tried to help her elaborate on her perspective further. I asked her if there were any other reasons or ways for people to love her. She denied this possibility. She then took out her makeup kit and asked me to do her makeup. I was very surprised by her request. I said that I was here to listen to her. Even though I answered her softly and clearly, I felt a little angry because I thought she was not taking me seriously, as she would other, more senior, psychologists on the unit. In retrospect, I understood that this was her way of relating to me: identifying with me as a woman, asking me to care for her, to connect with her around what she regarded as most important, and possibly for her to feel beautiful with me and maybe loved by me.

In the beginning, it was very hard for me to understand what Suzanne was saying. Her speech was very unclear because she was wearing dentures, and she spoke very quickly and "swallowed" her words. It was very frustrating and uncomfortable to have to ask her to repeat herself. Her appearance was an interesting contradiction to her behavior. I related to her mentally as one would relate to a young child, but she looked significantly older than her stated age. She used to fiddle with her dentures and had a childlike presentation.

Meetings with Suzanne were often draining in their rote repetitiveness. Every session was the same process of her wanting to "hang out." I thought to myself that this was not what I had come to do; I wanted to experience therapy and meaningful dialog. I wanted depth, and instead I got emptiness, boredom, and what often felt like babysitting. I was very frustrated. I felt that I had to make her talk. I also noticed that she "absorbed" everything I said. Any reflection I made, she adapted, to the extent that she changed her feelings in response to my words. For example, in one session she arrived in a very good mood, smiling and moving around in the chair in childlike movements. She then told me she had just spent a nice week with her daughter who had left the day before. I said that it must have been very hard to say goodbye after a week of being together (usually, visits were restricted for weekends). Suddenly, she became very sad and scrunched up her face as if about to cry. It was as if she had realized that the emotion of sadness was more appropriate and true. She then started crying. I felt bad. I thought to myself that it would have been better to have said nothing. I felt powerful, but it did not feel satisfying. The thought that she simply absorbed any content that I suggested made me worry that I was not doing my job properly. I thought that I needed to be very careful about what I said, which frightened me. It was as though she had such a limited sense of self; she was so disintegrated and detached, and dependent on me to *identify* and *integrate*.

The images that came to my mind in our meetings were of scattered islands in a big ocean. I often noticed that my reflections helped her make meaning of her experience. At times it felt superficial and was hard for me to regard or accept that this was therapeutic. I remember feeling consumed with responsibility to help her develop a coherent sense of self by "holding the islands together." Her dependency on me was overwhelming and made me want to reject her. I often experienced her as too "needy," which brought up anxiety about my ability to fulfill her needs adequately. This was surprising to me given that I typically gain a sense of security and satisfaction from relationships in which I feel needed. I wondered if this was in a way an enactment of her relationship with her mother, who rejected her needs and was neglectful.

The supervision I received was essential and helped me to understand Suzanne, my own reactions, and how to better help her. I remember feeling agitated, confused, and flooded with emotions. Through supervision, I came to understand how her illness impacted her emotional experience and expression, and related thinking.

It was difficult for her to generate her own ideas and conversation since her internal world was so constricted. Over time, I understood that she did not need me to interpret her words or give her advice. She needed me on a primal level: she needed my presence and nurturance, in the way that a mother nurtures her child. Unconsciously, she related to me as if I was part of her, an extension of her body, in which I was an object, not a subject. Like an infant that becomes less anxious in its mother's presence. It was difficult for me to completely detach from my own need for recognition and to let her "use" me as the container she needed me to be because I lacked the confidence and training at that point. Developmentally, Suzanne had an undifferentiated sense of self that required me to lend my own internal world, allowing her to find and understand herself *through* me. She needed containment and structure to understand her own emotional experience. I realized that I was valuable to her and that lending myself to this process created some change in her. It was rewarding to witness. Exposing myself to another person and fulfilling their emotional needs was a meaningful experience for me. To sit with the unknown and unexpected was initially very hard but as I allowed myself to be "in the moment" it became more manageable.

Being with her increased my curiosity and excitement to encounter further challenging clinical situations. Working with Suzanne taught me, in a very profound way, the impact that the therapeutic relationship has on me as a therapist and how demanding and yet rewarding this work is. I think that the inpatient setting and the severity of her symptoms amplified this understanding for me in a way that a higher functioning, more differentiated person might not have. This relationship opened my eyes to the potential conflict between my own narcissistic needs to be recognized and to have a "therapeutic impact," and the needs of the client. It made me more aware, open, and receptive to how a client may need to use me as an object in their own movement toward self-coherence.

Case Number 2: Janice

Janice was a 29-year-old woman diagnosed with schizophrenia who reported a sexual trauma history. She came from a religious household and was raised in a very strict setting. Her psychotic process was clinically fascinating. She had unique tactile hallucinations of being touched and associated paranoid delusions, as well as omnipotent thoughts of mind-reading and communicating with the dead. She felt disturbed by this (perceived) power of hers, was terrified, and wanted her mind "to stop thinking." Her tactile sensations of being touched reportedly started around the age of 19, which was also around the time she started having sexual thoughts, thoughts that were forbidden within the context of her cultural-religious background. She was also sexually assaulted around the age of 21, which likely further impaired her perception and tolerance of healthy sexual desires and boundaries. In one of our first sessions, she talked about her ability to change a person's mind, to make people "do things." She seemed to have a delusional sense of agency that was powerful yet destructive. For example, in one session she reported that she "brought down an airplane" just by thinking it. She was very distressed by these delusions and described these thoughts as debilitating and difficult to undermine and challenge. She often felt isolated and lonely, but at the same time worried about people looking at her and invading her space, assuming that others could penetrate her physical space as she could do to others. Her paranoia and anxiety were present in our therapy sessions as well. She often questioned my motives and asked me many personal questions about my background. She was often worried that I was part of the CIA and that it was unsafe for her to disclose her omnipotent thoughts to me. In those moments she experienced me as an intruder and potential threat to her, which I understood to be similar to the way she experienced others, particularly her mother. Her unpredictability made sitting with her stressful because it was not clear whether she would feel threatened and targeted by me, or regard me as safe and supportive. It made me feel hypervigilant as if I should carefully choose my words. I felt she was repeating a victim/perpetrator relational pattern with me, which made me wonder if this had been her experience with her mother. I often found myself in the rescuer position with her. At times I would help her communicate with the staff and walk her over to different parts of the hospital. I sensed that she needed protection and I felt for her, and thus sometimes provided that "protection."

Janice's family had a very low socio-economic background, and both her sister and her mother had struggled with mental health issues. Her mother would often make derogatory comments toward her and dismiss her attempts at recovery (e.g., finding a job). The sense of interpersonal boundaries in the family was very poor, and her mother was very controlling of her. Janice was ambivalent about her relationship with her mother. On the one hand, she felt very attached to her mother, and wanted her acceptance and approval; on the other hand, she was enraged with her mother for how she treated her in childhood (e.g., verbal abuse, neglect). This ambivalence would become intertwined with psychosis and emerge in therapy when she would push me away if she felt we were getting (too) close.

Although she was able to engage in some reality testing, Janice remained very vulnerable to delusional, particularly referential, thinking. She had some insight and self-awareness, noticing when she started having more delusional thoughts. Unfortunately, this awareness would (at times) increase her hopelessness and general distress. I provided some psychoeducation about her beliefs and gradually helped her to find meaning in her delusions. Together we examined some of the thoughts she captured in the thought record sheet we had created. We also did some reality testing (i.e., cognitive restructuring) by working collaboratively to refute her beliefs about controlling others' feelings and reactions and replacing them with more realistic alternate beliefs. We tried to think about things that would help her ground herself in reality, using external stimuli such as cold water, ice, or a stress ball. She began to notice that when she became more emotional, her thinking became more disorganized and delusional. Gradually, Janice became aware of her need to control me and our relationship and able to notice this feeling in her and check her behavior. This seemed to help her separate from me, and, gradually, to a greater degree, separate from her mother. She began to be more assertive and to communicate her thoughts and feelings to her mother. She even ultimately left the hospital for a group home without her mother knowing.

Her relationship with her mother was overly enmeshed and symbiotic, and she was never able to fully separate. Her needs for individuation (as well as her pull for enmeshment) came up in sessions, and since it took me a while to recognize them, we initially enacted her relationship with her mother. Although I was not controlling her through derogatory comments (as her mother often did), I took a more active and directive role in our relationship than I typically would with other patients. I recognized that I had a need to take care of her and possibly "rescue" her from her painful experiences. These attempts were at times interpreted by Janice as my way to control her, which made her push away, rebel against and reject my help; for example, by not completing the homework assignments or not showing up for treatment sessions on time. As I grew aware of her need for autonomy and control in the relationship, I started to provide more options so that she would not feel obliged to please me. I believe that structuring our relationship in a collaborative way allowed for autonomy within boundaries and empowered Janice in developing a realistic sense of self-control that helped organize and contain her. Her process of differentiation and push for boundaries (both physical and mental) helped her establish a sense of self. She was able to experience my presence, my mind, without being either consumed by it or needing to take control of it. I believe this was healing for her in some way; experiencing agency and control, and seeing herself as a competent adult allowed her to differentiate herself both from me and from her mother.

Janice taught me how to let go, to be led by *another*. Something about her growth process and separation–individuation capacity stayed with me. The concept of boundaries in relationships in general, and in my therapeutic relationships specifically, continues to accompany me, especially when encountering emotionally intense therapeutic relationship processes.

Case Number 3: Jorge

By the time I started working with Jorge, aged 31, he had been receiving treatment for his psychotic illness for several years. He had developed some insight and recognized his psychotic symptoms as part of a mental illness, and had come to accept this as part of his life that required ongoing treatment. Although he was taking his antipsychotic medication regularly, he continued to experience auditory hallucinations. He would converse with the voices on a daily basis, sometimes for a significant part of the day. In fact, the voices were his main source of social interaction, one that he generally found more interesting and entertaining than real-world interactions. Although he still preserved some awareness that the voices were "not real" he enjoyed bickering with them, especially defeating them in arguments. He would draw special satisfaction from humiliating them and making them feel "stupid," essentially offering counter-arguments that would confuse and anger "them." He had partial insight into his illness – he knew that the voices were not real, but at the same time he would derive satisfaction and power from insulting them. Working with him provided a fascinating opportunity to learn about the mind and its capacity to generate such ideas. Jorge expressed interest in working on managing how he related to the voices. He acknowledged spending much of his day talking to them, which limited his ability to engage in real conversations and activities. He even expressed interest in setting a few goals for his recovery, including going back to school and improving his physical health. On the surface, his interests appeared straightforward. I remember coming into sessions feeling motivated to work with him on reducing the voices' influence on him. I taught him different "cognitive behavioral therapy for psychosis" techniques related to monitoring his voices and using distraction skills to manage them. However, I soon learned this was not a fully shared goal. Jorge also liked having the voices around. He did not have much interest in engaging with his peers or hospital-based activities, including recovery and treatment groups. He felt discouraged, stuck, powerless, and in a way I also believe hopeless about ever being able to move past this stage in his life. Without his voices, he felt bored, disempowered, and sometimes lonely. He would often initiate and invite a conversation with the voices, thus contributing significantly to their maintenance by reinforcing their presence. His ambivalence about his voices soon became a topic of exploration for us, which he ultimately recognized, but resisted working on. This made it difficult to sit through our sessions. Jorge would not engage in much conversation, and I felt that I had to pull information out of him. My reflections were either ignored or dismissed by him. He told me once that his voices said I was "stupid." He would often forget to attend our sessions. His affect was typically constricted and detached. I felt self-conscious about what I wanted to say, often feeling as though my own mind was disorganized and out of my control, which in a way served as a window to his experience. Jorge had little experience of control or agency in his life. He was abused as a child by his father and was haunted for years by the relentless harassment of his derogatory and accusatory voices in the context of untreated psychosis, during much of his 20s.

A particular session highlighted for me his low sense of agency and control and provided a better understanding of his object relations. This session started with efforts on my part to talk about his motivation for treatment and to assess whether he actually wanted to work on managing his voices. Unexpectedly, I found myself telling him that I was feeling frustrated that he was not taking the therapy seriously (perhaps not taking me seriously), often forgetting sessions and not engaging. I said that I was putting a lot of effort into trying to be helpful to him, and needed him to show that he was interested; otherwise, I could not help him. He seemed quite taken aback by my comment, perhaps even overwhelmed. I did not plan this intervention, so I cannot say I skillfully created this situation, but I believe that my unintentional self-disclosure and expression of my emotional vulnerability showed him that he had an impact *on me*. Conceivably, that provided some sense of worthiness, agency, and control which made him feel more connected and interested. Jorge apologized and reassured me that he was interested in working with me. This was the first time we had a conversation as two individuals, rather than me holding back and trying to contain his emotions without revealing my own. I remember being afraid that I might have come across as demanding or maybe even shaming or punitive. I then took a step back and was more passive for the rest of the session, and he was able to be somewhat more active in the conversation. The following session he arrived on time and completed the symptom log I had given him. He was excited to show it to me, to be recognized by me, and to show that he recognized me as well.

Jorge never stopped conversing with his voices. Our sessions focused on developing our relationship, and his engagement with me seemed to increase. We also shifted to a more activity-based therapy in which we played cards and took walks together which appeared to support him in expressing a wider set of interests and emotions. This targeted his negative symptoms of schizophrenia and indirectly reduced the amount of time he felt bored, hopeless, and engaged with his voices. I also noticed that I was able to be more relaxed and relate to him more naturally. I still struggled to find meaning in our encounters and feared that without the imposed structure of the worksheets and other measures of success, I was not providing him with *meaningful* therapy. At the same time, I knew that I was meeting him where he was emotionally and relationally at the time, which felt *right*.

Case Number 4: James

"Oh my god, you were assigned to work with James? Wooow, good luck ... You know, he was smearing feces on the walls and throwing it at staff ...," said my colleague as she twisted her face in disgust.

The first time I met James, a 42-year-old man diagnosed with Bipolar I disorder with psychotic features, I was naturally worried. He extended his hand to shake mine, and I was hesitant because, aside from what my colleague said, I also learned that he was extremely violent, aggressive, and hypersexual. I was afraid to meet him. He came from jail on a detention order due to an increase in manic and psychotic symptoms. They wheeled him down in a smock suit and a spit mask. He spent most of his first few weeks in seclusion and at times in restraints. This must be the most dehumanizing aspect of mental health "treatment." It was scary to hear about, and I later learned from him how scary and humiliating it was for him. The amazing thing was that James turned out to be my favorite client. He was excited to meet with me (which made me feel valuable), and he would tell me all sorts of interesting stories about his love life and travel adventures. I looked forward to our meetings and had a sense of loss when he left. We only worked together for three months, and during those months I watched his affect become calmer, his thought process become more organized and focused, and his relational capacity deepen. As he was "sobering up" (as he described it) to reality, he started recalling and sharing with me difficult situations he had encountered. He told me about the correctional officers beating and humiliating him, and how painful it was to be isolated and rejected in his cell. James admitted he gave them a hard time, but it still seemed like unjust behavior toward someone who clearly was significantly ill. He often described his experience of coming out of the manic episode as an embarrassing and shaming experience. He shared that his psychiatrist, in an attempt to do some reality testing with him, would remind him of previous delusional beliefs he held when he was psychotic. James would describe these meetings as "stupid." He spoke about how uncomfortable it was to learn that he endorsed delusions about joining the CIA, and how much more uncomfortable it was to be reminded of that at every meeting. I was angry with the psychiatrist for not being sensitive to his feelings. I felt protective of James, which I now can see was an indication of the commonly occurring splitting among staff.

Initially, James was very tangential in his thinking; his speech was pressured, and his voice became silly, even childlike, particularly in moments when he was talking about emotional experiences, which was something he tried to avoid. As we worked together, he was more capable of sitting with difficult emotions and talking about some painful, traumatic experiences from previous incarcerations, and about losses that he had experienced. It was difficult to realize that his improvement in symptoms and stabilization meant that he would go back to jail. Since he was on a detention order, he was not allowed to leave the unit, when otherwise he could have gone on some outings and had more diversified and healing experiences. This often made me feel stuck, helpless, and frustrated, as I imagined he might also be feeling. When I asked him about this, he had an interesting view of this situation: he wanted to sleep off his time in the hospital, hibernate, and go back to jail. To him, being in the "nut house" (as he described it), and being surrounded by other male, mentally ill patients was "worse" than jail. It was a confirmation that he might be "one of them." Also, for James, jail had a definite release date, while at the hospital his discharge date was uncertain and, in his view, out of his control. The only thing he was able to control was when he would shower, and whether he would go to groups. For James, this was a difficult feeling because he described himself as a free spirit. He liked to travel and to enjoy life, and he had a somewhat a rebellious nature. On my part, I felt that I was becoming more and more aware of the restriction and limitation of the inpatient unit, perhaps identifying with his free spirit and need for independence, autonomy, and control.

I found that as an intern, especially when working within inpatient settings, I often felt a need to show that I accomplished something with the person, and that pushed me from the "being" into the "doing" mode. With James, I learned that making the person feel heard, validated, and valued was sometimes the most effective therapeutic intervention. I found that providing him with some agency within the therapeutic relationship was liberating even in this restricted setting.

I had a positive countertransference to James; somehow his grotesque behavior, aggression, and legal history no longer scared or disgusted me. We had playful interactions; I felt lighter, allowing myself to contain him, and allowing him to impact me. Even when he made a racial comment about being of the "White supremacy race," I was still able to see him as *whole* and have positive feelings toward him. I related to him. I found him to be a funny, vulnerable man, and I felt for him. It was easy to connect to him because he willingly connected with me, which perhaps fed my narcissistic need to feel valuable and helpful to someone else, particularly someone whom colleagues had avoided or harbored pessimistic feelings about. I think that his demeanor made me "softer," more open, and empathic, which allowed for a deeper, more holistic understanding of James as a person, beyond his symptoms.

At this point in my personal and professional development, I found that the most clinically challenging situations for me are with mistrusting and rejecting patients. They make me feel most insecure, incompetent, and vulnerable, all of which are feelings that are difficult for me to sit with. James, on the other hand, was willing and interested in working with me. My work with Alan would pose different challenges.

Case Number 5: Alan

Alan was a 64-year-old man who was admitted to the hospital following a suicide attempt. He had been the main caregiver for his mother whom he had lost a few years prior to his hospitalization. He was living with his younger sister whom he described as judgmental and dismissive of him. Alan worked as a clerk but had injured his back and became unable to work, which increased his depression and sense of hopelessness. Alan had many complaints. He was unhappy with other patients' behavior, with his social worker, and with the way the hospital functioned in general. He constantly felt as though people were failing him. I surely failed him too. Anytime I would try to make a point he would get angry and frustrated with me. He repeated: "Well this is how I am." Even though I was trying to be empathic and validate his feelings, my attempts were never received well. In our work together, I found myself struggling to maintain unconditional positive regard, as he often devalued and dismissed me. I did not get to say much, since he did most of the talking, leaving me feeling that he was not interested in what I had to say. Part of what created our dynamic in the room was that I often felt rushed and dismissed by him, which increased my need to show that I was valuable at any opportunity I might get to own the "stage." We enacted what seemed to be a familiar relational pattern for him, perhaps based on his relationship with his mother who was critical of him. His guardedness was related to his need to maintain control and appear self-sufficient. On my part, I connected my feelings to my own sense of vulnerability to rejection, particularly in the role of a trainee. Whenever I tried to make a reflection or join with him in his experience, he dismissed it by saying he was "all set." I felt like there was no space for me and my worthiness in the room, which pushed me to claim and prove it.

This dynamic initially created negative feelings in me, making it difficult for me to show up for our sessions. Supervision helped me explore our interaction more objectively, which increased my understanding of his rejection as an enactment of his longstanding narcissistic injury; this in turn allowed me to adapt a more empathic stance and be more compassionate toward his difficulties. This shift in my attitude helped me monitor my reactions and my need to prove my worthiness. I noticed that in moments that *I* felt insecure or incompetent, I shifted to a teaching role, a more comfortable role. It made me feel safer because it supposedly kept me in the *certain*, knowledgeable position. It took a lot for me to tolerate not having a voice in the relationship. I found that when I had empathy toward him it was easier for me to be more gentle and understanding, which reduced my need to prove my value. I think that in those moments I felt closer to him and our connection was stronger. I wanted to be able to talk with him about his impact on me because I believed it could have been an empowering and informative experience of an authentic *other* for him, but we did not have a strong enough rapport to do so during the short time we worked together.

Alan communicated his needs for differentiation in a more developed way than Janice was able to, but he was still very emotionally fragile. He had a greater capacity to communicate his feelings verbally. In a similar fashion to a teenager working through his separation-individuation process, he was defiant and pushed back against my comments, which allowed him to define boundaries for himself. He needed to be recognized, but at the same time he felt threatened by his relational needs, particularly his dependency needs. In those moments, when we got too close too fast, I experienced him as a hedgehog who in response to threat, protectively curls up into a ball and uses its quills to reject the connection. He was sensitive to rejection and learned ways to protect himself from needing others.

A Few Things I Have Learned

Thinking about the cases presented above, I feel a strong sense of gratitude and appreciation for the experiences gained in my inpatient training. Developmentally, the traineeship is a crucial and formative time that helps to establish and to cultivate an emerging professional identity and understanding of complex human experience. I found the inpatient internship experience exciting because of the opportunity to encounter patients in their utmost acute, raw mental state. In inpatient settings, the trainee is often confronted with the patient's needs in a way that makes it difficult to remain indifferent. Constant exposure to the unpredictable and unknown is exciting and scary at the same time. I found that for me, working in the inpatient setting provided an unexpected sense of calm, knowing that there might not be one "right way." This perspective allows for ruptures and repair in the relationship, which can set in motion a therapeutic relationship that is authentic and powerful.

I also had to confront uncomfortable feelings related to incompetence, which challenged my ideals about what it means to be "productive": or actively achieving something in therapy. Interestingly, despite the fast-paced environment in an inpatient unit, the therapeutic process could feel longer and slower. There is much value in learning to pace yourself as a trainee, as I think we often have omnipotent wishes to "fix" people. The disillusionment that we are all "only human," and that the patient is often not ready to change, can be painful. I find it an important learning experience to meet people where they are at, and adjust the treatment and, perhaps most important, one's approach to the therapeutic relationship accordingly. My definition of what constitutes "therapy" was broadened and became more flexible as I responded to what each person needed from me.

The psychologists I consider to have been my mentors were all comfortable and confident with making mistakes and with tolerating uncertainty. This made them human and admirable to me. I hope that I will become comfortable with the knowledge and skills that I have, while continuing to grow and develop through my experiences, without uncertainty or lack of knowledge threatening my perception of myself as a good (enough) therapist. I find that the most rewarding and memorable patients with whom I worked were the most difficult ones because they challenged and changed the way I think about myself and my limitations and vulnerabilities, which hopefully will make me a better clinician.

Even with the support of supervisors and mentors, inpatient work often feels like riding a bicycle for the first time without the aid of the stabilizing training wheels. There is no protection from the fall and the pain that comes with it, which is exactly why the experience is so powerful. The impact that my patients had on me made me more comfortable with the next fall, allowing me to acquire balance. I know I will survive the fall. In a way, much like learning how to ride a bicycle, the inpatient unit experience is ingrained in me like a procedural memory. Not in the sense that I can control the situation, but rather knowing that I will find a way to tolerate whatever I will encounter. In that sense, finding answers to the challenging emotional experience of training in an inpatient unit brings with it development and growth of ego capacity.

As I recognized, accepted, and worked on my needs in the therapeutic relationships, it became easier for me to be more attuned to my patient's needs. I became more comfortable with failing and not knowing. That made me braver, able to be more vulnerable and open to experience, and thus, I think, a better psychologist. This experience enhanced my understanding and capacity for empathy, especially when working with people with psychotic disorders, whose daily experiences are often so distinct from my own.

Whether or not I will continue working in an inpatient unit throughout my career, the experiences I have had as a trainee in this setting will remain an invaluable and deeply formative part of my learning experience and professional development.

20 The Benefits and Challenges of Clinical Psychology Internships in Psychiatric Inpatient Settings

Valerie Sims

Obtaining and successfully completing a psychology internship in the United States, particularly one accredited by the American Psychological Association (APA), is a significant accomplishment which follows years of professional training and preparation. By the time interns begin their internship, they have completed their doctoral studies, sometimes including a terminal master's degree, which takes between 8 and 12 years including undergraduate work. Interns are often still in the process of writing a dissertation and have accumulated between 500 and 1,000 hours of experience working in a psychological capacity in various treatment settings across different populations. The internship is considered pre-doctoral because it is the final requirement of doctoral-level training, and must be successfully completed before a doctoral degree will be awarded.

Following the completion of their doctoral studies, and practicum or externship training at several sites under the supervision of licensed psychologists, potential interns apply throughout the country to sites that meet their desired training goals. They travel to those sites that invite them to interview and then participate in a computer matching program. According to the Association of Psychology Postdoctoral and Internship Centers' (APPIC) website (www.appic.org/), the match rate for the 2017–2018 academic year was 95%. While a high percentage of applicants were selected at internship programs where they applied, 5% of applicants, or 169 individuals, did not obtain an APA-accredited psychology internship through the APPIC match process. Of the 3,881 internship positions offered in the 2017–2018 academic year, only a small percentage of the positions available were within inpatient psychiatric settings, making these settings among the most competitive in the match process.

Internship placement can significantly impact a psychologist's post-internship training choices, job opportunities, and credentialing throughout their career. In the United States, some jobs are only accessible to applicants who have completed their training in APA-accredited doctoral programs and internships. Requirements for licensure vary by state in the United States. Most states require the successful completion of the Examination for Professional Practice of Psychology (EPPP), or licensure exam, developed by the Association of State and Provincial Psychology Boards (ASPPB). Additionally, post-internship training, in formal post-doctoral training sites or supervised employment, is required by many states within the United States, usually 1 calendar year accruing between 1,500 and 2,000 supervised hours of experience or work.

Interns may arrive at their internship sites with strong backgrounds in some theoretical orientations and with little exposure to other approaches. For example, they may be trained in cognitive behavioral therapy, but not psychodynamic methods. Likewise, some interns are exposed to certain assessment methods and not others. For example, they may be trained to use the Minnesota Multiphasic Personality Inventory, second edition (MMPI-2) and not the Personality Assessment Inventory (PAI) or any projective measures, such as the Rorschach Inkblot Test. Furthermore, their individual comfort level working with patients, particularly those with severe and persistent mental illness, varies based on interns' past experience and opportunities. Such variation in pre-internship training leads to numerous challenges when selecting didactic experiences to provide intern classes, in matching interns with supervisors, and in providing individualized education and supervision.

Variations in graduate school and other pre-internship training experience means that at the onset of the internship, each intern has had a different type and amount of professional training. Some began working with patients during the pursuit of their master's degree, others not until beginning their doctoral work. Some have done the majority of their work in their doctoral program's outpatient clinic; others have trained throughout the community in outpatient mental health centers, private practices, inpatient psychiatric hospitals, medical hospitals, Veteran's Affairs hospitals, university counseling centers, and correctional facilities. Every intern presents with a unique set of experiences. The range of experience of incoming interns poses the first major challenge to inpatient psychiatric internship sites. Because of this variation in previous training, it is important to evaluate intern competence and experience level working with severely and persistently mentally ill individuals at the onset of the internship. These evaluations assist training directors to tailor the internship program to meet each individual intern's needs so that training experiences are at an appropriate level for all interns. It is also essential to continue this assessment for each intern throughout their training year in order to gauge progress.

In addition to these challenges coordinating training for interns with varied prior experiences and training foundations, basic logistical challenges often arise early in the internship. An APA pre-doctoral psychology internship is generally 1 year long. Interns' hours are generally equivalent to full-time positions, 40 hours per week, though in some instances the internship can be completed part-time over the course of 2 years, with interns working 20 hours per week. For many interns, this is their first experience working in a full-time capacity. Prior to the internship training year, the interns in most instances were practicum students who worked approximately 16 to 20 hours per week, without pay or benefits, while simultaneously attending their doctoral program classes. Once they begin their internship, interns have left the familiarity of academic life and are not afforded the time off that academic schedules allow. In addition, many interns are still working on their dissertations, requiring additional work on top of their workweek schedules. This shift from full-time student to full-time employee can be very challenging, particularly for individuals who have never previously worked full-time.

Managing a new role with less direct oversight and guidance than they were provided in prior training experiences encourages them to rely on their own knowledge and skills; however, this can prove overwhelming for an intern who does not feel well prepared for such an undertaking. In order to help interns adjust to their new role and work environment, it is important to set expectations up front and early. This includes discussions regarding hours, pay, and dress code as well as details like lunch breaks and office space. They should be made aware of their chain of command and be informed about whom to approach with concerns. They should also be made aware of other services and benefits available through the workplace, and whether or not they are optional, such as retirement programs, and opportunities or requirements to work overtime hours.

To add to the stress of beginning their first full-time job within their field, some interns have moved away from home, are separated from family and friends, sometimes even living apart from their spouse and children. These conditions can limit the support they have outside of internship. The limited vacation time available to visit family and friends can make this even more difficult. Often interns, particularly those relocating for internship, experience significant loneliness and social isolation. Many utilize their fellow interns or cohort as sources of support and companionship. When asked, one intern stated: "this is a built-in friend and peer group with whom I can get support for the transitions and vent about negative experiences." Some relationships established during the internship experience develop into lifelong friendships. Such sources of support are particularly important in this field, which can often be emotionally very strenuous. However, not all interns can rely on their cohort for support. Some interns may not have a cohort or their cohort may not be housed in the same location, making contact limited. It is also possible that individuals in the cohort will not relate well to each other and develop an unhealthy interpersonal dynamic that impacts their ability to engage in their work effectively. In facilities where the interns interact frequently, it is important to address major conflicts early on in order to prevent problematic issues from increasing in magnitude. If this happens, it is very possible that the negative interpersonal dynamics among the intern group will overshadow and distract from clinical work and training, or even pose safety concerns for the individual interns in the group. At our site, we maintain a cohort of three interns annually. In many cases, two interns become close, and the third is not as involved in the cohort. This can lead to communication failures, disorganization, and a general sense of displeasure for the interns, particularly on projects requiring the entire cohort's participation. Over time, the interns may become focused on their own relationships with each other more than they are on their clinical work, leading to a lack of training progress, and interfering with patient care. When this occurs, interns' supervisors may become distracted and focused on the interns' relationships with each other as opposed to addressing skills based issues due to the impact of strained relationships on the overall training experience.

During their internship year, some interns are also working on finishing their doctoral dissertation. They may be traveling back and forth to their graduate schools to meet with advisors and complete their dissertations and defenses. In addition, many interns are worried about what will come next and quite a few have accumulated excessive amounts of student loan debts due to the high cost of advanced degrees, and may not be sure if they will have a job after internship to help them make the large monthly payments. Upon starting an internship, interns may already be preparing to apply for post-doctoral positions. Others may be looking into potential work opportunities for the following year. Both post-doctoral positions and employment opportunities often include moving to another new location. It may sound dramatic, but we should never assume the internship will be "easy" or "fun." Though the overall experience may be positive, the internship year can be one of the most stressful years in the life of a psychologist-to-be.

Supervision

Supervision is the single most important factor in any internship program regardless of setting, resources, clientele, or past intern experiences. For the intern, good, solid supervision can help them develop previously underdeveloped skills as well as sharpen and solidify those that are already present. On the contrary, inadequate supervision can contribute to interns' failure to grow and progress as a psychologist. Sadly, this is not something in the control of the intern. Supervisors are not required by the American Psychological Association (APA – www.apa.org/) or by most internship sites to demonstrate specific training in supervision before supervising interns. The APA dictates that intern supervisors "are doctoral-level psychologists who have primary professional responsibility for the cases on which they provide supervision, and are appropriately credentialed to practice psychology in the jurisdiction in which the internship is located." Supervisor training can be completed through continuing education or informally within a consultation group among the psychologists. Supervisor training can be focused on approaches to supervision, and on recognizing and resolving problems in intern's work, as well as ensuring that specific competencies are established on which to evaluate interns, and processes are in place to enable supervisors to recognize if training expectations are not being met.

One common and effective way of increasing consistency among supervisors in an internship setting is through regular meetings held with intern's supervisors. In such meetings, the psychologists providing the supervision and the training director(s) meet to discuss the current status of each intern, successes, areas of growth, concerns that require addressing, the type of supervision being conducted, and how the intern is responding to supervision. An intern supervisors' meeting not only increases consistency of the supervision work but also provides opportunities for sharing of multiple opinions and methods of approaching situations so that the supervisors can consult and identify how to handle various situations. In addition, information shared during these meetings informs future supervisors of the interns' strengths and recommendations for further development. This is particularly important at sites where there are multiple rotations and supervisors. That being said, it is important that this meeting be used to constructively solve problems rather than to complain or vent, which can occur when there are significant concerns with the intern class.

According to the APA guidelines, an intern is required to obtain a minimum of four hours of supervision per week, two of which must take place in individual supervision. The other two hours can be carried out in group supervision, didactics, or through interactions with other psychologists or the training director(s). Intern sites fulfill APA's supervision requirements in a variety of ways. There are sites that provide a full four hours or more of formal supervision, including group supervision and supervision that addresses particular treatment issues or focuses on applying particular treatment models. How supervision is provided depends on factors such as the quality and number of available supervisors, time available to staff to provide supervision, productivity demands on interns, areas of expertise of supervisors, etc. In inpatient settings, it is very common for the extra two hours of supervision to be provided periodically during the work day in an informal manner. This often occurs on the treatment unit when situations arise that lead to interns seeking supervisory support, or that the intern and supervisor can approach together.

As mentioned above, didactic training is another primary component of a pre-doctoral internship and can consist of a variety of subject areas. These may include therapeutic techniques, theoretical orientations, program development and evaluation, forensic issues, diagnosis-specific training, psychopharmacology, alternative treatment modalities, and training on specific assessment measures. Time set aside for didactic training can also be used for group supervision on individual therapy cases, group therapy issues, styles of supervision, and specific assessment case consultation. Furthermore, other professionals including psychiatrists, social workers, nurses, recreation therapists, expressive arts therapists, and occupational therapists may educate interns about their areas of expertise. In order to allow for the most collaborative internship experience, it can be helpful to elicit didactic requests from interns early in their internship year. This helps faculty to tailor training to each intern class' training needs and interests while still maintaining a core curriculum in order to meet APA requirements.

Preparing for Long Term Goals

It is integral to a good internship program that supervisors help interns look beyond the internship year. Early on in the internship, it is helpful to identify interns' future goals and provide them with support in working toward those goals. Knowledge of interns' goals can help ensure that interns are provided with the exposure and experience that they need in order to pursue their goals. Examples include the provision of trauma treatment training, or neuropsychology training and experience if a formal post-doctoral position in one of those specialties is their intention. Preparing interns for life after internship also includes encouraging and helping them to update their curriculum vitae, learn up to date job and postdoc search techniques, and identify requirements that lay ahead, such as state requirements for licensure, preparation for the licensure exam (EPPP), and documentation of hours on internship. If an intern is planning to practice in a state that does not require post-doctoral hours for licensure, it may behoove the intern to consider studying for and taking the licensure exam prior to the completion of the internship. This may be a stressful and time-consuming undertaking; however, having a license to practice makes the process of finding a job significantly easier. Although ultimately researching and following through on these tasks are the interns' responsibility, such tasks are often not something within their awareness when beginning an internship as it can already be such an overwhelming time. Internship training programs can help provide interns with a basic overview of these topics and provide them resources to find the appropriate information, perhaps in didactic training. Although initially stressful for the intern, ultimately this prevents the panic that can occur later in the internship year, which can significantly distract interns from their training and assigned clinical work.

Interns are constantly under stress. Providing support and encouraging stress management are vital parts of supervision and the training program as a whole. Many interns can benefit from assistance in developing and utilizing skills such as time management and organizational techniques. Attending to self-care and coping mechanisms in supervision can help ensure that an intern is not allowing the stress of internship to build to an unhealthy level. Some hospitals offer wellness programs for staff, which include exercise classes or meetings with nutritionists. It can be helpful for supervising psychologists to model and encourage participation in these types of staff wellness activities. If stress and anxiety levels are rising to an unhealthy level or if personal or emotional issues are tapped into through the intern's clinical work, supervisors are in a position to encourage interns to seek additional help, such as personal therapy. This allows interns to process their own emotional responses and promotes ongoing personal and professional growth. Although this cannot be required, it can be discussed and suggested. It is helpful for internship sites to have a list of local resources, including low-cost providers for interns, to access if desired. Often, therapy services are available free of charge through an Employee Assistance Program and should be advertised at the onset of internship and periodically throughout the year.

Developing Autonomy and Professional Identity

The best way for a supervisor to prepare a pre-doctoral psychology intern for their career is to encourage them to develop independence and autonomy during their internship year. When interns begin their training, the assumption can be made that they most likely have at least a basic understanding of therapeutic and assessment techniques, as well as some degree of practice in both areas. However, it is unlikely they have had much opportunity to develop a professional identity or time to develop awareness of their professional presence within a multidisciplinary treatment team (MDT). Although interns require some training on the specifics of the site at the onset of the internship, once the basics are covered, it is important they are allowed freedom and autonomy in order to discourage dependence on others. Following several years of practicum training in which they were provided limited responsibility, interns may initially feel uncomfortable with this independence. It is helpful for supervisors to provide some initial structure and training, though also to allow the intern to experience independent structuring of their work, setting priorities, and functioning as treatment team members. For example, interns may begin consulting with the treatment team on specific patients, particularly those with whom they are conducting an assessment or providing individual therapy. As a major part of the MDT on an inpatient psychiatric unit, an intern acts as an extension of the psychologist. This includes providing individual and group therapy, conducting cognitive, personality, and risk assessments, completing intake evaluations, providing consultation, and sometimes providing supervision to other team members. Other duties may include conducting legal evaluations, writing court documents, and creating and implementing behavior management and reinforcement programs. Although all of these responsibilities are supervised by a licensed psychologist, the amount of direct oversight can vary based on the comfort level of the supervisor and the demonstrated skill of the intern.

Feeling as though they are truly part of a treatment team has been noted by past interns as a primary factor related to satisfaction with their internship. One intern stated: "it really helped me solidify my professional identity in who I was as a psychologist and what I have uniquely to offer to a team setting." Another intern stated: "being part of an interdisciplinary clinical team of skillful and experienced individuals who acted so effectively and seamlessly toward a common goal, particularly under pressure, gave me a sense of purpose and exhilaration."

A responsibility of a good internship program is ensuring technical knowledge and basic competence in psychology, including the provision of therapy, efficient and well-developed report writing skills, the ability to develop diagnostic formulations, and the administration and interpretation of psychological assessment measures. It is assumed that interns coming from an APA-accredited graduate school have received the required training experiences to provide them with a set of skills necessary to begin to function professionally as a psychologist. Through the selection process, we attempt to identify applicants whose basic competence in the field of psychology will not need to be addressed in depth during the internship. However, we will provide the necessary education if an intern demonstrates a significant deficiency in any aspect of the above-mentioned areas. This may include the creation of a formal remediation plan between the intern, their supervisor(s), and the training director in order to identify the deficiency and identify a remedy.

The primary focus of a successful internship program is on the development of professional competence and identity. Interns must take into consideration how they are viewed as professionals by patients and other staff. Are they seen as quiet and reserved? Are they considered knowledgeable? Do patients feel they can trust them? Supervision focused on the intern's presence in the therapy room allows for this type of professional development. One intern stated:

> it was hard because my supervisor was direct, but helpful because it was about developing awareness. At this level, the clinical stuff is down, it is learning about yourself in the room and how people view you as well as the unexpected pieces.

This focus on the growth of the professional rather than the training of a student creates a significant shift in the dynamic present within an internship training program. When interns primarily identify themselves as "students," they default to a state in which they are dependent upon their supervisor(s). In order to feel empowered to take on more responsibility and encouraged to develop their own professional identity, it is necessary that interns feel they can be open and honest in supervision without fear of repercussions. With a safe and open sharing environment, interns will have the best opportunity to learn from mistakes without the event feeling punitive.

In order to promote the development of independent professional competence, it is important to allow mistakes to happen during the internship year and to provide supervision around the issue(s) rather than to over-supervise protectively. It is better for interns to experience mistakes during their internship rather than during the first years of their career, when they may lack the advantage of access to a supervisor. Many interns fear making mistakes following years of overachieving in academic environments with little exposure to real-world crises and limited inpatient experience. It is not uncommon for students to leave school with the expectation that they know what they need to know and believe it is a sign of weakness to admit they do not know something. They then struggle to enter a supervisory experience in which they are encouraged to explore what they do not know and admit shortcomings. One intern stated: "I remember being terrified I was going to give a patient something they weren't supposed to have or do something that would result in an elopement." This fear can hold interns back from truly learning and growing during their training year as they may avoid situations and experiences that are more challenging to their skill set or outside of their comfort zone. It is vital that interns be encouraged and empowered throughout the training year to challenge themselves to the point of discomfort in order to take full advantage of what might be their last opportunity to try new techniques or learn and test new skills with a supervisor available for support and assistance. For example, an inpatient internship may be the first setting in which an intern can get experience utilizing the Rorschach Inkblot Test or try implementing Cognitive Behavior Therapy for psychosis (CBTp) with an individual diagnosed with schizophrenia.

The transition from student to professional occurs during this short, 1-year period and interns may not feel ready for this leap. Many experience a lack of confidence because they feel that they are "just an intern" and may find themselves experiencing "imposter syndrome." This generally refers to high-achieving individuals, such as pre-doctoral interns, who experience an inability to internalize their accomplishments and an ongoing fear of being exposed as fraudulent. As a result, interns may be hesitant to speak up in meetings, be anxious about working with patients, and become overly dependent on their supervisor. For example, the intern may sit quietly in treatment planning meetings while patients they are conducting therapy with are discussed, assuming the information they would share from therapy is not important enough. In this case, the underlying issue for supervision may be that the intern is coping with an issue of autonomy versus dependency, which is holding the intern back from developing self-confidence and a sense of identity as a psychologist. The supervisor should directly address this within supervision, empower participation, and remind interns of the knowledge and education they do have as well as how they can meaningfully contribute to meetings addressing patient care, specifically regarding their patients' care. At the other end of the spectrum are interns who appear overly confident in their abilities. For example, an overly confident intern may jump in, right away, seeming very comfortable with patients. Later, however, they may inappropriately argue with a patient about a paranoid delusion, causing the patient to become agitated in response. In this case, an underlying supervisory issue may be that the intern has an overconfident stance with regard to their knowledge and/or skill level. This could be rooted in the insecurity of their abilities, assumptions based in past experiences, or difficulty in meeting the patient's inner reality and feelings. It is important to distinguish what is happening with the intern, a skills deficit versus overconfidence when determining what requires supervisory attention. Regardless of the precipitant, it is important the supervisor addresses these issues in the supervisory relationship directly and in a timely manner in order to prevent a possible negative event, such as an intern getting into a dangerous situation with a patient. Addressing these issues is also important to promote growth critical for developing the intern's professional competence.

Supervision during the internship year can focus on the technical aspects of the job, such as therapeutic techniques and assessment methods. However, learning about systemic issues within inpatient settings and providing support around the frustration encountered in work within this setting can become a major focus throughout the year. Some of these issues include the lack of adequate community resources for patients upon discharge, insufficient discharge placement options, and the detrimental effects of institutionalization. An example of a frequent issue interns express concern about within a state-run psychiatric hospital is a longer length of stay in the hospital than is necessary due to a lack of available housing options in the community. Another example of a concern interns voice is the re-hospitalization that occurs when patients are not provided with adequate support and care in the community.

Although interns are sheltered from the majority of the bureaucratic problems during their training year, it is impossible to prevent them from having some exposure to systemic issues. Interns should be encouraged to share their concerns and experiences with the hospital or system as a whole in supervision. This does not mean that supervision should be focused on complaining about the system. Rather, supervision can provide opportunities for interns to reflect on situation(s) that raise concerns and to encourage interns to consider how they might handle a situation differently if they were the psychologist or an administrator within the hospital. It can be important for interns to consider how the system is impacting patient care and what needs to happen in order to facilitate productive and positive changes within the system. In addition, it is helpful to educate interns regarding methods of advocacy for patients within the system, and how they can use their position and skills to promote positive changes related to patient care and patients' rights during their internship and throughout their careers. Interns could be advised to become involved in local, national, or international mental health advocacy groups, or volunteer with mental health non-profit organizations. Positive ways they can assert themselves can also involve participating in board meetings or projects specific to their hospital in order to encourage positive change within their workplace. When possible, supervisors should try to bring interns to administrative and policy meetings in order to gain early exposure and develop their voice in an advocacy realm.

Challenges Specific to Internship in an Inpatient Setting

A pre-doctoral psychology internship in an inpatient setting can be extremely stressful and difficult. Not many days go by when a psychologist leaves a psychiatric inpatient facility and feels that they have made a significant change in a patient's life or accomplished all that was on their "to do" list for the day. The patients housed within an inpatient psychiatric hospital are often the most severely and persistently mentally ill individuals in the region. Most often, patients present with severe psychosis and/or mood disturbance. Often, primary psychiatric diagnoses are comorbid with substance abuse disorders, traumatic brain injuries, significant trauma histories, and medical issues. The severity of the patients' illness and symptom presentation creates a learning environment like no other.

In many cases, patients are admitted to inpatient facilities because they pose a danger to themselves or others, leading to civil commitment, or involuntary hospitalization. In forensic facilities, individuals who have been charged with a crime may be found "incompetent to proceed" to trial and require hospitalization in order to have their illness stabilized before proceeding to trial. Another reason for hospitalization at a forensic hospital would be if the individual is found "not guilty by reason of insanity" or "guilty but insane or mentally ill." This means the individual is not responsible for their actions at the time of their offense due to an episodic or persistent mental illness present at the time of the criminal act, the symptoms of which interfered with the individual's ability to distinguish that what they were doing at the time of the offense was wrong. Both of these can result in commitment to a psychiatric hospital for court-ordered inpatient treatment. Regardless of how the patients are admitted to the hospital, the mission remains the same: to provide patients with the highest quality psychiatric and psychological services in order to facilitate their recovery and help them return to their lives in the community, to the greatest extent possible.

However, many patients in psychiatric hospitals have limited community support and have damaged the relationships in their lives, including with their families. It is not uncommon for patients to have accused their families of crimes or to have previously harmed their loved ones. For many patients in this setting, treatment providers may be the only support that remains for them. Other obstacles patients face can include limited funds, lack of housing options, inappropriate levels of care, and limitations in community mental health treatment including frequent staff turnover leading to inconsistent support and treatment providers.

This reality can be extremely frustrating for staff at inpatient psychiatric hospitals, including interns. It is often the case that motivation to work in the mental health field, particularly in public service environments, includes a desire to help others to recover. Although this is the mission and goal in treatment facilities, it can be disheartening to experience the roadblocks that persist related to resources, support, and the community. One intern stated:

> I kept finding it frustrating ... I had trouble understanding why community mental health agencies that receive government funding were able to deny patients, forcing people to stay in a setting that is more restrictive than necessary. I was disheartened at the perception that the community mental health agencies did not want to take the responsibility of caring for the more difficult or high-risk patients ... I understand that the risk in caring for such a patient is high, but the risk of not caring for them is much higher.

In some cases, an internship at an inpatient psychiatric hospital is the intern's first experience working with individuals with severe and persistent mental illness. Often interns with prior experience in inpatient settings enter the internship expecting to know what the experience will be like. However, interns often quickly find out that during their part-time practicum experiences, they were sheltered from many of the realities of the work and only saw a small piece of the whole picture. One of the first noticeable issues within an inpatient setting can be the diverse levels of functioning among the individuals in treatment. Providing treatment, particularly in a group modality, can be very challenging when the participants' levels of functioning span from the level of an intellectual disability to a high level of cognitive functioning as well as from highly symptomatic to stable.

Another concern voiced by interns is the difficulty identifying an individual patient's baseline, or alternately, what their functioning looks like at their best. For one individual with severe and persistent mental illness, the baseline may include returning to a full-time job and living independently. However, for another individual, their baseline may include being free of self-harming behaviors for one week at a time and returning to live at an assisted care facility. Recovery is a very individual process, different for each person, particularly in an inpatient setting. Recognizing this can be very challenging for interns, who come into a practice setting with high aspirations for themselves and their patients.

When asked why they studied psychology, many interns' responses include their wish to help people. Within an inpatient setting, help is always needed and welcome, but it may not look the same as what the interns have envisioned for themselves and their patients. Interns are often unaware of how devastating years of untreated severe and persistent mental illness can be on an individual's cognition, physical body, emotional maturity, personality structure, and relationships. Consequently, interns might feel ineffective or hopeless when they are unable to observe a noticeable change in the patients for whom they provide care.

Furthermore, interns may attempt to apply the skills they developed through years of training only to find that these skills are not at a level appropriate for the current needs of their patients. Doctoral programs generally do not present material geared specifically toward the treatment of severely mentally ill individuals. Interns' previous training may have been in less restrictive environments requiring them to adapt their skills when working in an inpatient psychiatric setting. In supervision, it is important to address this throughout the year and help interns develop realistic outlooks and goals for themselves and their patients. For example, one intern attempted Cognitive Behavior Therapy (CBT) with a patient actively experiencing hallucinations and delusions and became frustrated when the patient returned session after session without completing the assigned Thought Records. The supervision then focused on how to adapt this modality for use in an inpatient setting.[1]

Interns may believe their goal is to increase a patient's ability to develop positive social relationships, but the more realistic goal may be to help the patient develop a strong working relationship with the intern. Supervision can help to mitigate the frustration caused by a perceived lack of progress and can increase the intern's sense of confidence and satisfaction through reframing gains that are often overlooked. Such gains include developing relationships, using a coping strategy, engaging in a reality-based conversation, or even maintaining eye contact for a period of time. Helping interns transition their treatment expectations via the supervisory relationship, and for them to learn to respect a patient's reality versus serving their own desire and need to be successful, can be a true test of professional humility.

A primary focus in helping mentally ill individuals work toward recovery is meeting the patient where they are, not trying to push information onto them, but finding a way to communicate with the patient in a way they will hear and understand the information. For example, if a patient believes the hospital staff is trying to poison them, instead of challenging this delusion, it is more therapeutic and productive to reassure the patient that they are safe and help them to engage in calming strategies in the moment.

Interns often come to their internship eager to apply the knowledge they learned in graduate school. However, it should be noted that therapy and assessment within an inpatient setting must be applied in a flexible manner allowing for variation. Manualized treatment protocols have become increasingly utilized for treatment in many settings, though strictly following manualized treatment or assessment techniques may not always prove effective in this environment. For example, groups utilizing Dialectical Behavior Therapy (DBT) may be more focused on coping skills acquisition rather than on the analysis of problematic behaviors, since some inpatient psychiatric units do not have the staff training and organization to fully implement a structured and manualized DBT program. Treatment and programs in inpatient hospital settings often function differently than similar programs in outpatient settings due to the need for a more flexible style of patient interaction. Supervisors can provide education and model how to alter structured or manualized approaches to treatment in order to address individual patient's needs and abilities. Furthermore, supervision can be a place where interns develop a deeper clinical understanding of their goals versus the patient's goals and gain understanding about differentiating and negotiating between the two.

Another challenge for interns within an inpatient setting is separating a patient and their mental illness in order to avoid the diagnosis defining the person. When we allow a diagnosis to define a patient, and as a result to define the treatment approach and goals, we miss the individual's nuances and their personality, which should be what dictates a psychologist's approach.

Another challenge faced by interns and others working in inpatient settings is recognizing and addressing in a therapeutic manner, individuals with mental illness who may say and do things that stem from distortions related to their emotional disturbance. For example, a patient may, in some encounters devalue an intern while idealizing other staff. In later encounters with the intern, this patient may act as though the event never occurred and treat the intern well. This shifting from devaluation to idealization may be related to the patient's personal history with whom he or she has sought to rely upon for care. These apparent shifts in perceptions of the intern may be based upon the damage to trust engendered by past abandonment, rather than an indication that something is wrong within the therapeutic relationship. Interns may take these fluctuations personally, particularly when the shift is toward devaluation and questioning the intern's skills or abilities, and may struggle to handle their own emotional response to a patient. Supervision can help the intern to learn how to understand the patient's apparent shifts in valuing the intern while also addressing their own feelings. The need to manage extreme emotions as well as strong personal reactions to such intense interactions is commonly evoked with patients in hospital settings. Supervision is a crucial vehicle to help interns understand and cope with the extreme situations and difficult countertransference situations that arise while working with this population.

Working with severely and persistently mentally ill individuals can elicit numerous emotional responses in staff, but interns are often especially susceptible due to their eager nature and general lack of professional experience. As mentioned above, taking things personally can create strong emotional reactions, which may not be a situation the intern has yet encountered. Interns might first encounter and learn to deal with such situations during their year of internship.

For many interns, their internship may be their first experience with the struggle to develop a relationship with patients in an inpatient setting. Supervision can be helpful in educating interns on the various reasons for difficulties inherent in such efforts, as well as providing assistance in finding methods to improve rapport. Supervisors may need to sensitize interns to patients' experiences of paranoia and the impact of histories that may include relational traumas. Traumatic experiences of all types can drastically impact patients' abilities and willingness to trust others. The majority of patients in an inpatient setting have experienced trauma in their lives, including experiences of abandonment and harm inflicted by trusted individuals. It should be noted that even being diagnosed with a mental illness, or admitted to inpatient treatment, can be exceptionally traumatic. Trust, therefore, may be damaged before contact with therapeutic staff, including interns, is even initiated. In addition, many patients understand that treatment with interns is time-limited since interns are not permanent employees. Therefore, patients may hesitate to develop a relationship with an intern and may avoid the risk of making an emotional connection. There are some occasions in which it may be important to supervise an intern on the need to respect a patient's reluctance to engage in a therapeutic relationship, due for example, to a patient's effort to avoid an experience of abandonment toward the end of an interns' training year, or when the patient's discharge is imminent. Encouraging the intern to address these issues early and upfront in therapy can potentially, however, assist with the development of a strong therapeutic relationship.

Many interns in inpatient settings have their first experience in which they need to share sensitive information reported by a patient. A patient's revelation of certain information requires reporting that information to appropriate authorities, or other staff. This includes suicidal and homicidal ideation, knowledge of child or elder abuse, substance use, and other potentially dangerous situations. It is not uncommon for patients to report this information to interns and ask them to keep it secret. Prior to engaging in any patient contact, it is imperative interns are made aware by supervisors that all such information need be reported to staff immediately. It is also extremely important for interns to provide informed consent related to these types of communications upon initiating contact with a patient. Specifically, patients should be made aware at the onset of the interaction that if they report thoughts of hurting themselves or others this will need to be reported to staff in order to ensure patient and staff safety. Sadly, there are numerous occasions in which a patient tells an intern they are feeling like hurting themselves or someone else, and then feels betrayed when that information is reported to the treatment team and supervisor. This damage to the therapeutic relationship may be repairable but can lead to a loss of trust and less disclosure of true feelings in the future of the relationship. In any such situation, interns should be encouraged to immediately report concerns to their supervisor or other available staff, and to document the experience. Although supervisors can provide support and ensure proper protocol is followed, it is often beneficial for the intern to take the lead in mandatory reporting and documentation of these types of events, as well as informing the client about their legal requirement to report to the appropriate authority. After the patient's and others' immediate safety is ensured, the event should be processed and reviewed with the intern. Supervision is an appropriate forum to help interns address their emotional reactions to situations that often include fear, anxiety, and doubt in their abilities. Some of these feelings arise due to the multiple roles assumed in inpatient settings with regard to treating or assessing the patient while also having an obligation to keep others, including the community, safe. Normalizing conflictual feelings and providing support for the intern are important aspects of the supervisor's role in these situations.

Similarly, it is not uncommon for mentally ill individuals to harm themselves or others in the course of an inpatient hospitalization, through self-injurious behavior, suicide attempts, or assault. After all parties' safety and well-being is ensured, debriefing with interns is important, regardless of the intern's connection to the patient or event. Even a suicide attempt occurring on a different treatment unit with no direct relationship to the intern can strongly impact an intern. It may be some interns' first or closest exposure to this type of event and may be traumatic. The event may trigger memories from a past experience in some interns' lives, creating powerful emotional responses. Whatever responses are evoked, these events must be addressed immediately and not saved for a later formal supervision session. Following a recent assault on a staff member, an intern assigned to the same unit was given the immediate opportunity to meet with their supervisor in order for the intern to vent concerns and fear of the patient as well as for the well-being of the assaulted staff member. The intern described having witnessed similar events before in a different setting but also left the impromptu supervision meeting feeling emotionally supported as well as reminded to remain vigilant and aware of her surroundings at all times.

Debriefing with an intern following an incident may include identifying motives for the actions, formulating ideas of what the patient's needs may be at this point, and reviewing appropriate, therapeutic boundaries. Debriefing may at times provide an opportunity to express emotional reactions. In the worst-case scenario of a patient's death by suicide, most parties involved will experience a form of trauma, interns being no exception. Interns may also struggle emotionally when experiencing their supervisor's emotional responses to such events, leading to an increase in the complexity of their response. In such a situation, a supervisor must maintain awareness of their own reactions and responses as well as their intern's, while at the same time remaining aware of their modeling and need to validate the intern's emotional reaction to the event. It may also be beneficial for a larger group, such as the treatment team or psychology discipline, to convene in order to process and debrief regarding a traumatic loss or event as well as provide support, and resources for additional supports as may be needed.[2]

Many emotional reactions interns experience during their internship stem from the interns' particular life experiences. Interns seek to become psychologists for a variety of reasons. For example, experiences such as a relative living with mental illness, or a friend's suicide are among the life experiences providing motivation for pursuing the study of psychology. An intern may have personally struggled with mental illness at a point in their own life. Interns may have powerful desires to help others for many reasons. Regardless of the motive for entering the field of psychology, every intern has his/her own personal history and reasons for entering the field and will be impacted differently by the patients with whom they work. In the case of an intern who has coped with their own mental illness or illness within their family, work in an inpatient setting can be especially rewarding while also complicated. Their own personal experience may allow them to better relate to the patients, but may also influence their approach to patients, in both positive and potentially negative ways. Although personal experience may increase empathy, being immersed in an inpatient setting may prove overwhelming for an intern with such personal experiences with mental illness. Continued education and supervision on the importance of self-care is imperative due to the high "burnout" potential for those working in these settings with mentally ill individuals.

Pre-doctoral psychology internships within an inpatient psychiatric hospital setting can be among the most challenging, but rewarding, experiences in a psychologist's life and professional development. It is the high quality of supervision that allows interns to truly grow as people and professionals. Therefore, the focus and emphasis of an internship program in an inpatient setting should not be solely on obtaining high-quality interns, but also on ensuring the presence of strong psychologists who are knowledgeable and well-versed in clinical supervision. The stressors present during the internship year are endless, but good supervision can make the stressors of the year feel like challenges that can be mastered rather than roadblocks in the interns' way to their career.

Notes

1 See Chapter 12 by Sally Riggs on CBTp, this volume.
2 See Chapter 21 by Daza and Sharma, this volume, on supervision regarding patient suicidality.

21 The Most Difficult Lesson

The Impact of Patient Suicide on Training in an Inpatient Psychiatric Hospital

Patricia Daza and Shweta Sharma

Suicide completion within psychiatric hospitals is fortunately rare but, when it occurs, can have deleterious effects on both patients and staff. For a trainee studying to be a psychologist, it can have a profound impact on their development as a clinician. Although graduate programs are now more mindful of core competencies needed in suicide assessment and treatment, training related to these competencies varies widely across different programs and facilities. This chapter focuses on several topics germane to working with suicidal young adults within an inpatient psychiatric hospital. It highlights an approach to suicide intervention that is collaborative and patient-centered. The chapter describes an approach in the training of psychology interns working with suicidal patients, which includes careful supervision with respect to risk assessment, clinical intervention, and reactions to loss. Case examples are provided to elucidate the difficulty in providing training and education during this challenging time.

The psychology internship year is a time to solidify interns' learning experiences in order to prepare them for entry into the profession. Although experiences vary based on the internship site, psychiatric inpatient settings may expose trainees to more situations that bring to light life's precariousness than what they might experience in other settings (Farberow, 1981; Gibson & Taylor, 2003). Approximately 4–7% of suicides occur within hospital settings (Wolfersdorf, 2000) and 11% of mental health trainees experience a patient suicide during their training years (Kleespies, Penk, & Forsyth, 1993). More specifically, one in six psychology interns experiences a patient's suicide during training (Kleespies, Smith, & Becker, 1990). Suicide among young adults is the leading cause of death (Heron, 2013). There are a myriad of hypotheses about the prevalence of suicide among young adults. Young adulthood is a time of significant transition and identity exploration. Key decisions about relationships, future careers, and political views become intensified in this period coined as "emerging adulthood" (Arnett, 2000). The Menninger Clinic in Houston, Texas, has a specifically dedicated unit for young adults to help address the issues pertinent to this significant developmental stage. Psychology interns are core members of the multidisciplinary treatment (MDT) team that provides treatment.

The Menninger Clinic is a not-for-profit inpatient psychiatric treatment center serving adolescents and adults with a broad range of psychiatric and substance abuse problem and offers specialty inpatient programs as well as diagnostic services. The treatment follows an integrated biopsychosocial model in which pharmacological, psychotherapeutic, and systems approaches are employed to assist patients in understanding and managing their symptoms. Treatment teams are composed of psychiatrists, social workers, psychologists, nursing staff, addiction counselors, psychosocial rehabilitation specialists, mental health associates, and trainees. Much attention is given to a careful and thorough diagnostic workup as well as a compassionate, client-centered approach to patient care. For the past 29 years and since the inception of the US World and News Report psychiatric hospital rankings, the Menninger Clinic has ranked in the top 10 of psychiatric hospitals for patient care in the United States (US World and News Report, n.d.).

At the Menninger Clinic, we have a longstanding tradition of training and professional development within a psychiatric specialty hospital. Training students has been at the heart of the Clinic's mission for over 70 years. Staff at the clinic train psychiatric residents, psychology interns and postdoctoral fellows, social work interns and fellows, and nursing residents, to name a few. A significant amount of time is spent organizing supervisors, deciding topics for our didactic series, and reading the evaluations from the previous group of trainees. We have a director of education who, in collaboration with clinical staff, develops a series of didactic seminars; orients the students to human resources policies; and gathers data at the end of the training year to assess potential changes for the following year. Trainees are given a broad overview of the history of the clinic; introduced to the longstanding and rich tradition of psychological testing at the clinic; and oriented to the ethos of client-centered care.

The core training experiences for the internship year are divided between two, six-month rotations on two separate treatment units. The intern integrates diagnostic formulations into treatment planning, meets with patients during weekly rounds, helps to co-lead therapy groups, and provides individual evaluation and therapy services within an MDT team. Every member of the treatment team has a different function and responsibility with the patient; however, all contribute to the diagnostic picture and treatment planning. Central to treatment planning is psychological testing. Testing provides additional information that not only aids with clarification of diagnoses but, more importantly, helps elucidate the patient's core issues (i.e., what is keeping them stuck in treatment). Testing generally includes a focus on personality dynamics and, in some cases, cognitive assessment.

Early in the training year, the interns are encouraged to attend clinical rounds and team meetings. In clinical rounds, the treatment team checks in with each individual patient. In team meetings, the core team discusses the patient and the progress they are making in treatment. If the patient's family approves, interns also observe a diagnostic conference family feedback session. A diagnostic conference is an extended team meeting where the team members formulate their understanding of the patient's struggles and share their recommendations for ongoing treatment with the family and the patient. The exposure to these meetings serves as a model for how to work in the "psychology role" but, more importantly, how to work in a family system with a member who experienced suicidal ideation and made suicide attempts. Interns learn how to discuss previous suicide attempts, how to discuss chronic risk for suicide, and how to decrease fear from dominating the family system. The psychology interns, in combination with the licensed clinical social workers and the nurses, help contain the patient's and the family's anxiety about future attempts and support a stance of "curiosity" about the patient's suicide. For example, if a patient is curious about their suicidality, it suggests they are trying to understand it and what may have led to the event. It implies that the patient is not actively trying to avoid the topic. We encourage them to decipher what led up to the event, whether support could have been accessed, and whether other factors may have exacerbated their emotional experience (e.g., substance use). In addition, we encourage patients to be mindful of the impact of this event on their family, their friends, and significant others. The goal of this process is not to induce guilt, but to help patients understand the suffering and stress in people around them. It helps them understand why families may try to "hover" or "watch me like a hawk" after a suicide event. Our hope is that the patient can begin to see their own role in this dynamic and why their family's behavior might have changed so radically.

Clinical Challenges for the Psychology Intern

All clinical work at the clinic is done with sub-acute patients who are admitted from across the United States, and, at times, from abroad. One of the primary populations with whom we work are patients diagnosed with borderline personality disorder (BPD). Working with patients who have symptoms of BPD can be challenging for any clinician, but may be especially difficult for an intern. Knowledge and awareness of the importance of boundaries, a holding environment, and self-regulation skills are needed. Self-destructive behaviors and suicide attempts can become the focus of internship supervision. These topics often elicit anxiety from the trainee. Trainees may also have heightened fear surrounding patients' non-suicidal self-injury and suicidal ideation and may be more likely than experienced staff members to be affected by patients' interpersonal challenges. Without the necessary training, interns may take slights from patients more personally. For example, a patient may refuse to have an intern present in their clinical rounds. The patient may assert that the trainee is not qualified to contribute to their care. Although this is the patient's right, the intern might take this personally believing they are not wanted or do not have the skills to help the patient. Supervision might involve understanding the concept of projective identification (Ogden, 1979) and how to manage one's own emotional experience. The following vignette provides an example of supervision in such a situation.

Experiencing Rejection

Caroline was a 20-year-old female who had been hospitalized several times in her life. She had a complicated attachment history and much difficulty trusting others. Every week the team would meet with Caroline for treatment rounds. Staff included her psychiatrist, psychologist, social worker, nurse, and the psychology intern. As soon as Julie introduced herself as the psychology intern, Caroline had a negative reaction. She looked at her with disapproval and quickly stated, "I don't want her here. Please leave!" The team tried to encourage Caroline to be curious about her reaction though she remained adamant. The intern politely left the room, and this seemed to calm Caroline. During supervision, Julie was honest and said that the interaction had been very difficult for her. She felt "less than" in the team and even felt some anger, although also was understanding toward Caroline. In supervision, I (the first author) tried to have Julie reflect on Caroline's experience. Caroline had also majored in psychology in college but was unable to finish college due to her frequent hospitalizations. Julie was older than Caroline, married (something that Caroline desperately wanted), and was close to completing her psychology doctorate. Julie's presence was too much for Caroline to bear: Julie represented everything Caroline had failed to achieve. This perspective-taking allowed Julie to empathize with Caroline's reaction, which subsequently improved their relationship.

Avoiding and Mentalizing the "Split"

At the clinic, we frequently use the term "mentalization," which refers to the ability to understand actions both by oneself and others in terms of intentional mental states such as beliefs, desires, feelings, etc. (Allen & Fonagy, 2014). In working with patients with BPD, frequently a split occurs within the team where some staff members may feel protective of the patient while others may experience frustration. For interns, in particular, it may be harder to "hold the hate" or be a recipient of the patient's anger. In our training, we focus on keeping an open, curious mind about the patients and our feelings about them. As early career psychologists, we need continued reminders to not get caught up in a split within the team. Recognizing and remembering at all times that staff observe different aspects of the patient is of utmost importance. As Sharma and Daza (Chapter 18, this volume) address, we are all trying to understand the patient by sharing our different perspectives – encouraging a mentalizing stance. Early career clinicians, like interns, often harbor doubts about their competence in their roles; they desire to carry out their work well and wish for their work to be acknowledged and appreciated; and they experience some trepidation about working with challenging patients.

At the Clinic, all work occurs within MDT teams. One important role within the team is that of the individual therapist. The individual therapist meets with the patient twice per week during their time in the hospital. Psychology interns see two therapy patients twice per week and are supervised during the process. In almost all instances, the individual therapist falls on "the good side" of the split. Patients often present wishes concerning treatment, such as wanting to increase therapy sessions to three times per week, to discuss their frustrations with their psychiatrist or social worker, and at times to "fire" their team. These challenges are difficult to manage without good supervision concerning the dynamics of working in a team. Supervisors work to increase the intern's own curiosity about the split (i.e., How did I fall on the good side? Is there a part of me that likes being put on a pedestal? What is it like for my colleague doing the family work or the psychiatrist who is tapering medications that the patient wants to continue?). Sometimes falling on the "good side" of the split can feel intimidating for the interns. They worry that they are not as skilled as the patient believes they are and worry that the team will discover the truth.

Interns learn how to encourage and develop curiosity and help patients understand that they too are members of the team. "I was part of the team that made the decision to disapprove your opportunity to have a pass with your family." More importantly, supervision addresses the inevitable consequence that the intern will eventually experience "the bad side" of the split over time and how to be prepared for it. Much of this experience consists of trial, error, and reflection, with much support (and educational material) from supervisors provided to help interns through the process.

Demoralization: How Best to Contain It?

Working with patients who physically harm themselves (e.g., burning, cutting) and engage in suicidal behaviors can be both frightening and demoralizing. Interns begin to experience growing frustration and a sense of hopelessness when they witness patients who struggle to improve over time. They begin to wonder if they are doing enough in treatment; if they have the clinical knowledge to help the patient; and it can leave them feeling unskilled and unsure about their career path. A supervisor is critical in this process by modeling vulnerability and sharing their own stories of "clinical impasses." As we often also discuss in our psycho-educational groups with patients, we may not always have the exact roadmap but we know there is a road and that road generally leads to improvements in quality of life. Interns need guidance on how to navigate the doubts and disappointments that may arise with certain patients, including ways of understanding both the good and "not-so-good" outcomes with patients. This is crucial as interns begin the daunting task of working with a patient with suicidal thoughts and plans.

Working with Suicidal Patients

Suicide and suicidal ideation are both nebulous and vacillating. Many of our young adult patients are admitted to the clinic with long-standing histories of suicidal ideation and multiple suicide attempts. Approximately 50% of the young adults in our program are diagnosed with a personality disorder based on the Structured Clinical Interview for DSM-IV (First et al., 1997). Many have made one or more suicide attempt, and have ongoing ideation concerning suicide (Madan et al., 2016). The presence of a personality disorder or traits can be problematic for young adults. Patients with personality disorders can pose a high risk of harming themselves. They have difficulty regulating emotions through healthy attachment relationships. This may contribute to being more susceptible to feelings of being overwhelmed. While most people diagnosed with personality disorders do not commit suicide, the presence of certain personality disorders or traits, under certain circumstances, increases both the risk of suicide attempts and completed suicides. In a longitudinal study assessing predictors of suicide among depressed, adult individuals, the presence of cluster B personality disorder symptoms was the most robust finding (May, Klonsky, & Klein, 2012). During the interviews for the internship, the staff is frank about our patient population and the families we serve. We openly discuss the diagnostic complexity of our patients and the severity of their clinical presentation. One question I frequently ask interns is, "Have you ever lost a patient to suicide?" Almost invariably, interns respond that they have never experienced the loss of a patient. My goal in asking the question is not to frighten them, but to underscore the clinical challenges they may face while on internship.

Currently, there is much debate in graduate programs regarding how to address suicide training and prevention during supervision. Interns are eager to begin their clinical work when they arrive. They have completed several practicums, and have taken courses in assessment and clinical intervention; they have begun practicing the art of psychotherapy. However, many interns begin the internship year with minimal exposure to didactics and research in suicide prevention. The dearth of exposure is shifting with the development of core competencies in suicide risk assessment and management (American Psychiatric Association, 2003; Suicide Prevention Resource Center, 2006) as well as key elements to keep in mind for supervision (Rudd, Cukrowicz, & Bryan, 2008). Topics such as attitudes and approaches to suicide; understanding suicide; collecting accurate information; understanding risk; developing treatment plans for suicide; managing care (documentation, consultation); and understanding legal issues related to suicide are being targeted to help better prepare graduate students in psychology. At the clinic, we actively work to address these topics in supervision and especially in the work with our patients. The case examples below will help elucidate our work. It should be noted that the cases described are a composite of many patients that we have worked with over the years and are not about one particular individual.

Case Study: Intervening with Suicide

Henry was a 26-year-old man who was admitted to the young adult program after increasing suicidal ideation with plans. He was not a traditional young adult patient: he was older, in medical school, and had no history of substance abuse. From the beginning, he felt as if he did not fit in with our patients and he wondered whether a transfer to our executive treatment program (i.e., treatment for working professionals) would be a better fit. He was born into a family system where, in his opinion, his parents were not invested in his development. He sought comfort in other relationships, mainly those he developed with his therapists. Prior to admission, he had worked with a therapist near his medical school and was aware that he was growing increasingly dependent on him. He felt this therapist was attuned to him and was trying to actively understand his suicidal thoughts and desires. He felt nurtured and cared for by the therapist. In one example he provided of his therapist's care, he noted that he had been taken to the ER after a suicide attempt and his therapist had stayed with him until he was released. His therapist, however, had become overwhelmed with the patient's crises and, while the patient was hospitalized, suggested he find another therapist when he returned home. The therapist's decision to end the therapeutic relationship was a focus of our work together. The termination of the relationship with his outpatient therapist led Henry to have frequent thoughts of suicide, abandonment, and a general distrust in humanity. I was faced with a dilemma: how to engage him in therapy and let him know I also had his mind in mind, but also be mindful of his potential dependence and overreliance on me. Our initial work focused on containing his grief around the loss of his therapist (aka parent) but also helped him be curious about his therapist's struggle. In treatment, we often discussed that as clinicians, we have the "H factor": we are human. We get angry, fearful, and frustrated. We encourage patients to be curious about what their therapists may have been feeling when they suggested the patient be hospitalized. In Henry's situation, the therapist wanted to help but had also become overwhelmed in the process. The therapist was seeing the patient frequently, responding to crisis phone calls, and essentially had become the patient's case manager. The patient felt great shame about being asked to find a new therapist upon discharge. He had thoughts of suicide and self-harm, and we approached our work together through the Collaborative Assessment and Management of Suicidality (CAMS: Jobes, 2006). Henry had never participated in CAMS but was eager to try this approach. CAMS has been reviewed extensively in the literature, and a summary of the work being done at the Clinic is available (Ellis, Daza, & Allen, 2012).

Briefly, CAMS-M is a collaborative approach between the therapist and the suicidal patient. It recognizes that suicide is one way, though not an adaptive one, to cope with insurmountable stress. The therapist tries to introduce alternative ways to help the patient cope with the stress while also validating the pain they are experiencing. Together, the duo work to develop an alliance, the cornerstone of this approach; to develop a realistic plan for treatment that addresses the urge to commit suicide; and to reduce vulnerability for future attempts. The general objectives of CAMS-M include: a) ongoing assessment of level of suicide risk; b) resolution of acute suicidality; c) education of the patient through functional analysis of previous suicide attempts; d) development of adaptive coping responses; e) improvement of the drivers (to be discussed below); and f) relapse prevention plans (Ellis, Daza, & Allen, 2012). Coping skills are taught in sessions based on the patient's clinical presentation. This approach includes coping cards, safety plans, and the Hope Kit. The therapist relies on the Suicide Status Form (SSF; Jobes, 2006) to assess the drivers of the patient's current suicidal state. Drivers include Pain, Stress, Agitation, Hopelessness, and Self Hate. Other domains assessed include the patient's current wish to live and die, completed on a Likert scale; a section addressing the patient's reasons for living and dying; and a question that directly asks about the "one thing" in the patient's life that makes life worth living. Because patients at the Clinic are hospitalized for an average of 6–8 weeks and are seen in individual therapy twice per week, the SSF was administered once per week with Henry.

Henry was initially hesitant to discuss his suicidal ideations and attempts. He shared his concerns that these discussions might lead to the imposition of restrictions on his freedom and monitoring of his behavior. He found these possibilities onerous although their purpose was to keep him safe. He had experienced episodes of unit restriction in other settings (i.e., not being able to leave the unit to go to crafts, to the cafeteria, or to off unit appointments) and had also been placed on a one to one observation in the past (i.e., having a staff member present and at arms-length, and at all times, to monitor his safety). He shared his discomfort about the intimacy of the subject matter (suicide) and how private it was for him. The collaborative and nonjudgmental stance taken with him appeared to calm him as he slowly began to share his thoughts with me. He reported he was fearful of feeling hope, and also fearful of being disappointed by future periods of hopelessness and desires to end his life. Consistent with the CAMS-M approach, we began discussing relationships and the impact they can have on suicidal thinking and behavior. His relationship with his therapist was central to this work, in light of his attachment to the therapist and subsequent "loss" of him. Our relationship also served as a bridge for the development of other relationships on the unit (e.g., nursing staff, peers, and the delicate relationship with his parents). I tried to help foster a more curious stance regarding his difficult relationships with others and why he often felt so alone. Addressing isolation was important because of its link to his suicidal thinking and because of what it reminded him of in his childhood: being alone. He benefited from the structure of the milieu, his relationship with peers, and the ruptures and repairs that frequently occurred in the therapeutic setting. As discharge approached and the next level of care was discussed, Henry became suicidal, worried that he would be unable to relate to a new set of peers and clinicians. He also wondered if the suicidal thoughts would ever cease. I was honest with him, acknowledging that suicide might always be an option for him; however, it did not have to be his primary option during times of despair. Although this is difficult for some clinicians to discuss, it is imperative that we recognize why this work is difficult: that ultimately, the patient has the final decision whether to live or not. In our sessions together, we worked to develop other, more adaptive options that would make suicide a less probable outcome. I think he valued my ability to walk this difficult path together with him. During these sessions, we discussed how to provide a safer environment, without items and objects that would make suicide more feasible. He seemed invested in developing his Hope Kit, and we generated ideas of what to put in his kit (e.g., an encouraging letter from his therapist; pictures of his friends' kids; a poem of his that was published). At times, even creating the kit can be therapeutic (i.e., choosing how to decorate it, what to include in the kit, etc.). Before Henry was discharged, he noted that, over time, our direct discussions about suicide and drivers to his suicide attempts provided a sense of comfort for him. He appreciated working with a therapist who was not afraid to directly and openly discuss suicide with him. He gave me a touching note that suggested our work was helpful to him: "I have to admit that I was hesitant to start CAMS, but I could tell you were not scared of this topic and, over time, I was able to speak about it more directly. You saw this as a strength in me, and that gave me the courage to continue this work."

Such a case can be invaluable for a number of reasons. First, it serves as a reminder that empirically supported treatments are available for suicide assessment and prevention, and can be taught to psychology interns and other trainees. In supervision, I often discuss these types of cases; I speak about my initial fears as an early entry psychologist working with suicidal patients, and the value of continued supervision and collaboration when working with psychiatrically complex patients. I think it is important to highlight initial and ongoing fears of suicide prevention work and how these fears, if not discussed directly in supervision, can impact both the assessment of suicide and the subsequent treatment. Students need instructors who can model vulnerability, who can verbalize what they do not know, and who make use of consultation. Unfortunately, not every patient has the outcome that we want.

Case Study: Losing a Patient to Suicide

Andrea was a 19-year-old woman admitted to our young adult program. She had a longstanding history of depression and substance use and had been in and out of psychiatric hospitals for most of her adolescent life. She, admittedly, questioned whether our facility could help her as she had grown tired of treatment and treatment providers. During her eight-week stay with us, she was guarded with staff and peers and had difficulty adjusting to the milieu. She felt disconnected from her peers and believed that others could not fully understand her plight. Family work was also challenging. She felt she had disappointed her parents by not "succeeding" and also felt pressure to make this treatment work. She often noted that her peers outside of treatment were "leaving me behind."

During our initial therapeutic work, she questioned whether she should invest her energy in giving it "one more try." As is true with many suicidal patients, she seemed significantly ambivalent about suicide. Although she had thoughts of not engaging, she was always on time for her sessions and participated actively. Her investment with treatment waxed and waned but, at times, she appeared future-oriented, experiencing curiosity about a life worth living. She wanted friendships and intimate relationships but had been disappointed in the past. The treatment focused on both validating her internal experience and encouraging her to take risks to reach out to others again. Andrea was able to do well in treatment. She developed a core group of friends, attended groups more actively than before, and improved communication with her family. However, approximately two months post-discharge, we learned from her peers that Andrea had completed suicide. The program director announced the news during our morning meeting where the staff convenes to review every patient. The staff, especially the trainee who had worked extensively with her, completing her psychological testing, was stunned. How did this happen? Why did it happen? I glanced at the trainee who had tears rolling down her face. After the meeting, I asked to speak with her in my office. She was visibly shaken. She had never, to her knowledge, worked with a patient who subsequently completed suicide. She began the ruminative process of considering things she may have missed, wondering why Andrea did not contact her for help, and speculating about what Andrea may have been thinking about during her last day of her life. The conversation about suicide completion is difficult and requires great care and concentration. It is a conversation that may need to be repeated on more than one occasion, as the reality of the event doesn't settle in for some time. I encouraged the trainee to take some time off and spend time with people who were important to her. When the time was appropriate, we worked to understand what might have led to the suicide. This is difficult, as the supervisor needs to take great care to not instill blame, and is often struggling with his or her own emotions at the same time. A knowledgeable supervisor carefully navigates between knowing how to soothe and comfort while also allowing the intern to question and work through her own emotions (e.g., anger, sadness, and fear).

Our supervision together focused on grief, fear of working with suicidal patients again, and uncertainty about her career choice, as well as other topics. We also discussed how, as a group co-leader, she might manage the questions asked of current patients who had heard the news about Andrea. This was difficult as it involved managing her anxiety and sadness in the midst of the patients. After some time, there were also requests from staff to assign "easier" patients to interns (i.e., not suicidal or diagnostically complex). In theory this would have made sense; however, at the Clinic, many patients come with intensive suicidal histories and challenging diagnostic histories. The decision is not as easy as it would seem. Tied into our supervisory meetings were more practical discussions about administration sequelae after sentinel events.

As clinicians and supervisors, we did our best to learn from this catastrophic event. Initially, the treatment team was asked to join the "root cause analysis" (RCA). I notified the intern about the RCA and what might be involved in this process. For those unfamiliar with a RCA, it is a framework used in psychiatric hospitals to understand systemic factors that may have contributed to an adverse event (e.g., patient suicide). The purpose is to prevent the recurrence of other adverse events within the hospital and to improve hospital safety. A RCA is required by the Joint Commission for any sentinel event (Percarpio, Watts, & Weeks, 2008). The Joint Commission is a US-based agency that accredits health care organizations and programs. The staff complied with the RCA request and, likely, given their own anxieties about the meeting, did not contact me (the trainee's supervisor) to be present for the meeting. The intern felt a need to comply and attend the RCA and later told me about the meeting. She appropriately shared her anxiety about the meeting and worried about what it would mean for her internship and career. She also worried about other staff and wondered whether they would lose their jobs. However, she felt better after understanding the structure and purpose of the RCA. After the completion of this RCA, staff at the Clinic began drafting a protocol to implement in the event a suicide following discharge occurred in the future. The need for a post-discharge adverse event coordinator was discussed. This point person, selected from the executive team, would be an experienced clinician who would ensure the protocol was being followed. The clinician would:

a. Serve as the primary contact person in cases of the death of a former patient (inpatient or outpatient), regardless of the time elapsed since discharge, and determine whether additional action was indicated.
b. Serve as the designated point person for staff to receive information or hear rumors regarding the death of a former patient.
c. Obtain additional information, when needed, to determine the validity of any such information.
d. Make determinations as to whether and with whom such information should be shared. Those to be notified immediately would include the CEO, Chief of Staff, Medical Director, and Office of Risk Management.
e. If appropriate, in consultation with the executive team, make arrangements for staff relief, including meetings that allow for information sharing and emotional support for directly affected staff members.
f. In consultation with program directors, determine what information, if any, to share with patients who knew the deceased patient or were known to have information regarding the same.
g. Serve as contact person for affected family members, as appropriate.
h. When appropriate, and after emotional needs of affected staff members were addressed, coordinate the process of a non-blaming clinical and administrative review, the purpose of which would be to determine what might be learned that can be used to enhance treatment of future patients.

We continue to assess ways to improve the experiences of our patients and our trainees. Each year, in collaboration with the director of education, we take time to reflect on the experience of the previous training class and decide how to make improvements that will most impact our students. All psychology trainees now obtain training in CAMS. They learn about drivers for suicide, the use of the SSF, and the importance of a collaborative stance when working with suicidal patients. All staff members, including trainees, are required to attend a live training program addressing suicide risk. The training format includes a series of vignettes to encourage discussion about suicide assessment and prevention (C. Mulder & T. Ellis, personal communication, February 23, 2016). In addition, a mock sentinel event is organized to educate trainees about what to do in the unlikely event of such an occurrence. Details such as: who would notify the family (if the patient were still in the Clinic); how to discuss the event with current patients; how to plan a memorial service for the current patients; and preparing the trainee for an RCA, are all included. Recently, the trainees also participated in training called "Collateral Damage." The trainees watched a video of senior clinicians who lost patients to suicide and how they coped with the aftermath. The trainees were then placed in small groups with senior clinicians to discuss and process any questions or comments that they had. The event was well received by both the trainees and the staff and is now part of the scheduled training every year. In addition, the psychiatry residents collaborated on a quality improvement project with the goal of developing resources for residents who have lost a patient to suicide. They developed a "contact support list" with senior clinicians who had a patient complete suicide. The goal was to find a space to share their thoughts and fears around this loss in the event they wanted more containment than the setting could offer at the time. The training program was, in part, developed to better prepare our students for working with suicidal patients.

None of us can ever be prepared to lose a patient to suicide, and yet all of us must be prepared for the possibility, especially when working in a hospital setting. The challenge of training and supervision is to prepare the trainees for work with this high-risk population but also protect them from severe stress reactions. Consistent with the findings of other researchers (e.g., Hendin et al., 2004), it is our experience that trainees tend to be more vulnerable to severe distress reactions like intense guilt, self-blame, or questioning the choice of their decisions. We find that being part of a treatment team and having the support of the whole team, in addition to the supervisory support, may allow a potential crisis to be turned into an opportunity for growth. Hendin et al. (2004) note that experience alone does not protect clinicians against intense emotional responses, like feelings of inadequacy and self-doubt. Instead, it is the emotional support to process such an experience that allows for the occurrence of learning, growth, and resilience in the midst of doubt and despair. We find that this is also true at the institutional level, as continued efforts in the hospital to not only improve but to invest in ongoing training for all employees are beneficial for all staff. In conclusion, we believe that the inpatient internship work is crucial to the training and development of future clinicians who are interested in working with high-risk suicidal populations. The hospital setting, with the treatment team approach, may be the ideal setting for this crucial but challenging professional training experience.

References

Allen, J.G., & Fonagy, P. (2014). Mentalizing in psychotherapy. In R.E. Hales, S. Yudofsky, & L.W. Roberts (Eds.), *Textbook of psychiatry* (6th ed., pp. 1095–1118). Washington, DC: American Psychiatric Press.

American Psychiatric Association. (2003). *Practice guidelines for the assessment and treatment of patients with suicidal behaviors*. Washington, DC: American Psychiatric Press.

Arnett, J.J. (2000). Emerging adulthood: A theory of development from the late teens through the twenties. *American Psychologist*, *55*(5), 469–480.

Ellis, T.E., Daza, P., & Allen, J.G. (2012). Collaborative assessment and management of suicidality at Menninger (CAMS-M): An inpatient adaptation and implementation. *Bulletin of the Menninger Clinic*, *76*, 147–171.

Farberow, N. (1981). Suicide prevention in the hospital. *Hospital and Community Psychiatry*, *32*, 99–104.

First, M.B., Gibbon, M., Spitzer, R.L., Williams, J.B.W., & Benjamin, L.S. (1997). *Structured clinical interview for DSM-IV axis II personality disorders, (SCID-II)*. Washington, DC: American Psychiatric Press.

Gibson, J., & Taylor, D.H. (2003). *The dangerous detour*. Washington, DC: US Department of Health and Human Resources, Agency for Healthcare Research and Quality. Retrieved from https://psnet.ahrq.gov/webmm/case/20.

Hendin, H., Haas, A.P., Maltsberger, J.T., Szanto, K., & Rabinowicz, H. (2004). Factors contributing to therapists' distress after the suicide of a patient [Electronic version]. *The American Journal of Psychiatry*, *161*, 1442–1446.

Heron, M. (2013). Deaths: Leading causes for 2010. *National Vital Statistics Reports*, *62*(2), 1–95.

Jobes, D.A. (2006). *Managing suicidal risk: A collaborative approach*. New York, NY: Guilford.

Kleespies, P.M., Penk, W.E., & Forsyth, J.P. (1993). The stress of patient suicidal behavior during clinical training: Incidence, impact, and recovery. *Professional Psychology: Research and Practice*, *24*(3), 293–303.

Kleespies, P.M., Smith, M.R., & Becker, B.R. (1990). Psychology interns as patient suicide survivors: Incidence, impact, and recovery. *Professional Psychology: Research and Practice 21*, 257–263.

Madan, A., Frueh, B.C., Allen, J.G., Ellis, T.E., Rufino, K.A., Oldham, J.M., & Fowler, J.C. (2016). Psychometric reevaluation of the Columbia-Suicide Severity Scale. Findings from a prospective, inpatient study of severely mentally ill adults. *Journal of Clinical Psychiatry*, *77*(7), e867–e873.

May, A.M., Klonsky, E.D., & Klein, D.N. (2012). Predicting future suicide attempts among depressed suicide ideators: A 10 year longitudinal study. *Journal of Psychiatric Research*, *46*, 946–952.

Ogden, T.H. (1979). On projective identification. *International Journal of Psycho-analysis, 60*, 357–373.
Percarpio, K.B., Watts, B.V., & Weeks W.B. (2008). The effectiveness of root cause analysis: What does the literature tell us? *The Joint Commission Journal on Quality and Patient Safety, 34*(7), 391–398.
Rudd, M.D., Cukrowicz, K.C., & Bryan, C.J. (2008). Core competencies in suicide risk assessment and management: Implications for supervision. *Training and Education in Professional Psychology, 2*, 219–228.
Suicide Prevention Resource Center. (2006). *Core competencies in the assessment and management of suicidality*. Newton, MA: Author.
US World and News Reports. (n.d.). Best hospitals for psychiatry. Retrieved from https://health.usnews.com/best-hospitals/ranking/psychiatry
Wolfersdorf, M. (2000). Suicide among psychiatric inpatients. In K. Hawton & K. Van Heeringen (Eds.), *The international handbook of suicide and attempted suicide* (pp. 457–466). New York, NY: Wiley.

22 An Intern's Experience on an Acute Closed Ward

From a Shadow to a Bird: The Psychotherapeutic Process of Mr. B.

Karin Reddie[1]

I began working in a closed acute ward after completing 3 years of my clinical psychology internship program in an outpatient clinic. I found the encounter with the various psychotic patients hard to describe in words. These patients differed greatly in the intensity of their suffering and distress from the patients I met with in my outpatient work. Today, after working for a year as an intern on the ward, I understand that where words have lost their meaning, a new channel of experience has evolved; a channel that involves willingness to be lost, to surrender to emotional intensities and to recognize them as a matrix, that enables the therapist and the patient to be transformed and emerge anew.

The description of Mr. B.'s treatment presented in this chapter demonstrates the fluctuating intensities that arise with psychosis. The therapist must "fade" into her own and her patient's ancient province of suffering because the annihilating mechanism of psychotic defense has to meet someone willing to bear the burden and destruction without any hope for cure; and still, somehow, the therapist must hold on to a vague belief that something can be built together. A world of professional knowledge acquired through years of training is about to be tested. Paradoxically, we therapists are required to relinquish our ability and the need to know, in favor of the belief that we may be able to heal the wounded mind of the patient that we are now able to discover within ourselves.

In the introduction to his book, *Damaged Bonds*, Eigen wrote:

> When we think of damaged bonds, we think of ties to one another, parent-baby bonding, links to self, other, universe. No one escapes damage to these bonds or to one's linking capacity. Yet we live with our damaged relational capacity and sometimes live well. We make the best of damaged selves with a mixture of pushing past, ignoring, transcending, and trying to heal our sense of injury.
>
> It may be that psychological damage is an intrinsic part of bonding processes, just as a certain amount of physical damage is a natural

> part of birthing. We take for granted violence attached to hatching processes but we play down the role of violence and loss in forging links. We are damaged by bonds that give us life, disabled by connections that help us to grow, succored by damaging processes.
>
> (Eigen, 2001, p. 1)

From the outset, Mr. B.'s treatment began too late. His God failed him.[2] He disjointedly and relentlessly made internal and agonizing indictments. He repeatedly claimed that he was not a bad person, not guilty. Not a junky. We must believe him, that he was good.

I felt that in my attempt to understand him, I annulled him as I imposed order and meaning on the incomprehensible agglomeration that he put before me. I filtered out what my mind could not relate to or understand. As we ordinarily perceive reality in a framework of space, time, color, and size, it is hard to imagine a world without categories. With Mr. B., everything was random. There was no large or small, no distant or close. Everything was now and never. That was how talking with him felt; cruising the galaxy with supernova debris floating around, with no gravitational force and no direction. There was nothing to grasp and hold onto.

Mr. B., 27, was single, with no children. He had no one in the world except for his brother S., with whom he had lost contact. According to his medical record, Mr. B. was sometimes diagnosed with paranoid schizophrenia, sometimes with schizoaffective disorder, and sometimes with "plain" schizophrenia.

Mr. B.'s file was one of the thickest and heaviest in the filing cabinet. Despite his young age, there were countless admissions, psychiatric committees, hospitalization orders, and long-term hospitalizations. At the end of the file, there was a drawing that he drew from who knows when. It was there as if to add some color to the paperwork, to help the reader experience the person behind all of the pages.

Mr. B. began using hard drugs at an early age and made several suicide attempts. When he was 17 years old, he was hospitalized after he jumped in front of a passing car. To this day, he suffers from the many broken bones in his body, the damage evident through his awkward movements.

His most recent hospitalization was about 18 months ago. He disappeared from the hostel for several days and returned in poor condition. He talked in fear about the devil lurking in the bathroom for him and about the wires connecting him to the moon. He was disturbed by the belief that his internal organs were falling out of him.

It could be said that we were admitted to the ward at the same time. For him it was the millionth hospitalization; for me, it was my first ward experience. On my first day working on the ward, I saw him lying on the floor in the lobby like a bundled up lump of flesh.

His appearance told of the horrors he had endured. No part of his body was free of scars. I tried to glance beyond what seemed like a shadow of a human being. I saw a bruised young man, piles of hair hiding his face, and I felt sorrow. However, I could not yet fully comprehend or feel that sorrow. I continued walking.

On my second day on the ward, the senior psychologist suggested that we see Mr. B. together. Mr. B. entered the room holding an orange, dispersing the aromatic smell of citrus fruit. He sat down and immediately started to talk in an associative stream that was impossible to understand. I was preoccupied with his appearance, with the black and blue marks around his eyes, his thinness, the bruises on his skin, and I thought to myself that he must be in pain. Mr. B. appeared untroubled by any of it and even seemed satisfied. He threw the orange peels and pits on the table and asked me to make him coffee. I was shocked and fascinated at the same time.

Mr. B. ate his orange while giving his psychotic speech, and sat down comfortably in the chair. He belched and immediately apologized with his sweet and silly grin. He looked like a small child to me.

The conversation with him was terrible. I did not understand anything, and I do not remember even a word of what he said; only how he looked, which was seared into my consciousness, apparently forever.

A week later, Mr. B. asked for a session with me. He waited for me at the ward's locked door at the appointed time; a door that separates worlds. As the door opened and he entered the corridor, a furious, aggressive patient pushed his way in. I tried to understand what had happened, but the patient was agitated and rushed into the doctor's room. Mr. B. stayed close to me, as if to buffer me from that patient, and said in a calm tone, "There are all sorts of people, sometimes people do not act nicely."

Only later did I understand his gesture toward me. He was protecting me. During the session, Mr. B. eyed my bottle of diet coke. "It is tempting me," he said. "Just a sip." "My throat is dry." "If you're not giving me any of your diet coke, then at least make me some coffee." In between, he told me that he is a prophet and gave his explanation of light, divinity, and mysticism. He explained to me that as a child he was enchanted by the moon, and since then he can see things that others cannot.

At our next meeting, Mr. B. entered the corridor angrily and shouted at me, saying that we wanted to put him in jail. In the room, he went berserk and screamed, and I felt afraid. I opened the door to signal distress, so that at least someone would know if he attacked me. He instantly took advantage of the opportunity to leave and burst into the next room, which was the office of the ward director. The scene was surreal. Mr. B. was wild and screaming, and the ward director was yelling back at him and threatening with theatrical movements as he dialed the nurses' station. When he did so, Mr. B. left, only to return. It seemed to me as though I were in a slapstick movie. I stood there like a golem; I was unable to initiate a meaningful intervention. A male nurse appeared suddenly and calmly said: "Mr. B., come with me," and Mr. B. immediately obeyed. Magic, just like that. I admired the nurse at that moment. After the tumultuous meeting, I brought to supervision my experience of confusion and shock. I understood my feelings as reflecting Mr B.'s experience in a world where we are all fragments of an object in a bizarre and grotesque internal theater.

During supervision the question arose of how and where would it now be possible to meet Mr. B.? I found myself wandering with him throughout the ward, in tune with his changing moods. When there was danger, we met in the nurse's room or the morning report room. When he was calm, I brought him to my office. Before each meeting, I arranged the room for him as if it was being arranged for a baby. Suddenly, each item in the room required my attention. Scissors, which I had previously not noticed, had to be hidden in a drawer, as did every stapler, pencil, and ruler. I forgot to hide some decorative painted stones. Mr. B. noticed one and picked it up, and said that the stone seemed complete on the outside, but inside it was hollow. When he noticed a drawing on the wall, he explained to me that it was the shadow of a bird that has already died, but one could see the path it took on its way to death.

At first, I did not give myself to his intensities. I was preoccupied with his words; I forced myself to remember them, to remember his sentences. I found myself listening and memorizing in order to remember, so that I would have something to bring to supervision. Perhaps afterward I would be able to understand what he said. At the same time, I understood how my need to remember interfered with my being with him. I gradually allowed my mind to wander, to dissipate into his spaces; spaces that always felt as if they were a monument to what was once magnificent and full of hope.

The process of creating a relationship or vanishing along with him proved overwhelming and impossible. Mr. B. showed me how

> ... relationships break as they are forming. Something is always on the verge of breaking, beginning to break, actually breaking, and, finally, broken.
>
> (Eigen, 2001, p. 14)

I discovered to what extent Mr. B.'s encounter with his inner world was painful and unbearable; "the womb keeps breaking apart" (Eigen, 2001, p. 43). Sessions which he entered calmly and smiling, ended in disintegration, with him screaming and crying. His psychotic speeches always converged somehow on themes dealing with good and evil, the evil that threatened the good, and the good that was pillaged.

A haunted and terrifying world emerged from the tone of the conversations with him. Relationships were malicious and harmful. I began asking myself what I was for him – was I good or was I bad. Is there a "me" when I am with him? Who is that "me," and what does it represent? I think that at least during the first two months, there was no "me." I understood that for him, I was he. In one of the sessions, he cried and asked me why I was crying. When he screamed at me, he was screaming at himself.

It was amazing how at some later stage of the treatment Mr. B. approached me in the ward's lobby and reminded me that he had attacked me. You shouted at me; I corrected him. True, he replied. He explained to me that sometimes he confused himself with others. He asked for forgiveness. There was a festive feeling at that moment. I do not know whether we celebrated our survival or our birth; a celebration of our being.

In retrospect, it is difficult to explain what made it possible to survive, to be born, how we continued to meet. We were destroyed so many times; he destroyed the possibility of being in touch, bringing him to the room, getting to know him. After all, he signaled to me in every possible way that these talks were dangerous for him. Dangerous for us. They tore us apart. The inner world was infected and cancerous. Sometimes I felt it was abusive to get him to talk. Why did I continue to abuse him? Why was I not destroyed?

However, "Complete destruction – that's idealism," wrote Eigen (2001, Introduction).

> Most are stuck somewhere partly destroyed. They've no suspicion there's a knack to letting destruction do good work. They tense up, protect themselves, find ways of getting through. They miss out.
> (Eigen, 2001, Introduction)

Mr. B. did his best to survive. Psychosis enabled a type of survival for him and repeatedly took apart his ability to experience and process destructiveness. The arousal of threatening emotions triggered the dismantling annihilating mechanism of psychosis. I asked myself how we could dream the destruction without destroying the dream.

In the next meetings with Mr. B., he returned and accused me of imprisoning him, and demanded free leave from the ward. I promised him that I would relay his request to the doctors. To God.

With a sense of futility, I brought his request to the morning report. To my surprise, Mr. B. was granted free leave on the hospital grounds. Magic. In the first weeks, it worked quite well. Mr. B. wandered around the hospital freely. I saw him walking around, and I was both worried and happy for him. He seemed happy and was calmer.

Suddenly, one day he disappeared. He did not return from a free leave, and the next day his absence was noted in the morning report. At first, I regarded it with a degree of humor. Where could he have gone? However, gradually, I began to feel a pervading sense of dread. I walked by the lake and was afraid that he might have drowned, or committed suicide. My imagination summoned various types of horrible ways of dying. He must be cold; he was wearing flip-flops with no socks. I had a weekend with nerve-wracking worries. On Monday, during the morning report, I rushed to look for his name on the list and saw that there was no Mr. B.. A police officer came and took my testimony about his disappearance. I told him what he was wearing. "Green hospital pants and a red fleece top with a picture of Mickey Mouse. Very thin. Brown hair. It is impossible to miss him," I told him.

The testimony itself made me feel paranoid. I only wanted to say what he looked like; why did the officer need all of my personal details? If Mr. B. did something to someone, I would be called to testify against him. That would be a tragedy. I felt like all of the internal police forces were after me. Nevertheless, I wanted him to be found; to be alive. The police could wait.

That same day, Mr. B. was found wandering in one of the cities. He was alive. The police brought him back to us. Mr. B.'s magical mystery tour was cut short after five days. Indeed mystery encompassed the five-day disappearance. Mr. B. would not know how to tell exactly what had happened, what had occurred.

It was like seeing events through their cracks. He came back with two black eyes and a huge open sore the length of his finger. On the day he returned, part of my car's fender came loose. It seemed symbolic. In the garage, I was told that a few screws had been loosened, and then I realized that my defenses had loosened too, and the encounter was now more exposed, more accessible.

Mr. B. returned as if his light was extinguished, as I had never seen him before. There had always been something alive within him; crazy, insane, and alive. However, he returned dead, injured, and wounded. Just like on the first day in the ward, I saw him lying on the floor, again with black eyes. This time I looked at him and felt a deep sorrow. I stayed with him for a few moments on the floor. I put my hand on him. It was the closest as I could get to caressing him. One of the veteran patients in the ward passed by. He looked at him, and I saw the pain in his heart. At that moment, my eyes filled with tears and I had to leave, so they would not see that I was crying. I went … and left him there.

In supervision, I told everything and could not stop the tears. Later in the week, I met with Mr. B., and he cried and cried; if only he knew how much I cried and cried too. I told Mr. B. that I was worried about him and how happy I was that he returned. It was hard for him, but he allowed me to care for him. It tore him apart, but less so as time passed. His destructiveness diminished. We continued to meet with our "fenders" loosened, and at the same time, something was happening beyond our sessions in the room. In the lobby, Mr. B. told me while I was rushing to the morning report, "I will never forget you." Another time, he stopped me in the lobby and said, "I miss my mother." Parallel to the primary maternal preoccupation (Winnicott, 2012) going on between us, the relationship between Mr. B. and Miss N., a patient in the ward, also became stronger. In one of our meetings, Mr. B. burst into tears when he spoke of her. He said that women always harm. How could he fall in love?

Alongside the crying, dreaming about destruction became possible, it was possible to talk about how dangerous it is to love, how frightening and painful it is. When he cried, he asked me to stroke his head. I told him that I, too, felt a closeness. He kept asking to be caressed, and my heart ached with pain. I could only be with him there in that unbearably painful moment and tell him how much a caressing hand was missing. I felt bad. I remained with that moment for a long time.

Mr. B. brought poems he had written to our next sessions. The poems expressed the courses of his soul, and I found myself relishing every word. He asked that we draw together, and I discovered how beautifully he could draw. In one of the sessions, I found myself drawing for him the bird from the picture on my office wall. The one that was a shadow and that had already died. Mr. B. was interested in the drawing and said that it was a "bird that was being set free." For a moment, we were able to forget that we were in a closed ward. In some of the sessions, he asked me to play music for him. He liked Pink Floyd and Eric Clapton, especially the song with lyrics that describe tears in heaven. He explained that he had lost his heaven long ago. I told him that he was not at fault. During some of the sessions, he lay on the carpet in the room in a fetal position. He tried to dismiss the voices that he heard in his head. He asked me to hold his hand. He said, "thank you."

Mr. B. gradually began to approach additional staff and patients on the ward. One day he noticed we had the same color of eyes – "Is that why you are my psychologist?" I was able to see it as well and suggested that he was perhaps asking what connects us. I understood that via the connection and the similarity, he was able to begin differentiation. The sessions during this period were magical, and through the shared experiences, I began to hold more and more parts of him, hoping that perhaps I could give him something back from this holding, something that might in the future be able to become his self-experience.

I empowered his growth, and in parallel during the days of despair, I experienced the slippery slopes with him. I coped with the difficulty of holding his various parts, in order to enable him to have a more coherent experience. In one of the sessions, he explained to me

> if you bring a baby to the world he talks to you without a voice, and that is how you raise him. You need to see his fragility and his development, and then you need to understand the magic because you owe him his security.

I found myself admiring his depth and sensitivity and suggested that security and growth become possible when we feel held when we are not alone.

The therapeutic holding enabled Mr. B. to grow stronger, and the ward staff began to discuss the possibility of Mr. B.'s moving back to the hostel. I was busy separating from him and wondering which one of us would leave first. There were two months until the end of my internship, and I was concerned that my departure would be experienced as a destructive abandonment. I felt guilty and sad about being only a partial and temporary good object. I wondered what would remain of us. When I raised the issue of separation, Mr. B. ignored it, and his speech became incoherent. I noted his difficulty and told him that it was hard for me as well. I found myself torn between hope for his hospital discharge and anxiety regarding the possibility that the freedom would be dangerous for him. I considered the possibility that perhaps my desire for his discharge might be mixed with guilt because I was soon to leave him. In one of the sessions, he asked that we pay attention and see when the hospitalization is killing him. I asked myself what is right for him. What will "kill" him less? I accompanied him to the rehabilitation committee. On the way back his thought process began to break down, and he expressed paranoid thoughts about his brother. Later in the week, his condition deteriorated. He did not return on time from leave, and he attacked another patient. The hostel was no longer an option. I understood the regression as a reaction to the imminent separation. Separation was considered death. During sessions, I tried to process the events with Mr. B., but he was busy with the coffee cups that he plotted to steal from the psychiatrist's room. His life was stolen from him, and he had to steal too.

That month I received a job offer from the hospital that would enable me to continue working in the ward. I stayed, and he also remained, but something died. The sessions became heavy and exhausting. Mr. B. reverted to talking in bits and pieces, and I began to feel less invested in him, empty of thoughts, and even wondering about the contribution of the therapy. I understood that death entered our relationship the moment that separation entered as something tangible and was experienced as emptiness and loss of love. In one of the sessions, Mr. B. asked that we be quiet. "Give me some quiet." I asked him what we were quiet about and he answered; "I miss my mother." I felt that trauma entered the relationship as I also let him go. In the following session, he said that he doesn't need anyone, not even me. Later in the week, he asked for a different psychologist. He avoided me when I called him to come for a talk. It hurt me, but thanks to the supervision I received, I managed to contain my anger and insult and to tell him that I was there if he wanted me. I reminded him of the dates and times of our appointments. When we finally met, he said that the therapy was worthless if he is still here. I reflected his disappointment; he wanted something but did not receive it. He was filled with rage and shouted at me that I was avenging him, that I was evil and that because of me he was imprisoned. The words were hurtful, and I told him how much they hurt me to hear. I debated whether to end the session and decided to stay and absorb the anger. I felt that he needed me to stay with him. Two weeks later, he said that despite all, there was a connection between us. That I have a soft spot for his madness. "There is love, even if it has a price."

The next sessions were full of grief. He expressed a longing for lost relationships, and for the first time Mr. B. began to talk about his past and his parents. He told of his girlfriend who died of an overdose. He talked about guilt and the "internal prison." He asked that we light a memorial candle and deal with the devil together. I was touched and told him that perhaps we could endure this hell together. His life story is saturated with death. His parents died when he was young, his older sister committed suicide, and he too was a "shadow of a bird that was already dead." Death was always there, but he ran away from it. I enumerated for him the things he had lost, what the illness had taken, and the fragility of the relationships. I felt his death with a sense of despair in me. In one of the sessions, he asked me "What do I have to live for?" I wondered what I had to offer him instead of the psychosis. I could only be with him in his pain. To tell him that it is not his fault.

During that period, Mr. B. did not receive free leave to go out alone, and at every session he asked that we go outside. In my supervision, I discussed the dilemma this raised regarding therapy and decided that one of the two weekly sessions would take place outside the ward, on the hospital grounds. I understood his request and my response as an attempt to survive the death, to create an intermediate space between inside and outside, between death and life. When he went outside, he was blinded by the sun and mentioned how good it was to be outside the walls for a moment. "Walls of hope," he said and laughed. I reflected on his vitality and was happy for him. One day he asked to look at my identification tag. He noticed that my name was Karin. He asked if I, like him, also liked to climb trees. If I also had childhood traumas. I pointed out that his interest in me was a way to get to know himself, and I understood that I was beginning to be for him the other through whom he could see himself reflected. He began to create a self-experience that could hold the nothingness, the loss, and the suffering. In one of our last sessions, Mr. B. explained that he was a bird that flew out of the cage but always returned because in the cage he was protected, and then he said – "I'm happy with you, and it seems to me that you are also happy with me."

Mr. B., I am grateful for the opportunity given me to get to know you, to be with you in hell and to see you slowly emerge. You entered my heart. When I came home after my sessions with you, I could not stop crying. The pain, the suffering, and the agony. You gave me precious moments of joy when I saw you laughing, calm, free, so loved, helping others, sensitively caring for them. I hope you know how important and significant you became for me. I will never forget you.

Your treatment would not have been possible without the emotional support I received from the wonderful team of psychologists I worked with in the hospital. Thanks to them, I succeeded in thinking about you, cultivating emotion, connecting to theory, and putting all this into words.

The therapeutic encounter with Mr. B. helped me shed my own defenses and connect with raw and primal feelings; feelings with which I had previously not been in touch. This encounter was difficult and frightening. A kind of initial horror, as Winnicott described in his article "Fear of Breakdown" (1974). Thanks to the guidance I received through supervision, I was able to stay with the difficult emotions and give them a place within me.

In addition to my therapeutic encounter with Mr. B., work in the hospital enabled me to meet a spectrum of patients who suffer from severe mental disorders. The work required that I adapt to each patient in order to meet them in their own unique places. This meeting with the ward's patients generated my developmental and maturational processes as a clinical psychologist, contributing to growth that was not possible in prior settings, and in the earlier stages of my professional development.

Over time, I was able to see beyond the severe symptoms and breakdowns and recognize the richness and uniqueness of each patient. I was able to see each patient I worked with as a person with hopes, dreams, desires, and yearnings for a relationship. Work in the hospital is fascinating for me and repeatedly engages me with basic questions about life, the mind, and the therapeutic relationship. I feel that working on the inpatient unit has contributed much to me, on both professional and personal levels. I am grateful for the opportunity provided by this experience.

Notes

1 Translated from Hebrew by Mrs. Rena Kurs.
2 Paraphrasing (Eigen, 2001, p. 22).

Reference

Eigen, M. (2001). *Damaged Bonds*. New York, NY: Routledge.

Winnicott, D. W. (1974). Fear of breakdown. *International Review of Psycho-Analysis, 1*(1–2), 103–107.

Winnicott, D. W. (2012). Primary maternal preoccupation. In P. Mariotti (Ed.), *The new library of psychoanalysis. The maternal lineage: Identification, desire and transgenerational issues* (pp. 59–66). New York, NY: Routledge/Taylor & Francis Group.

Editors' Perspectives and Closing Remarks

23 Weaving with a Relational Thread

The Clinical Psychologist's Use of Empathy in Work in the Mental Health Inpatient Setting

Meidan Turel

The mental health inpatient setting can be home to the most severe and distressing mental disorders encountered by mental health professionals. Persons receiving treatment within these settings are frequently at the extreme of human emotional and mental suffering. Debilitating psychotic and affective disorders, as well as severe personality or reactive disorders, may render the person dependent on the mental health inpatient system and its professionals to contain, understand and take appropriate action in aid of support and recovery, and at times to sustain life itself.

As the chapters in this book demonstrate, clinical psychologists working in these settings can have a crucial role in helping the mental health inpatient system and its professionals achieve these goals. Whether involved in systems level work, psychotherapeutic interventions or psychological assessments, the attention and understanding that psychologists' work brings to psychological phenomena holds the potential to support an integrated application of the biopsychosocial model of treatment in the inpatient team's work with its patients. Throughout the book's four parts, chapters demonstrate the humanistic and person-centered approach inherent in psychologists' practice, principles consistent with the humanistic vision of the biopsychosocial model of mental health inpatient care.

Competing Models of Treatment: The Biomedical versus the Biopsychosocial

Mental health professionals working with the biopsychosocial model of treatment, an important and influential model within modern psychiatric inpatient care, seek to understand and treat mental illness through a holistic and individualized perspective toward the suffering person. Illness is perceived as the result of a complex and idiosyncratic interaction between biological, psychological and social factors operating in the past and the present in a person's life (Engel, 1980). Introduced by Engel in the 1970s, the model offered a humanistic alternative to the dominant biomedical model, criticized for its dehumanizing and disempowering approach in which patients were reduced to the sum of their symptoms and diagnostic labels, and cast in the role of passive recipients of a dictated and impersonal medicalized treatment.

Engel's biopsychosocial model, in contrast, offered a treatment approach that placed the patient as a unique and autonomous individual in the center of the therapeutic endeavor. In this model, the person's ailment is contextualized within the person's historical and present life's circumstances. Treatment, accordingly, is geared to address in a multi-disciplinary and integrated manner, the particular configuration of biological, psychological and social factors operating in the individual's life and current predicament. Furthermore, the therapist's participation and investment in the therapeutic relationship is enlisted as part of the therapeutic endeavor, allowing an involved and human encounter with the treated person to evolve (Borrell-Carrió et al., 2004).

Undoubtedly, such a holistic and integrated perspective within the psychiatric inpatient system opens the door to the person-centered and humanistic approach driving clinical psychology. Such a vision of the biopsychosocial model of psychiatric inpatient care offers the psychologist a shared language with which to communicate with the multi-disciplinary team. It invites the clinical psychologist to serve as an active and contributing partner in the team's collaborative effort to provide an integrated, humane and person-centered treatment.

However, in reality, this vision of the biopsychosocial model and psychiatry's professed commitment to it, have never fully realized. As various writers observed, the biopsychosocial model of psychiatric care is "fighting a losing battle" in the face of the historically entrenched and reductionist biomedical model (Benning, 2015; Pilgrim, 2002). According to Gabbard and Kay (2001), the biopsychosocial model of care is paid "lip service" by the dominant biomedical approach, and at best, multi-disciplinary psychiatric team members tolerantly co-exist, functioning side by side without disturbing each other's separate agendas.

Alluringly, the biomedical model, with its endorsement of impersonal and coercive medicalized methods of treatment, can make the difficult management of persons suffering from severe mental distress and illness, appear as if easier to cope with.

I first became aware of the inherent tension between the biopsychosocial and biomedical modes of practice through my work in a closed acute unit in a large state psychiatric hospital, in what was the final part of my clinical psychology internship program. From the beginning of my work there, in the mid-1990s, I observed the opposing tendencies between these two modes of practice, as they came to influence and bear on the unit's treatment of its patients. While the unit strived to incorporate some measure of the biopsychosocial perspective in its work with the patients, in practice, this was difficult to achieve. The biomedical model appeared to be the unit's "default" mode of operation in addressing its intensive and challenging daily heavy workload. It was usually with some effort and struggle, undertaken by one or the other of the multi-disciplinary team members, and centering on some particular patient treatment issue, that briefly a more integrated and person-centered biopsychosocial perspective would emerge. However, this perspective was difficult to sustain over any length of time, as it would soon dissipate and "vanish," enveloped by some urgent issue coming up and requiring the unit's immediate attention and response.

During my many years of work in that unit and hospital, I have progressed from the position of intern to that of a licensed clinical psychologist, followed by the role of a licensed supervisor and more recently as director of the hospital's psychology department. Throughout these years, and in my different roles and capacities, I have endeavored to decipher the underlying issues challenging the mental health inpatient system's endorsement of a more integrated and person-centered biopsychosocial model of care for its patients. I have been engrossed in finding ways to support the system with these challenges, initiating interventions sensitive to my understanding of the system's difficulties in implementing such a model.

In closing this book, I present some of my understandings of these underlying difficulties and describe one approach I have used in my effort to therapeutically respond to them. I will end the chapter with some thoughts on the important role clinical psychologists can have in the future development of the mental health inpatient system, supporting its movement toward a more integrated and person-centered treatment of the individuals under its care.

The Painful and Fragmented Mind

The severity of the mental distress that leads to inpatient treatment includes a splitting and fragmenting impact on the mind of the person who is suffering. The ability to cogently organize one's thoughts and feelings, to mentalize and understand one's own mind's inner workings, all these are compromised and challenged by the severity of the person's mental disorder. Difficulty symbolizing, relating to and meaningfully being in touch with painful or difficult aspects of internal life, may lead to the evacuation of such mental content and its externalized expression through symptomatic and maladaptive behaviors. Such a concrete behavioral expression of mental life shows the damaging effects of the splitting and fragmenting forces present in severe mental states. It is the inpatient unit and its staff that serve as a receptacle for these processes, as they contain and deal with their behavioral consequences.

Confronted by a devastated and painful inner reality, the severely distressed person may lack the ability to tap inner emotional meanings and sensitivities from which to generate a coherent and consistent sense of self and identity. Facing a threatening void in the sense of self, the person resorts to a functional mode of behavior, split off and disconnected from the underlying emotional experience, with which to adaptively define some sense of self and fill relational spaces.

For example, a patient who seeks constant proximity and physical closeness with, or comfort, from a staff member may be behaviorally expressing profound dependency needs that are split off and otherwise unacknowledged within a precarious sense of self. Such split off and unacknowledged needs cannot be represented or touched upon in a more meaningful relational mode. In this example, the patient's maladaptive behavior on the unit might actually be the person's most adaptive way to express deep dependency needs to be awakened toward the staff. Expressing his or her dependency needs in such a "maladaptive" manner, allows the person to survive and sidestep the impact of revived painful and mind-shattering traumatic experiences with thwarted dependency needs originating in other relational contexts. Such a behavior affords the patient escape from a shattered and confusing inner sense of self, substituting for it a self-experience anchored in concretized behavior, disconnected and alienated from the underlying threatening inner emotional need.

Offering respite from the frightening experience of discontinuity and loss of the sense of self, such a disconnected and de-subjectifying behavior (in the example above, the proximity and comfort-seeking behavior), provides the person with an alternate means of organizing a sense of selfhood and identity. Behavior comes to define modes of being and relating vis a vis the other through concrete functions and roles. In this way, some measure of the necessary sense of inner control and security is obtained. Thus, psychological space collapses, its elements dispersed, with their meanings obliterated, substituted by a mentally emptying scaffolding of the person through externally defined roles and functions.

In many of this book's chapters, examples of such intrapsychic and interpersonal dynamics in the lives of persons suffering from severe mental disorders and treated in mental health inpatient settings can be found in the psychologists' descriptions of their work. Whether in examples describing the work of early career intern psychologists (e.g., chapters by Daria Mamon and Karin Reddie), or describing work of highly experienced and expert practitioners (e.g., chapters by Marilyn Charles and Hilik Peri), such dynamics can be seen to abound in mental health inpatient settings, adding unique difficulties and challenges to the therapeutic work.

Paradoxically, the mentally distressed person's compromised ability to process and contain distressing emotional content and its meaningful communication in a relational context is echoed in the medically oriented mental health inpatient system's disposition to avoid delegating underlying psychological significance to a person's presenting symptoms and illness, for which the inpatient treatment is required.

Parallel Processes

In some ways, the present day medically oriented mental health inpatient system can be viewed as both a reflection and a therapeutic adaptation of the psychic processes described above. The various mental health professionals that in many units make up the multidisciplinary team (i.e., psychiatrist, psychiatric nurse, social worker, occupational therapist, psychologist and others), each address different functions and therapeutic needs of the hospitalized person, as defined by their respective disciplines' perspectives. The patient's treatment is compartmentalized according to these different functions of the multidisciplinary team, and expectedly, when the team's efforts are coordinated, the person is "held" appropriately and treated toward his or her potential recovery.

Such a model lends itself well to the deconstruction of the patient from a whole, subjectively contextualized mentally distressed person, into a patient having disparate objective therapeutic needs and defined functions that are attended to separately. Parallel to the fragmenting and alienating processes operating in the patient's mental world, such a functional division of treatment among the staff offers a way to bypass the impact of emotional contact with the mental plight underlying the patient's state. Performing concrete duties and functions toward part aspects and therapeutic needs of the patient allows to create a distance and avoid connecting with overwhelming aspects of the patient's emotional and subjective reality. This inner reality is replaced by an operationally defined and professionally ordered mode of therapeutically responding to that which is fragmented and unbearable to realize.

Thus within the mental health inpatient system, there can be a hidden collusion of underlying parallel processes, operating within both the mentally distressed person and the system entrusted with receiving and treating that person, working together reciprocally toward the annulment of psychological space. Such a process works to replace the distressing subjective psychological essence of the person's being with a phenomenological and role-attributing definition, put in place according to presenting symptoms and behaviors, together with their defined and indicated treatments.

In line with the biomedical model's perspective, the patient's subjective identity and inner psychological life are cast aside as irrelevant to the task at hand. Instead, the patient's symptoms, diagnostic labels, and concrete treatment needs, are used to identify the person and define who he or she is within the inpatient unit.

The Psychologist's Use of Empathy as a Therapeutic Tool

Needing to find respite from the intense mental distress of a pained and fragmented mind, the patient enters the therapeutic milieu of the inpatient unit. Here the patient can find succor in being held and treated by the various members of the multi-disciplinary team. The formalized therapeutic roles and functions of these team members as well as the unit's ordered setting offer a way to organize and survive the internal mental turmoil.

The clinical psychologist is a part and partner of this multi-disciplinary team. However, beyond being recognized through the more formal and well-versed role as the provider of assessment and psychotherapy, the clinical psychologist holds an additional position within the multi-disciplinary professional matrix. Through the systematic and scientific studies in human psychology and the rigorous training regimen that all go into the making of the clinical psychologist, the clinical psychologist holds expert knowledge and understanding of mental phenomena, personality and behavior.

In many of this book's chapters, authors emphasize the psychologist's important role in finding and imparting psychological and emotional significance to their patient's stressful behaviors and symptoms. This is a common theme uniting psychologists' work in these settings, beyond differentiating theoretical and technical orientations or the mode of intervention used. Chapters describing systems-level interventions, individual psychotherapy, as well as assessment work, emphasize the important role the psychologist's formulation of the patient's predicament has for understanding and contextualizing the patient's behavior. All of these chapters show how such a formulation promotes a person-centered tailoring of the patient's treatment. Whether driven by cognitive behavior theory (e.g., chapters by Sally Riggs; Parswani and Stewart; Walker and Li) or psychodynamic approaches (e.g., chapters by Beatriz Sanchez Curtis and Dione Johnson-Williams), such a formulation provided by the psychologist imparts unique psychological and emotional meanings to the individual patient's behavior and predicament.

The psychologist endeavors to meet and come in contact with the patient's inner psychological world, in an attempt to subjectively contextualize the person's condition and predicament. Such an approach works toward (re)creating psychological space within which emotional meanings and needs, driving so much of the person's mental distress can be recognized, acknowledged, and as therapeutically appropriate, validated and acted upon. In the face of rigid and stultifying mechanisms and processes working on deadening mental reality and emotional truth, the psychologist strives to discover and enliven these assets through benign communication with the patient and staff alike. Using psychological knowledge and clinical acumen, coupled with an empathic stance, the psychologist works toward giving structure and meaning to the patient's hitherto hidden mental reality.

Empathy, a universal human phenomena, is used by the psychologist as a mental tool with which to "hear" and come in contact with various layers of the inner mind. Much as the physician's use of the stethoscope allows the patient's heartbeats to reverberate within him through his auditory senses, so the psychologist's use of empathy allows the patient's inner layers of the mind to reverberate within him through his experiential senses. Empathy is a connection. Opposite mentally destructive forces working to attack and disconnect links within the mind, empathy is a mental process working to promote links in an interpersonal context.

Using empathy, the psychologist experientially discovers and connects to more hidden aspects of the other person's mind, and using psychological acumen, strives to meaningfully contextualize them within that person's life. This understanding of empathy as a tool used by the psychologist for therapeutic means is perhaps a variant rendition of Freud (1912) famous recommendation to the practice of psychoanalysis in which he states that "the doctor … must turn his own unconscious like a receptive organ toward the transmitting unconscious of the patient" (p. 115), and so "from the derivatives of the unconscious which are [thus] communicated to him, to reconstruct that unconscious …" (ibid., p. 116).

To allow such a process to unfold, the clinical psychologist must be a willing and able partner for an emotionally uncensored meeting with damaged aspects of the patient's mental life. The psychologist gains some sense of these parts of the patient's mental life, as they may impact and reverberate within him. Being in touch and listening within himself to the experiential repercussions of such a meeting, the psychologist can then process, think, and bring some sense and understanding to that which was previously not possible to think about or make sense of. Reminiscent of Bion's description of the maternal reverie function (Bion, 1962), the psychologist's ability to experientially sense, contain and think about these disturbing elements, enables those elements to gain mental significance and emotional meaning within a personalized subjective context.

Case Example

Forty-year-old P. is diagnosed with unremitting paranoid schizophrenia. He is continuously psychotic and has spent many years in the acute closed ward where I meet with him for twice-weekly psychotherapeutic sessions. On the unit, the staff are puzzled and disconcerted with P's behavior of secretly removing food from the dining room, hiding and hoarding it under his bed and other places in his room. This unhealthy behavior troubles the staff, especially as the food spoils, spreading a foul smell. Although this behavior was repeatedly addressed in the multidisciplinary teams' interventions with P., no lasting change could be achieved. In our relationship as well, it was not possible to deal with this behavior as P. would get agitated and enraged if I attempted to bring it up. Well into our relationship, P., who having been orphaned as a young child was raised by his aunts, proudly confided in me his exploits as a gifted young basketball player on his school team. He bemoaned the "fact" that he could have become a great national league player but for the reality that he always came home from ball practice to an empty home, hungry and thirsty, never finding anybody waiting for him with food and drink. Although he grinned as he recounted and shared with me these thoughts and memories, I could feel the pain underlying his tale, and a feeling of sorrow filled me for the young orphaned, and deserted child revealed in him. In one of our sessions, as he turned once again to this narrative, he delved deeper into a real life-like account of these events, vividly describing how throbbing with hunger pangs he expectantly opened the refrigerator door to find it empty except for some stale and rotting non-edible food remains. As we were both engrossed in his tale, the scene experientially came alive in the room. For a fleeting moment, I somewhat visualized it and was filled with an unrecognized sensation, with a raw emotional impact difficult to put into words, that I immediately sensed as replicating some unrepresented mental elements of the harsh experience being lived in the room. While "holding" on to our shared dyadic experience, in the back of my mind I associated to Bion's concepts of unassimilated beta elements and the therapist's alpha functioning (Bion, 1962), and found this inspiring and moving, as well as adding to my compassionate stance toward P. At the end of our session, as always, I escorted P. back into the locked unit. As we entered the unit and my senses were impacted by the overwhelming stimuli filling the place, I was reminded of P.'s troubling behavior of hoarding stagnating and foul-smelling food in his room, and felt a strengthened compassion and connectedness to that lost and abandoned child I could recognize within him.

This example demonstrates the psychologist's use of his own mental space in an effort to find connections and meanings allowing for the creation of a psychological perspective within which to "hold" the patient's mind. Such work goes to show the libidinal element involved in the therapeutic endeavor, in working through an emotionally empathic attitude to form links and connect together elements of the patient's inner mental life, by allowing these to connect within a caring other.

The psychologist's empathic stance, coupled with understanding and knowledge of mental processes, is used in work with the inpatient multidisciplinary team as well, helping to work through difficult situations encountered on the ward. For example, when dealing with a complex treatment situation with a patient, unconscious and forceful defensive mechanisms can come into play within the team, and processes such as splitting, over-identification, and others, may work to hamper the team's therapeutic potential. Understanding the dynamics at play, as well as team members' difficulties in dealing with these, enables the clinical psychologist to connect with the staff, and intervene in a manner that helps create a shared mental space in which to observe, think, and get in touch with the underlying processes rather than blindly play them out.

Case Example

Staff were increasingly expressing frustration at the unit's inability to end P.'s behavior of hiding food in his room and its harmful and unhygienic consequences. Some described their uneasiness in rejecting P.'s requests during mealtimes for any extra portions of food because of this behavior. Feelings of antipathy as well as an aversion to what was explained away as bizarre psychotic behavior typical of schizophrenic illness were taking hold. An attitude of detachment and aloofness toward P. was developing as the staff were increasingly distancing themselves from P., limiting interactions with him to the basic management of life on the unit and occasionally clearing the room from the cached food, to which he would react passively and without resisting. Underlying this attitude within the team, one could sense less acknowledged and unrecognized feelings of helplessness and of being at a loss toward P. and his behavior. In one of the morning reports following the session described above, as the team was once again briefly discussing the futility of their work with P. while venting some anger at his behavior, I found an opportunity to wonder out loud about the possible connection between P.'s obsessed behavior with food and his early-life background. As I met with some curious gazes, I continued and reminded the team of P.'s childhood circumstances, well known anamnestic facts, about his being orphaned as a young child, to be raised by his aunts amidst poverty and neglect. While within me holding on to the shared experience with P. of his overwhelming feelings of deprivation and hunger, I described to the team something of a child's possible harmful psychological and emotional consequences in the face of parental loss and abandonment. For a moment, the atmosphere in the room changed and softened.

In the coming days during morning reports, P. received additional attention, as staff would give more details of his daily doings and activities. In the next weekly patient treatment-planning meeting, time was given as P.'s turn to be discussed came up. A more concerned and involved attitude developed, as the participating team members reflected on their perspective of

P.'s unrelenting concern with food. From a more empathic stance toward what was now recognized as possibly signifying deep and traumatized underlying needs, new ideas came up of dealing with P.'s behavior, and a plan was put together by all the multi-disciplinary team members present. The plan included, among other things, involving P. in aiding staff in the dining room during meal times, as well as allowing P. out of the locked unit to visit the hospital canteen, whereby the social worker assumed the responsibility for finding the funds to enable his purchase of goods there.

The psychologist's creation of psychological space helped the team members realize and get in touch with possible underlying emotional meanings of the patient's behaviors, allowing for a more compassionate and empathic attitude to develop. Replacing a constricting enactment staged by the patient's dissociated and split off painful elements of mind, with staff and patient bound together in a hidden and repetitive script, such a space allowed for a more integrated perspective of the patient and the multi-disciplinary team's therapeutic efforts. From such a perspective, the multi-disciplinary team could observe their differentiated therapeutic modalities as serving differentiated aspects of the whole person, rather than as serving disconnected functions and needs, split off from each other and alienated from the person as a whole.

Promoting such a holistic approach toward persons treated in mental health inpatient settings accords well with Engel's original vision of the biopsychosocial model of treatment, as well as with more recently developing social attitudes regarding treatment of persons suffering from mental disorder. Seeing the patient's mental predicament within a contextualized and subjective perspective rather than mainly through diagnostic lenses, and enlisting the patient as an active partner in the therapeutic alliance rather than being the passive recipient of a formalized treatment plan, are goals that psychologists working in inpatient settings strive to achieve and that are congruent with such modern trends.

These goals, derived from basic humanistic tenets, underlie the practice of clinical psychology and can be identified in all of the psychologists' work described in this volume. Finding and validating the person in the patient, and having a deep curiosity and respect for the individual and his or her psychological life, are factors that feed much of the motivation driving the clinical psychologist's work in these difficult and strenuous settings. The patient, on thus being discovered and validated, can better connect and take ownership over disparate elements of his or her mind, allowing for a more integrated and grounded sense of self to grow. Paraphrasing Loewald (1960) on this issue, it is an element of love and respect for the individual's growth that the patient needs to find in his or her therapeutic relations, in order to develop beyond his/her present binding predicament. The clinical psychologist, promoting an empathic and integrative stance in the inpatient unit's containment of its patients, promotes the creation of psychological space where the potential for such an opportunity can arise.

Concluding Remarks

For the fragile mind of the severely mentally distressed person, experiencing the painful emotions involved in relating to the world becomes unbearable. The mind's function as a generator and container of an emotionally meaningful subjective and relational experience of living in the world collapses. Disorganization and escape to illness and disturbed behavior ensue.

As much as a patient's damaged body requires the hospital to protect, treat and allow survival, so does the stricken mind of the severely mentally ill. The psychiatric hospital as such a place can become the protective container for these persons. The structured order and organization inherent in the psychiatric hospital's medicalized setting, together with the multi-disciplinary team's treatment, may serve as the "life-supporting" systems replacing the damaged relational and mental functioning of the "injured" mind. For the multi-disciplinary team members as well, the psychiatric hospital's defined structure, roles, and functions can provide the "safe ground" from which to therapeutically reach out to their patients while safeguarded from the potentially disturbing impact of meeting with a pained and fragmented mind.

Through an empathic attunement coupled with psychological understanding, the clinical psychologist can be sensitive to the presence of these underlying protective needs. The psychologist can be aware of the influence these needs exert in pulling away from a more personalized biopsychosocial mode of work, and toward the impersonal and alienating biomedical one. Through the use of his or her own psychological space, the psychologist can recognize and be in touch with these emotional needs and creatively and flexibly initiate interventions with patients and team members accordingly. Using empathy as a relational thread, the psychologist strives to weave together in an integrating manner, the unit's structured therapeutic resources with the subjective and emotional reality and needs of the persons involved. In this way, allowing a person's hidden emotional truth to surface and imbue the unit's therapeutic work with newfound meanings can provide a fulfilling and rewarding experience for all involved.

In our present era of evidence-based driven practice, it is encouraging to learn of some recent research findings supporting the beneficial medically therapeutic impact of interpersonal and relational variables, such as empathy, in the physician's relationship with the patient (Del Canal et al., 2012; Hojat et al., 2011; Kelley et al., 2014). Such present age empirical findings echo the wisdom of the ancient Greek philosopher and physician, Hippocrates (c. 460–c. 370 BC), who 2500 years ago urged physicians to treat their patients within a relational framework and recognize the subjective context in which their illness appeared. Hippocrates viewed the physician and patient as partners, working together in a common bond, with their relationship in itself being a therapeutic factor (Havelka et al., 2009).

Modern day social and cultural trends emulate these ancient directives, emphasizing the need for a more person-centered and humane approach to be integrated into modern psychiatric inpatient care. Psychologists have an important role to play in aiding such a shift, helping the inpatient system move toward a more person-centered and humanistic biopsychosocial mode of work, where the medical, psychological and social aspects of treatment are brought together and integrated in a manner that can best serve each individual's situation and needs.

All of the work presented in this book demonstrates the clinical psychologist's aptitude for fulfilling such a role. With an expertise in intrapsychic, interpersonal and relational psychological processes, the clinical psychologist can initiate interventions that are attentive and calibrated to the complex multiplicity of needs and dynamics operating within the inpatient setting. Trained to "work" with one's own psychological space, the clinical psychologist has use of empathy to connect and join together frayed threads of human experience into a whole and meaningful communication. Such communication can be heard, shared and therapeutically responded to on the unit, promoting integrative processes in the work.

It is hoped that this book, describing clinical psychologists' work in a wide and international variety of mental health inpatient settings, will allow a growing recognition of their contribution in promoting a humanistic and person-centered biopsychosocial mode of work. Hopefully, in turn, such recognition will encourage a widening inclusion of psychologists' practice in mental health inpatient settings for the benefit of all involved.

References

Benning T. (2015). Limitations of the biopsychosocial model in psychiatry. *Adv Med Educ Pract.* 6:347–352.

Bion WR. (1962). The psycho-analytic study of thinking. *Int J Psycho-Anal.* 43:306–310.

Borrell-Carrió F, Suchman AL, Epstein RM. (2004). The biopsychosocial model 25 years later: Principles, practice, and scientific inquiry. *Ann Fam Med.* 2 (6):576–582.

Del Canal S, Louis DZ, Maio V, Wang X, Rossi G, Hojat M, Gonnella JS. (2012). The relationship between physician empathy and disease complications: An empirical study of primary care physicians and their diabetic patients in Parma, Italy. *Acad Med*. 87(9):1243–1429.

Engel G. (1980). The clinical application of the biopsychosocial model. *Am J Psychiatry*. 137:535–544.

Freud S. (1912). Recommendations to physicians practising psycho-analysis. *The Standard Edition of the Complete Psychological Works of Sigmund Freud, Volume XII (1911–1913): The Case of Schreber, Papers on Technique and Other Works*, 109 120. London: Hogarth.

Gabbard G, Kay J. (2001). The fate of integrated treatment: Whatever happened to the biopsychosocial psychiatrist? *Am J Psychiatry*. 158:1956–1963.

Havelka, M, Despot Lucanin, J, Lucanin, D. (2009). Biopsychosocial model – the integrated approach to health and disease. *Collegium Antropologicum*. 33(1): 303–331.

Hojat M, Louis DZ, Markham FW, Wender R, Rabinowitz C, Gonnella JS. (2011). Physicians' empathy and clinical outcomes for diabetic patients. *Acad Med*. 86(3):359–364.

Kelley JM, Kraft-Todd G, Schapira L, Kossowsky J, Riess H. (2014). The influence of the patient-clinician relationship on healthcare outcomes: A systematic review and meta-analysis of randomized controlled trials. *PLoS One*. 9(4): e904207.

Loewald H. (1960). On the therapeutic action of psychoanalysis. *Int J Psychoanal*. 41:16–33.

Pilgrim D. (2002). The biopsychosocial model in Anglo-American psychiatry: Past, present and future. *J Ment Health*. 11(6):585–594.

24 Concluding Thoughts

Past and Present Trends, Future Directions

Michael Siglag

The past, present, and future co-mingle in inpatient mental health treatment. This is true for psychologists' work, many other aspects of such treatment, and even the facilities in which treatment takes place. This volume demonstrates this through chapters by a wide-ranging assemblage of psychologists who describe current and changing treatment emphases and issues in their work in such facilities.

Shifts in the terminology used to describe those receiving treatment, and designations of inpatient mental health facilities themselves, suggest the ongoing transformation that is taking place in treatment carried out by psychologists and others in such facilities. For example, during the twentieth century, the term 'psychiatric hospital' replaced terms such as 'asylum' and emphasized facilities' identities as medical treatment centers. However, the term 'psychiatric hospital' is now becoming outdated and has been replaced in many facilities. Newer terminology reflects changing attitudes and conceptualizations about treatment. Many of the facilities described by chapter authors in this book are called 'clinic,' 'institute,' 'mental health center,' 'psychiatric center,' or simply 'center.' Few facilities use the term 'psychiatric hospital' in their current official monikers. Yet, on their web sites, most of the agencies whose work is described in these chapters still use that term. A transformation is taking place. An old model is being shed, but the old and the new co-exist. Both literally and figuratively, the new continues to contain the old, and the old incorporates the new, in name and in practice.

The work described in this book provides evidence that a transformation is taking place in inpatient mental health treatment by psychologists in particular. To accomplish the goal of portraying the kind of work that psychologists currently carry out, and the transformation taking place in psychologists' work, the current volume provides a broad sample of current work carried out by psychologists in a variety of inpatient mental health settings. The type of work described here includes therapy, assessment, training, and systemic oriented work. The type of settings represented include public psychiatric and forensic settings, and privately run facilities.

Many aspects of the psychologists' work presented in this book are grounded in approaches that were initiated in the early twentieth century. Some date back to the mid-nineteenth century. Illuminating the continuity of such services, some of the treatment described here takes place in the same facilities that were originally established in the mid-1800s, during the height of the Moral Treatment era. Current treatment described in some facilities, including both public and private settings, explicitly incorporates psychological assessment approaches that stem from approaches developed by some of the pioneers of psychological evaluation. In some settings, psychoanalytically based models of treatment formulation and psychotherapeutic work, most prominent during the early to mid-twentieth century, continue to evolve and to be carried out as vital aspects of assessment and treatment. Much of the work presented in this book demonstrates how current inpatient services by psychologists are grounded in the past and have been adapted to current needs in modern settings. Chapters in this volume by Marilyn Charles and Beatriz Sanchez Curtis are among the chapters that highlight this type of adaptation.

The psychologists' work described in this book occurs within systems that are simultaneously local, regional, and international in nature. The local system described in most chapters includes the unit and treatment facility in which psychologists provide services. Each inpatient mental health treatment facility is also part of a larger system, the mental health treatment system in the particular region and country where they are located. Most broadly, the facilities in countries represented in this book can be seen as an international system linked by the type of work done, commonalities of populations served, and shared challenges and global shifts that are taking place in treatment. Among the most notable observations made evident throughout this book is that, as the systemic scope expands, remarkable similarities stand out in the work described by the authors of this book's chapters. While a variety of facilities in countries spread around the world are represented, and work by psychologists ranging from interns to experienced practitioners subscribing to a variety of theoretical orientations and practice approaches is represented, many common issues and trends are apparent.

One shared aspect of psychologists' work across systems is the tremendous expansion of this work in inpatient settings since the mid-1900s. When psychologists began working in inpatient settings, their work was primarily limited to psychological assessment. In most settings, this meant evaluating patients' intellectual and cognitive functioning. Psychologists earliest contributions to inpatient treatment consisted of providing assessment input that was incorporated into the predominant treatment approach, which was largely medically driven. Over time, the types of services provided and roles carried out by psychologists in inpatient settings have grown well beyond this seminal assessment role. Psychologists have greatly expanded their functions, influencing and helping to shape treatment approaches and paradigms, and applying psychological perspective, theory, and practice. Psychologists have influenced inpatient treatment through application of treatment models based on developmental theories, including those grounded in behavioral and psychodynamic understanding (Beck, Rector, Stolar, & Grant, 2009; Karon & Vandenbos, 1981; Kingdon & Turkington, 1994), humanistic, existential, and client-centered work, system-oriented interventions, treatments specifically addressing psychological dimensions of severe emotional disturbance, treatment addressing impact of emotional trauma including emotional dysregulation, and treatment addressing psychosocial aspects of treatment (Mueser, Deavers, Penn, & Cassisi, 2013). Many of those influences and approaches are represented in the treatment described by authors in the current volume.

The chapters of this book provide numerous examples of ways in which assessment and therapy work, done for decades by psychologists in inpatient mental health settings, continue to be central roles for psychologists. At the same time, the work described throughout this volume demonstrates ways in which the methods psychologists carry out these roles continue to evolve. Ways in which psychologists have expanded and adapted existing treatment models to fit the needs of specific populations with particular needs are repeatedly made apparent in the book's chapters.

Adaptation of established approaches and methodologies in order to meet presenting treatment needs may be a common characteristic of psychologists' work in these settings. Early versions of both therapy and assessment approaches established by pioneers and innovators in the mental health field have been adapted in order to remain relevant and effectively meet treatment needs of changing populations.

The assessment section of this book provides several examples of current approaches to cognitive, personality, and diagnostic psychological assessment. These chapters demonstrate how approaches initiated during the early years of the psychology profession have been refined and updated to meet current needs and paradigms. Early assessment tools such as the Rorschach Inkblot Test, and the Minnesota Multiphasic Personality Inventory continue to be updated, while new and specialized modes of psychological assessment continue to be established, researched, and expanded. Chapters by Biedermann, Ridenour, and Biel, by Paul Saks, and by Shweta Sharma and Patricia Daza, each detail current assessment approaches to traditional testing questions, using many assessment tools that have evolved over several decades.

Contemporary and important additional emphases in assessment work include assessment of suicide risk, violence risk, and sexual violence risk. Assessment of neuropsychological functioning and legal competency and sanity are among the aspects of functioning that have developed well beyond the original scope of psychological assessment. These and other aspects of psychologists' work reflect expanded application of skills and knowledge that have a link to inpatient work; for example, neuropsychological evaluations assessing functional and cognitive consequences of neurologically based dysfunction, and legal sanity evaluations distinguishing between individuals whose legal violations were generated by genuine emotional disturbance versus those who make efforts to portray emotional disturbance in order to limit or avoid legal consequences.

In addition to such expanded assessment roles and activities, psychologists have built on early therapy and treatment models. They have created and participated in applying innovative approaches to treatment. For example, psychologists have played significant roles in the development and implementation of updated and specialized versions of psychoanalytic, psychodynamic, and cognitive therapies. Chapters by Sally Riggs, Mark McFetridge, and Jimmy Kim and Peter D'Amico are among the authors in this book whose work exemplifies psychologists' expanded applications of such established treatment approaches.

Therapy approaches grounded in a variety of models have been developed to provide treatment addressing people presenting with depression, emotional dysregulation, traumatic experience, and other specific psychological issues. These include Cognitive Behavioral Therapy (CBT) approaches developed specifically for people presenting with psychosis (e.g., Sally Riggs' chapter in this volume), a Dialectic Behavioral Therapy (DBT) approach for individuals diagnosed with Borderline Personality Disorder, and approaches to treating traumatized individuals that incorporate psychoanalytic and other theoretical models. Examples in this book describing such work include chapters by Dione Johnson-Williams and by Beatriz Sanchez Curtis. Short term, modular, and scripted therapies have also become accepted and carried out by psychologists as well as other treatment providers. Chapters by Manish Parswani and Malcolm Stewart, and by Kim Griffiths, Hannah Green and Suzie Lemmey in this book provide examples of such work.

That effective psychological therapies do not need to be tied to a specific theoretical orientation has been widely recognized. For example, common factors seen as important for effective psychological therapies include the quality of the therapeutic alliance, and empathy (Duncan, Miller, Wampold, & Hubble, 2010; Hubble, Duncan, & Miller, 1999; Wampold, 2015). The chapters of the current volume provide many vivid examples of many of the crucial role of such common factors in various approaches to inpatient treatment.

Several chapters describe efforts made by psychologists to innovate and create new treatments, and efforts to ensure effectiveness through patient feedback, as well as measurement and research. Enav Or-

Gordon's chapter provides a compelling example of an innovation which, though apparently simple, demonstrated potential to be transformative on her unit. Or-Gordon's innovative approach provides the patient with a way of actively guiding their own treatment and provides a model that could transform the effort to engage patients in treatment in many settings. The chapter by Kim Griffiths, Hannah Green, and Suzie Lemmey also provides an example of psychologists' addressing the need to establish empirical as well as experiential validation. While most clinical psychologists working in inpatient settings don't have the opportunity to conduct empirical research and validate the innovative work they are doing, psychologists have become leaders in carrying out research on therapeutic work. Inpatient psychologists can at times collaborate with researchers, and help carry out research with direct relevance to their work (Lu et al., 2011).

In some chapters, psychologists describe engagement in broader trends such as the Recovery model. In the context of such trends, updated and innovative treatment models can emerge, and efforts may be made to reframe treatment approaches that have been carried out for decades (Leamy et al., 2011). Such reframing may include adding new components to treatment or reviving aspects of treatment that have been de-emphasized, forgotten, or marginalized. For example, several chapters of this book refer to the implementation of a modern 'Wellness' or 'Recovery' approach to treatment that incorporates ideas about treating patients humanely and with respect characteristic of the Moral Treatment era, as well as other treatment dimensions. The 'Wellness' approach also brings to the forefront aspects of a client or patient-centered model that psychologists are familiar with, and which in modern times has been advocated most strongly by an increasingly influential consumer movement. In the context of broad treatment movements such as the 'Recovery' movement, psychologists have been involved in introducing and applying new treatment approaches, incrementally expanding and refining established methods, combining existing treatment approaches in new ways, and evaluating the value of treatment approaches. Among the chapters in this book that demonstrate psychologists' involvement in these roles are those by Michael Siglag, Peter Walker and Sophie Li, Enav Or-Gordon, Manish Parswani and Malcolm Stewart, and Kim Griffiths, Hannah Green and Suzie Lemmey.

Current approaches to inpatient treatment described by psychologists in this book include empirically based therapies, as well as approaches that are innovative and have not yet been scrutinized through research. This includes cognitive behavioral therapies that are generally recognized as supported by research and psychodynamic, psychoanalytic and other approaches that have been supported by empirical research as well, though their empirical grounding may be less recognized (Shedler,

2010). Current psychological therapies in inpatient settings include treatments addressing traumatic and other developmentally disruptive life experiences that can contribute to the manifestation of severe emotional and behavioral disturbance. In addition, programmatic and unit-wide or systemic interventions including behavioral interventions and approaches, and an increased attention to 'patient-centered' or 'client-centered' treatment are common aspects of modern inpatient treatment. Thought provoking chapters in this volume addressing such issues, and providing examples of relevant work include those by Peter Walker and Sophie Li, and by Marilyn Charles.

Issues repeatedly emerge in the chapters of this book concerning the challenges posed by some subsets of patients. For example, treatment approaches with individuals presenting as aggressive, and those experienced as difficult or resistant to treatment are described in both civil and forensic treatment settings. A subset of these individuals have serious legal charges, but many do not. Though not the subject of this volume, it is notable that there are many people similar to those being described here who are housed in criminal justice facilities or who move back and forth between such facilities and mental health facilities. Several chapters in this book discuss treatment models carried out by psychologists with individuals who exist on the cusp of these two systems, including chapters by Hilik Peri and by Dione Johnson-Williams.

Several chapters in this volume present ways psychologists are impacted, and ways psychologists can help address problems that have emerged due to trends in the broader mental health treatment system. For example, the closure of many public psychiatric hospitals due to deinstitutionalization and reduction in the population of those that remain hospitalized has resulted in numerous consequences. One result of the closure of many hospitals has been a shift of treatment to more community-based options. However, there has also been 'trans-institutionalization' to other institutional settings such as correctional institutions, settings housing elderly or aging populations, and other facilities. Lack of continuity of care between hospitals and the community has long been recognized as an impediment to the successful transition of hospitalized individuals back to successful functioning in the community. Such a lack of continuity, followed by fragmentation of community services, has also been seen as contributing to repeated hospitalizations for many. The chapter by Kim Griffiths, Hannah Green, and Suzie Lemmey in this volume addresses the issue of continuity of care. The authors of this chapter describe a process intended to facilitate the transition from the hospital to the community. The approach they describe includes psychological treatment that starts in the hospital and continues in the community, which they assert could help many with that transition.

Another consequence of decades of hospital closures and reduction of the number of patients in hospitals, particularly government-run facilities, has been an increased concentration in remaining facilities of people who have particular difficulty reintegrating into the community. This includes individuals who are difficult to engage in treatment due to the severity of their emotional and social difficulties, and sometimes cognitive impediments. Also among these are highly disturbed, aggressive, and emotionally volatile individuals. The increased concentration of a more disturbed, self-injurious, aggressive, and 'difficult to treat' population in inpatient facilities creates dilemmas in many inpatient settings. At a time when more patient-centered oriented approaches are becoming predominant and seen as beneficial and desirable, and even required by accrediting agencies, this population shift can be particularly problematic. Providing patients with greater control, and greater input into their own treatment may generally be desirable, but can be difficult to reconcile with the dangerous behavior of some patients. It is difficult to predict how treatment trends that seem incongruent in some ways will unfold over time, and in relation to specific treatment populations. Among the chapters that specifically address working with patients who have been violent and may be volatile or threatening, while still maintaining a therapeutic stance and addressing psychological issues such as mentalization, are Dione Johnson-Williams's and Hilik Peri's chapters.

Approaches that emphasize greater patient engagement in their own treatment, increasing recognition of patient rights, reduction of coercive approaches to treatment, and pressures to lessen external controls such as seclusion and restraints on patients appear to be gaining particular strength in the broader treatment world. These trends are largely consistent with psychologists' approaches to treatment, though not always congruent with the treatment cultures in particular institutions. These trends also appear to be supported by a consumer movement that is increasing in recognition and developing a greater voice. The emphasis of treatment defined more by collaboration rather than control is the predominant direction generally in inpatient facilities, but it is likely that this shift will take place at different rates and in a variety of ways in individual settings. Psychologists have been and will continue to be impacted by the ongoing shifts and most likely will frequently play roles in facilitating the shift to more collaborative treatment approaches. Several chapters in this book describe ways in which psychologists are impacted and are navigating such changes in their settings.

The kind of relationship psychologists have with members of other mental health disciplines and with administrative leaders is another topic addressed in a variety of ways throughout this book. Though there are exceptions, psychologists most often describe working in collaborative and complementary ways with colleagues, including frequently providing consultation for other disciplines. Sometimes such consultation is formalized, but often it is more informal. Specific and compelling examples of this are presented in Mark McFetridge's and Amit Fachler's chapters.

Chapters in this book that describe treatment with an emphasis on treatment engagement generally include psychologists playing an active role not only with patient treatment but in facilitating team engagement. Regardless of theoretical orientation, these psychologists emphasize the crucial role of therapy as a kind of partnership between patient, therapist, and treatment team. These professionals do not work independently in 'silos.' Rather, their work is characterized by a collaborative approach addressing the multiple and complex factors patients present. Psychologists' validation of other professionals' and team members' engagement in collaborative treatment approaches may be among the most powerful dimensions of treatment.

As members of interdisciplinary treatment teams, psychologists frequently make unique and valued contributions to the team process. Many of this book's chapters describe the impact of psychologists' roles as both therapists and treatment team members. Authors describe multiple benefits generated from therapy interactions in the context of inpatient treatment. For example, in addition to therapeutic benefits directly derived by patients through therapy interactions, psychologists develop insights and understanding of patients that can be communicated to other team members. Insights arrived at in therapy can help psychologists provide input and guidance for other treatment team members treating the patient, helping the entire team better understand patient communications and behaviors in ways that can be used to facilitate treatment approaches and decisions that take into account both staff and patients' perspectives.

Treatment team members' success or failure to function in a genuinely collaborative manner can be seen as related to difficulties of ease in the engagement of patients in treatment. In addition to the influence of treatment team coordination, successful engagement of patients at a deeper level generally requires a degree and type of listening that is consistent with psychologists' training. Psychologists are educated and receive extensive supervision emphasizing the importance of considering the history of circumstances that brought individual patients to treatment, the patient's general life situation, important aspects of their background, triggers and vulnerabilities, capacity for resilience, and strengths that can be built upon. Several chapters in this volume describe treatment that highlights psychologists' skills in facilitating patients' active participation in the treatment process.

However, as also described by a number of authors in this book, for psychologists working in inpatient settings, conflicts with team members and other hospital personnel can emerge due to a number of factors.

Among these factors are psychological processes that generate distortions in staff members' perceptions in intense inpatient environments (Shur, 1994). Conflicts also emerge in response to very real ethical dilemmas, and in response to discrepancies in priorities between psychological, medical, and administrative leadership. Amit Fachler and Heidi Camerlengo, from very different perspectives, address these topics in some detail in their chapters.

Organizational leadership hierarchies can support psychologists efforts, but are described in some chapters as posing obstacles or agendas that conflict with psychologists' efforts. For example, psychologists sometimes take on leadership roles in treatment provision, and within the structure of interdisciplinary treatment teams. In addition, psychologists have taken on many other formal and informal leadership roles within inpatient settings. Despite being in such roles, psychologists in many settings describe experiencing being in a 'second tier' role in relation to psychiatry. This is especially evident in settings where treatment is driven by a predominantly biologically oriented medical model, where symptom reduction is seen as the primary goal, and medication is seen as the primary treatment. While many psychologists are able to work comfortably within this treatment model and hierarchical system, other psychologists can better be described as tolerating or adapting to work within the system. Some psychologists, for both personal reasons and in response to aspects of the treatment environment find things so intolerable that they exit the system. Jim Geekie's and Michael Siglag's chapters are among those that describe personal and professional impacts of such issues.

A related topic that comes up in several chapters in this book concerns psychologists' perceptions of the role of biological factors in the disturbances experienced by patients. Genetic and biological factors are widely perceived as factors in the etiology of the disturbances that contribute to inpatient treatment. Biological interventions, mostly in the form of medication, but via electroconvulsive therapies in some settings, are seen by many as important and effective aspects of treatment for people who suffer the extreme emotional disturbance that frequently leads to inpatient intervention. However, for many years there have also been critiques about the emphasis on medically based interventions. Specific critiques exist concerning risks and potential harm associated with pharmaceutical interventions and electroconvulsive therapy, questions about the need for continued medical interventions over time, and concerns about the long term effectiveness of such interventions. The broad use of such interventions for the great majority of those being treated for serious emotional distress or disturbance is questioned by mental health professionals, consumers, and others (Whitaker, 2010). Prominent psychiatrists have responded to these critiques. Along the continuum of this debate are the stances that: (1) for individuals with severe psychiatric disturbance, psychiatric interventions such as medication are the most effective and best available interventions we have to offer; (2) there are many people suffering severe emotional disturbance who either do not respond well to currently available psychiatric interventions, or do not persist with them due to the unpleasant side effects and other factors. However, improving treatment 'compliance' and/or new discoveries related to genetic and other biological factors will provide relief to these individuals who suffer severe emotional distress and disturbance; (3) there may be some for whom short term use of medications may be helpful, but for whom long term use may be unnecessary and may even impede full recovery; (4) there may be some for whom medications may be contraindicated; (5) medication and other biologically based interventions such as electroconvulsive therapy do more harm than good and impede the recovery of many who might otherwise improve.

On this oversimplified continuum, psychologists' do not have a monolithic point of view. Each psychologist's point of view is likely to be influenced by their particular training and experiences. Psychologists' perspectives may fall at different points on this continuum when considering different patients and considering different possible etiologies for disturbance manifested by particular individuals. In medically driven inpatient systems, however, tolerance of the full range of positions on this continuum may be limited. Many psychiatrists and administrators have genuine respect for their interdisciplinary colleagues and those colleagues' treatment conceptualizations, even when professional disagreements arise. That respect may be extended broadly within many inpatient cultures, contributing to healthy, collaborative treatment. However, this is not always the case. Where there is less respect, the assertion of hierarchical medically led leadership may be more overt and strongly enacted. One of the many ways these issues influence psychologists' work is related to their relative and actual importance in the treatment process – for example, whether their treatment contributions are seen as 'supportive' or more central. Among the many chapters addressing this topic are Peter Walker and Sophie Li's chapter, and Michael Siglag's chapter.

Despite potential and sometimes very real schisms in the professional views of treatment team members, many factors exist that support greater engagement and collaboration. Among these factors has been the effort to establish a genuine interdisciplinary biopsychosocial treatment approach in many settings. An additional factor has been the promotion of more engaging, collaborative relationships and interactions among staff, as well as between staff and patients, in inpatient treatment settings. In many facilities, these changes may require a significant paradigm shift in the way treatment is conceptualized and carried out. Psychologists' training prepares them well to play a significant role and to take leadership in facilitating these conceptual and practical changes in treatment.

What might psychologists' roles in future inpatient treatment look like in light of current trends? Psychologists are likely to become more valued and influential for a number of reasons. It is likely that agencies where a rigid application of the medical model still prevails will change. Psychiatrists who attempt or are empowered to apply a strict hierarchical leadership model are likely to move at different paces to more collaborative models. Facilities with treatment models or medical staff putting less value on non-medical interventions are likely to increase recognition of the value of all treatment contributions and promote work that is genuinely collaborative. Many psychologists already promote such values and are in positions to increase their influence. Within many settings, psychologists already frequently take leadership roles in treatment teams. In many facilities, psychologists hold management positions and help shape facilities' policies and approaches to treatment. Psychologists' traditionally collaborative approach, along with their emerging leadership, may be significant factors advancing the shift to a more genuine interdisciplinary biopsychosocial treatment approach within inpatient facilities.

The content of many chapters in the current volume provides clues about other ways inpatient treatment may progress. For example, the many chapters in which psychologists provide interventions based in CBT approaches, including CBT specifically designed for people with psychosis, indicates that CBT oriented therapies are being adapted to meet the needs of inpatient populations, and suggests they will continue to expand in such settings. At the same time, the work presented here suggests that psychoanalytically oriented therapies will continue to be found useful and provide unique benefits, and will continue being used in many settings as well. This is particularly evident in settings with long histories of psychoanalytically oriented work. Increasing emphasis on conceptions such as 'mentalization' suggests that psychoanalytically oriented treatment and assessment approaches are evolving in recognition of a need to conceptualize and work with patients in newer ways. New and revised versions of other treatment models are likely to also make inroads into current inpatient treatment. Shifting hospitalized patients to treatment based in small community-based settings, including group homes and apartments with varying degrees of monitoring and support, has been carried out as an alternate approach to large institutional facilities for many years. Versions of this type of facility exist in many countries. As inpatient facilities continue to attempt to discharge patients, and more and more patients are discharged to community-based settings and assisted by community-based treatment teams, increasingly specialized versions of community housing may be developed or expanded in order to accommodate the many people who continue to reside in inpatient settings. Psychologists' involvement in such initiatives would be valuable, and participation in outpatient/community-based teams may grow. As described specifically in one chapter of this book, there is evidence that continuity of psychological treatment is a factor contributing to the success of people who are discharged. Other models of treatment, such as Finland's Open Dialogue approach, which is recognized as successful there and in several other countries, is a treatment model gaining international recognition (Seikkula, Alakare, & Aaltonen, 2011). A key aspect of Open Dialogue is bringing in family and other participants in the psychotic person's life to be involved in that individual's recovery. Many other treatment approaches are also becoming integrated into treatment. Recent job postings for psychologists describe a variety of therapeutic approaches applicants should be prepared to utilize, including Dialectical Behavioral Therapy, Acceptance and Commitment Therapy, Motivational Interviewing, Solution Focused Therapy, Cognitive Remediation, Cognitive Processing Therapy for PTSD, and neuropsychological services, including rehabilitation psychology for individuals who have experienced a brain injury. Other approaches developed in specific countries, but with growing international followings could become applied more broadly in inpatient settings. Examples of such approaches are Paul Gilbert's Compassionate Mind approach (Gilbert, 2010), and the CBT based recovery oriented Comprehend, Cope, and Connect approach (Clarke & Nicholls, 2018), both developed by psychologists in the United Kingdom. The scope of treatments being incorporated into treatment with individuals treated in inpatient facilities is growing. Psychologists are trained and well situated to participate and take leadership roles in such treatment.

Psychology trainees in graduate school and post-graduate training learn a variety of theoretical and treatment orientations and utilize a variety of therapeutic approaches in their work. Throughout their careers, clinical psychologists typically continue to obtain training in approaches they find useful in their work, specialize in diverse techniques, and expand from specific theoretical orientations so as to have a flexible and broad conceptual base and skill set. Such training prepares psychologists to provide interventions better matched for each patient, including adjusting for phases of treatment when appropriate.

Chapters in this book addressing psychology internship training indicate steps that are particularly important in order to support interns obtaining professional training in hospital settings. Suggestions are provided that are also relevant for psychologists in general to support their resilience in the face of the challenges that psychologists may face throughout their careers. Interns may face situations for the first time that they will deal with throughout their careers, particularly if they continue to work in inpatient settings. For example, when encountering the degree of restriction and loss of personal freedom encountered by patients, and other aspects of the setting that are related to the compulsory nature of hospitalization for patients who are committed, it is likely for personal reactions to be evoked. The psychological and physical aggression that one can encounter may also provoke strong reactions. The realization of patients' vulnerability and the possibility of patients harming themselves or losing their lives due to suicidal acts is another aspect of inpatient work that provokes strong personal reactions, as well as professional and administrative responses. Chapters by Daria Mamon and by Karin Reddie provide insightful examples of early career psychologists describing the impact of inpatient internship experiences that evoke strong personal reactions and influence their approach to working with patients in inpatient settings. Valerie Sims, and Patricia Daza and Shweta Sharma, in their chapters, describe structures and supports, and aspects of supervision they utilize to ensure that interns, who can face such destabilizing and difficult encounters, are able to emerge from their internship training as professionals prepared to practice more independently.

Ultimately, chapters in this book convey a range of personal, clinical, administrative, systemic and other challenges that psychologists face working in inpatient settings. Many aspects of inpatient mental health treatment and many of the challenges involved in such treatment described in this volume are likely to persist in the foreseeable future. For some, as described by Jim Geekie in one chapter in this book, aspects of the work can elicit personal, professional, and ethical quandaries that can rise to a level that makes working in such settings intolerable, and leading to decisions to discontinue working in the hospital setting. Some, as described in Peter Walker and Sophie Li's chapter, become sensitized to such issues and make addressing human rights issues or reducing potentially traumatic aspects of such settings a part of their work. Many psychologists persist in their work in such settings through maintaining focus on the professional tasks of providing therapies, establishing team interactions, and carrying out other clinical practice aspects of the work, and are sustained through the rewards of the work itself, and the collegial and supportive personal connections they establish.

Yet working in such settings can entail very real costs, including the risk of physical injury and emotional trauma. The threats and genuine physical risks psychologists encounter are very real sources of stress in many inpatient settings. Psychologists are not immune from the impact of the emotional suffering and distress they encounter engaging with patients in inpatient settings. They may experience such effects as vicarious traumatization and compassion fatigue. They are not immune from feelings of frustration or even hopelessness that may be evoked working with many people who may recover slowly if at all, or whose continued progress following 'stabilization and discharge' they will never see once the person moves on from their care. Frustration over challenges working with colleagues or administrators who may fail to recognize the hurdles psychologists and their colleagues face, in some settings, can impact the psychologist as well. Working with members of other disciplines or for administrators who may not share one's values and priorities, and whose actions or leadership may create ethical and personal dilemmas can add to the stress of the inpatient setting. In some settings, the predominance of a biologically based medical model, in contrast to a genuine biopsychosocial model results in a devaluing of psychologists' work or contributions, and of psychologists' influence in the treatment process. As described in several of the chapters in this book, psychologists must find ways of coping with each of these aspects of hospital work in order to persist in such settings and remain effective. Such challenges and stresses pose difficult obstacles to psychologists who work in these settings.

Despite the challenges and obstacles, and the difficulties inherent to psychologists' work, as described in many of the chapters of this book, many psychologists persevere, accomplish much, and find satisfaction working in these settings. Psychologists find and develop personal and professional support, and experience satisfaction knowing that they are helping the people they work with and come in contact with. Some psychologists derive satisfaction through their efforts to make the hospital system a healthier place. Inpatient work has undeniable risks and potential costs, but the work described by the psychologists in this book indicates that many find value in the work they carry out in such settings, make important treatment contributions, and often make a positive impact on patients and facilities themselves. The work described in this book provides a diverse and rich picture of psychologists' current inpatient work. In the context of current international trends in the mental health treatment field, psychologists appear poised to continue building on a rich history, to make unique contributions, and to participate in expanding treatment and leadership roles in inpatient mental health treatment settings.

References

Beck, A. T., Rector N. A., Stolar, N., & Grant, P. (2009). *Schizophrenia cognitive theory, research, and therapy*. New York, NY: The Guilford Press.

Clarke, I., & Nicholls, H. (2018). *Third wave CBT integration for individuals and teams: Comprehend, cope and connect*. London: Routledge.

Duncan, B. L., Miller, S. D., Wampold, B. E., & Hubble, M. A. (Eds.) (2010). *The heart and soul of change: Delivering what works in therapy* (2nd ed.). Washington, DC: American Psychological Association. http://dx.doi.org/10.1037/12075-000.

Gilbert, P. (2010). *The compassionate mind: A new approach to life's challenges.* Oakland, CA: New Harbinger Publications.

Hubble, M. A., Duncan, B. L., & Miller, S. D. (Eds.) (1999). *The heart and soul of change: What works in therapy.* Washington, DC: American Psychological Association. http://dx.doi.org/10.1037/11132-000.

Karon, B. P., & Vandenbos, G. R. (1981). *Psychotherapy of schizophrenia treatment of choice.* New York, NY: Jason Aronson.

Kingdon, D. G., & Turkington, D. (1994). *Cognitive-behavioral therapy of schizophrenia.* New York, NY: Guilford.

Leamy, M., Bird, V., Le Boutillier, C., Williams, J., & Slade, M. (2011). Conceptual framework for personal recovery in mental health: Systematic review and narrative synthesis. *The British Journal of Psychiatry*, 199, 445–452.

Lu, W., Mueser, K. T., Shami, A., Siglag, M., Petrides, G., Schoepp, E., & Saltz, J. (2011). Post-traumatic reactions to psychosis in people with multiple psychotic episodes. *Schizophrenia Research, 127*(1–3), 66–75.

Mueser, K., Deavers, F., Penn, D., & Cassisi, J. (2013). Psychosocial treatments for schizophrenia. *Annual Review of Clinical Psychology*, 9, 465–497.

Seikkula, J., Alakare, B., & Aaltonen, J. (2011). The comprehensive open-dialogue approach in Western Lapland: II. Long-term stability of acute psychosis outcomes in advanced community care. *Psychosis: Psychological, Social and Integrative Approaches, 3*(3), 192–204.

Shedler, J. (2010). The efficacy of psychodynamic psychotherapy. *American Psychologist, 65*, 98–109.

Shur, R. (1994). *Countertransference enactment: How institutions and therapists actualize primitive internal worlds.* Northvale, NJ: Jason Aronson, Inc.

Wampold, B. E. (2015). How important are the common factors in psychotherapy? An update. *World Psychiatry, 14*(3), 270–277.

Whitaker, R. (2010). *Anatomy of an epidemic: Magic bullets, psychiatric drugs, and the astonishing rise of mental illness in America.* New York, NY: Crown Publishers.

Index